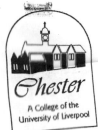

Inside the caring services

Inside the Caring Services
Second Edition

David Tossell, Head of Community Studies Section,
College of North West London.

and

Richard Webb, Lecturer in Social Care and
Social Work, Parkwood Centre, The Sheffield College.

Edward Arnold
A member of the Hodder Headline Group
LONDON BOSTON SYDNEY AUCKLAND

Edward Arnold is a division of Hodder Headline PLC
338 Euston Road, London NW1 3BH

First published in the United Kingdom 1986
Second edition 1994

8 7 6 5 4 3 2
99 98 97 96 95

British Library Cataloguing in Publication Data
Available on request

Typeset in 10/11 Erhardt by
Hewer Text Composition Services, Edinburgh
Printed and bound in the United Kingdom by
Mackays of Chatham PLC, Chatham, Kent

Contents

Acknowledgements   vii

1. **A review of recent changes**   1
Changes in legislation. Language and terminology. What the book sets
out to do. Anti-discriminatory/anti-oppressive practice. Community care.
Who the book is written for.

2. **The personal social services**   8
Local authority social work – a brief history. The work of local authority
social services authorities. Field social workers. Types of difficulties
presented to SSDs and SWDs. Preventive social work. Specialist
services. Children being looked after by the local authority. Services to
older people. Conclusion. Appendix. Exercises. Questions for discussion.
Further reading.

3. **The Probation Service**   92
Introduction. History. Anti-oppressive and anti-discriminatory practice.
Equal opportunities. The organisation and structure of the Probation
Service. What the Probation Service does. Conclusion. Appendix.
Excercises. Questions for discussion. Further reading.

4. **Other statutory services**   151
Introduction. The National Health Service (NHS). Local authority
education departments. Local authority housing departments.
Community work. Community police work. Interagency co-operation.
Conclusion. Appendix. Exercises. Questions for discussion. Further
reading.

5. **The independent sector – the voluntary sector in a mixed
   economy of care**   210
Introduction. What is a voluntary organisation? Origins of the voluntary
sector. The range of activity. The changing nature of the voluntary
sector. The private sector. 'Not-for-profit' organisations. Some examples
of voluntary organisations. Conclusion – what is the independent sector's
future? Appendix. Exercises. Questions for discussion. Further reading.

6. **Good practice – client rights and choices**   234
Influential reports, codes of practice and charters. The right to receive
anti-discriminatory/anti-oppressive care. The right to confidentiality and
privacy. The right to have individual rights and personal choices

respected. The right to have personal beliefs and identity acknowledged
and acted upon. The right to support through effective communication.
Conclusion. Exercises. Questions for discussion. Further reading.

7. **Qualities of an effective carer**   253
Anti-oppression. Personal qualities. Basic courtesies. Communication and
interpersonal skills. Knowledge. Conclusion. Exercises. Questions for
Discussion. Further Reading.

8. **Strategies for helping**   265
Introduction. The origins of helping strategies. Power in the caring
relationship. Anti-oppressive/anti-discriminatory practice. The 'process'
of helping. Three case studies. Groupwork and some other strategies for
helping. Community social work or community work. Radical social
work. Feminist social work and woman-centred practice. The social
systems model. Six-category intervention analysis. Conclusion. Appendix.
Exercises, Questions for discussion. Further reading.

9. **Some developments in the caring services**   296
'New Right' Conservative Government ideology. The common good.
Some recent developments. Working in the caring services. The wider
social setting. Anti-discriminatory/anti-oppressive practice. Conclusion.
Appendix. Exercises. Questions for discussion. Further reading.

Annex 1   **Training for work in the caring services**   313
Introduction. GNVQ/vocational A levels. National Vocational
Qualifications (NVQs)/Scottish Vocational Qualifications (SVQs). The
Diploma in Social Work (Dip.SW). Employment in the health service. A
range of other occupations. Further information. Appendix. Exercises.

Annex 2   **Practical work placements**   332
Broad aims of a practical placement. Observational placements. Types of
placement. Organisation of placements. A guide to practical placements.
Placement supervision. Visits from college tutors. Assessment.
Conclusion. Appendix. Exercises. Questions for discussion.

Index   345

Acknowledgements

We would like to thank the following people for the help and insight they have given us into the nature of their work within the caring services: Helen Barrett, Pat Benavithis, Sheena Campbell, Melanie Cawthorne, Nol Coppens, Vaun Cutts, Anita Dell, Jim Donoghue, Bill Downie, Johnathon Epps, Mike Fowler, Rosemary Fry, Colin Hall, Richard Johnstone, Jan Kemp, Stuart Kemp, Jeremy Kendall, Dr. Timothy Lambert, Peter Latham, Liz Leng, Sue Maisfield, Dr Gill McIvor, Howard Millerman, Joy Mitchell, Dr Claire Murphy, Helen Nettleship, Robin Parker, Julie Philips, Julia Rimmer, Abdul Galil Shaif, Norma Slimmon, Mike Tossell, Duncan Tulip, Hilary Walker, Chris Walton, Norman Watling and Maggie Woonton.

Finally, once again, we would wish to thank Joyce Tossell for the hard work and long hours she devoted to deciphering the sense of the original manuscript. In addition, we should like to thank staff and students of both the college of North West London and Parkwood College, Sheffield, for their ideas and support.

David Tossell
Richard Webb

Acknowledgements

1

A Review of Recent Changes

Changes in legislation

It has become necessary to produce a second edition because of the many changes that have taken place in the spheres of health, social care and social work since the book was first written. Most of these changes have been brought about by the implementation of recent legislation, namely the Children Act 1989, the National Health Service and Community Care Act 1990 and the Criminal Justice Act 1991. This edition describes the effects of these changes and retains all that is still relevant from the original edition.

Language and terminology

Progressive changes in both language and terminology have taken place within a relatively short period of time; some of the language and terminology in the first edition may therefore now be taken as unfashionable, if not obsolete. For example, the term *mental handicap* is no longer used because of its stigmatising effect on people who prefer to be referred to as having a *learning difficulty* or *learning disability*.

The term *ethic minority* is offensive to some groups even when it is reversed to read *minority ethnic groups*, but it is still commonly used. The word *black* now seems generally preferred when referring, in a political sense, to people who are likely to experience racial discrimination on the grounds of their skin colour or the way that they speak. People of Afro-Caribbean origin and from the Indian subcontinent will obviously be included in this category. However, Chinese, Southern European, Jewish and Irish people also experience racial discrimination and therefore may be included under the umbrella term *black*. The word *black* is also used to describe, specifically, only people of African or Caribbean origin in order to emphasise the cultural differences between African or Caribbean people and Asian people. The term *Asian* is imprecise, but generally refers to people from the Indian subcontinent, including Indians, Bangladeshis, Pakistanis and Sri Lankans.

The practice of using the prefix *the* with reference to groups of people, for example, *the homeless, the disabled* and *the unemployed* is now unacceptable because it distances people and stereotypes them as a distinct and homogeneous group. Terms such as *handicapped* and *elderly* are viewed as being disrespectful and are therefore discouraged.

What the book sets out to do

This book takes a different approach from that of traditional texts. It looks at the caring services from the practitioner's point of view and aims to outline their tasks, roles and responsibilities. It also examines the actual work of the caring services and the inter-relationship between them.

Chapter 2 looks at the work of local authority **social services authorities**. This is currently undergoing great change as the role of the local authorities diminishes. The work of the various specialised services is also explored.

Chapter 3 examines the work of the **Probation Service** which has also undergone great change following the implementation of the Criminal Justice Act 1991. An up to date version of the service is presented.

Chapter 4 returns to the local authorities to look at the functions of other caring sectors: education, housing, community work and the police. It begins with an outline of the workings of the National Health Service (NHS) which is not part of the local authority set up, but is a major statutory service.

Chapter 5 moves away from the statutory sector to focus on the **independent sector**, made up of voluntary organisations, private and 'not-for-profit' agencies. Each is described in detail, along with their inter-relationships with other statutory and non-statutory organisations.

Chapter 6 explores the value base of social and health care and the rights and choices of service users. It looks at some of the charters and codes of practice that contain client rights and attempts to categorise them in a helpful way.

Chapter 7 discusses the qualities required in an effective carer and explores their basis in fundamental humanistic principles.

Chapter 8 takes a wide-ranging look at the strategies used by carers to enable their clients to confront their difficulties and maximise their independence, dignity and self-respect.

Chapter 9 summarises the essential issues in the book, discusses the impact of change and looks toward future developments.

Annexe 1 briefly discusses ways of training for work in the caring services. **Annexe 2** gives information and advice about work – based placements undertaken by pre-service students, including those on GNVQ vocational A-Level, nursing and nursery courses.

Anti-discriminatory/anti-oppressive practice

This has come to the fore in recent years and is now a central and permanent part of good practice. It respects a person's individuality while recognising her or his history and social make-up. It aims to ensure equality and to counter the effects of unfair discrimination based on the following:

> Age, class, caste, creed, culture, gender, health status, HIV status, marital status, mental ability, mental health, offending background, physical ability, place of origin, political beliefs, race, religion, responsibility for dependants,

sensory ability, sexuality and other factors (such as lifestyle) that result in discrimination.

(Integrated Project Second Phase Consultation Document,
November 1991, p13, NVQ)

Community care

The term *community care* has two different but related meanings. Firstly, it refers to discharging people from existing and former psychiatric hospitals and other large scale institutions so that they may be cared for in the community. They may live by themselves, in small group homes or in other homely settings, with or without live-in support. The second definition refers to the relatively recent policy, encouraged by the NHS and Community Care Act 1990, of maintaining people in their own homes within the community for as long as possible. The emphasis now is for services to be provided for people in their own homes, in order that they may function more independently and avoid the necessity of entering permanent residential care.

Purchaser/provider functions

The NHS and Community Care Act 1990 separated the functions of **purchaser** and **provider** of services. Social Services Authorities are no longer the major provider of services. Instead they perform the combined role of assessors and purchasers of care. Increasingly, services are being provided from outside the statutory sector.

There is also a purchaser/provider split within the Health Service. Some hospitals have become *independent trusts*, and *budget-holding* GPs may now buy and sell treatment and health care from and to each other. Other hospitals and GP practices remain within the traditional NHS relationship.

Care management

This is undertaken by a named *care manager* who is appointed to co-ordinate the assessment and purchasing of appropriate care. This is most commonly a local authority social worker who may have the job title of 'care manager'. Alternatively, this function may be carried out by another care professional, an informal carer, a relative or the clients themselves.

Mixed economy of welfare

The NHS and Community Care Act 1990 imposed a duty on local authorities to create and develop a 'mixed economy of welfare'. This has been brought about by a split in the functions of purchaser/provider. Local authorities are currently required to spend 85 percent of all funds on care provision from the independent sector. 'Arms length' inspection units within the local authority have a statutory duty to inspect all registered care homes including those run by the local Social Services Authorities.

Statutory sector

A statutory service is one which is provided by law – by statute of Parliament. Examples include the National Health Service, Social Services Authorities and Departments of Education. For example, each local authority has a statutory responsibility to ensure that fulltime education is provided for all children between the ages of five and 16 (or between the ages of two and 19 if the child has special educational needs).

The independent sector

The independent sector consists of **voluntary, private** and **'not-for-profit' organisations.** All independent agencies are **non-statutory.**

Voluntary organisations   Are non-profit making organisations whose management committees provide their services without remuneration. However, they often employ paid staff, in the same way as the statutory sector. They have regularly emerged to make up for gaps in statutory provision and may operate exclusively at national level, local level or at national level with regional groups.

Private organisations   Provide care for which they charge in order to make a profit for the owners (or shareholders). They are often small scale and therefore more flexible in their response to need.

Not-for-profit organisations   These organisations are trusts which feed back surplus income from charges into the organisation. Whoever is in overall charge may also draw a salary for her or his services. This is a relatively new type of body and is expected to expand in influence.

Contracting

The relationship between the statutory and other sectors is now being shaped by the drawing up of contracts which determine costs and delivery of services. Quality assurance is expected to be written into the contract and care managers are encouraged to obtain value for money.

Care settings

Health care, social care and social work take place broadly within four settings: residential/hospital, domiciliary, day care and field. None should be considered superior, as each makes a different contribution to service provision. Within these settings there are a variety of occupational roles and titles, some of which overlap.

The residential sector is made up of nursing and care homes, hostels, sheltered housing and warden controlled accommodation. As a result there are a number of

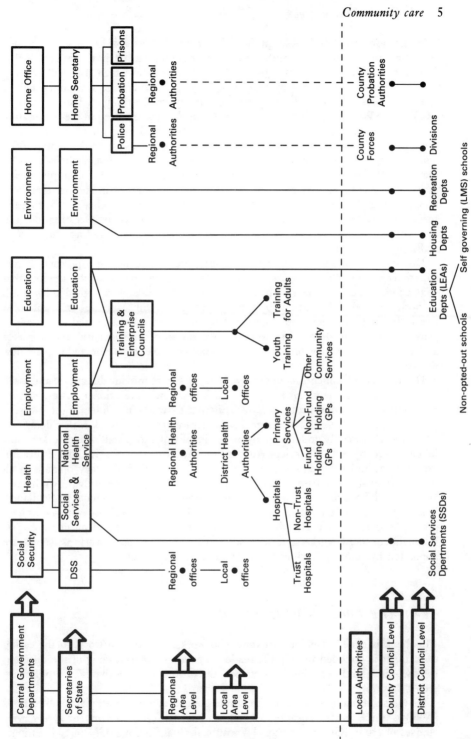

Fig 1.1 The administration of the statutory agencies.

differing job titles and descriptions. All residential establishments are graded according to function, size and number of residents and it is these factors that determine the number of posts, their titles and the way in which staff will be paid.

Care homes are managed by an *officer in charge* and their *deputy*, supported by *assistant officers in charge*. These posts are filled by senior residential social workers (RSWs). RSWs provide direct care and as *keyworkers* are involved in the preparation and delivery of individual care plans. Some organisations refer to non-senior residential social workers in different ways. For example, assistant residential social workers, care officers, care assistants or general assistants. Although their job titles may be different, their duties and responsibilities may merge; for example, a care assistant in one home may have the same role as a care officer in another establishment. A chief distinction between RSWs and care officers and other staff is that the former are paid a salary while the latter are remunerated weekly. Organisations can demonstrate how they value their employees by the status and grading they offer to staff.

Domiciliary services, as the word suggests, are carried out in a person's home. Recent community care legislation has encouraged the provision of services that enable individuals to remain in their own homes. Services may be provided by health authorities, local authorities or by the independent sector. Since fewer people now live in institutions, there are generally fewer posts in the residential sector and a growing number in domiciliary work. New posts such as *community support worker* and *home carer* (an extension of the former *home help* role) have emerged to meet new demands.

Day care establishments may employ *centre workers* to provide direct care and assist with skills development; *instructors* to work in Social Education Centres; *nursery officers* (nursery nurses) and *welfare assistants* to work in Under Eight Nursery Centres or Day Nurseries; and *care assistants/care officers* to work with elders.

Fieldwork is mainly undertaken by professionally qualified staff. Fieldworkers may be employed by Social Services Authorities, the Probation Service, the Education Department and voluntary organisations such as the NSPCC; they operate in all settings from an office base. Their work involves visiting people in their own homes. Within Social Services Departments (and Social Work Departments in Scotland), fieldworkers are often employed as social workers who specialise with one client group, or as care managers who are responsible for assessing and purchasing care. Unqualified social workers, trainee social workers and social work assistants are appointed by some authorities to undertake restricted caseloads.

Who the book is written for

This book is aimed at helping anyone who works, or wants to work, in the caring services. It is intended to help the reader to gain an understanding of the different roles within, and the relationship between, the various agencies that make up the care sector.

It is a useful resource for candidates undergoing National Vocational Qualifications (NVQs) and Scottish Vocational Qualifications (SVQs), students on pre-service courses of study (General National Vocational Qualifications (GNVQs)/Vocational A Levels), students on the Diploma in Social Work (Dip.SW) and students on other professional training courses. Medical and nursery nurses will also find it of benefit, as will informal carers. We feel that the interested general reader may also find it helpful.

The variety of material in the book

In addition to the expository text, the book contains other types of material:

(a) **Illustrations** These are intended to focus the reader's attention on the textual material and hopefully, to lighten it.

(b) **Diagrams** These interpret complex material pictorially in a precise and easily accessible way. Many are deliberately simplified in order to facilitate 'at a glance' understanding.

(c) **Appendices** These are found at the end of some chapters and contain case material from practitioners' working experience. They expand on the text and so enhance the reader's understanding of what carers actually do. The names quoted are fictitious. In some cases, a typical day's work is presented to enhance the reader's knowledge of what particular jobs involve.

(d) **Exercises** Almost all chapters include practical or role play exercises for people to undertake in a small or large group setting. Some roles are prescribed, others are more open, thus leaving interpretation to those involved. The role play settings are based on real work situations, and again the names are fictitious. The non-student reader will find the exercises informative and they will highlight dilemmas frequently faced by carers.

(e) **Questions for discussion** Most chapters contain six of these. Decide yourself on how best to use them. Some build on the text, others introduce topics not mentioned in the text. Many are included for their controversial nature.

(f) **Further reading** We have carefully selected a number of interesting and accessible texts. Each selection includes a very brief indication of the topics that the text covers. You will notice that throughout the text of this book we have used information from a number of sources: textbooks, reports, journals, periodicals, magazines, newspapers, television and radio programmes. We would encourage you to derive your own information from as wide a range of sources as possible and to seek up to date commentary on social and health care issues. We would specifically suggest reading weekly journals, such as *Community Care*, *Care Weekly* and magazines such as *New Statesman and Society*, as well as quality newspapers such as *The Guardian*, *The Independent* and *The Observer*.

Finally, much of the material in the book has been drawn from our own experience as a practising social worker or probation officer and as teachers of social care and social work in further education. In order to obtain authentic information about areas of work with which we are less familiar, and to up-date practice, we have sought the help of a wide range of fellow professionals who have provided up-to-date useful material concerning their specific fields. Any inaccuracies or shortcomings are, of course, our own responsibility.

We hope you will enjoy this book and that it will help you to build on and extend your own knowledge and personal resources and assist in your intention to become a more effective carer.

2

The Personal Social Services

Local authority social work – a brief history

The development of the personal social services was gradual and it was not until the passing of the Social Services Act in 1970 and the Social Work (Scotland) Act 1968 that a uniform and integrated service was finally established. Before this, older people, those suffering from mental illness and learning disabilities, disabled people and families with children were provided with services by different local authority departments. Consequently, it was possible for a child care officer and a welfare officer to visit the same family – one of these social workers being concerned with the child, the other focusing on the parent – without there necessarily being any liaison between them. In Scotland, probation was also a function of the new Social Work Departments whereas in England, Wales and Northern Ireland, social services and probation have always remained distinct.

The nineteenth century

Social work had its origins in the Poor Law and the voluntary organisations of the nineteenth century. The Poor Law Act (1834) was based on the idea that people were poor largely through their own fault and that to help them would only encourage idleness and intemperance. The Poor Law stated that those capable of work were no longer to receive any financial assistance in their own homes; instead, support was to be provided only in the *workhouse*. Proof of a person's destitution was that they were prepared to leave home, together with members of their family, to live and work in the workhouse. Conditions were made deliberately harsh – families were split up, labour was long and tedious and the rules were uncompromising. As a further deterrent, the wages received by inmates were always set lower than those of the lowest paid agricultural labourer outside. Thus it was hoped that only the truly needy would be assisted by the State; the others would be encouraged to help themselves.

What this moral attitude of the Poor Law administrators failed to take into consideration was the contribution made to poverty by such factors as low earnings, irregular employment, large families, sickness, widowhood and old age. Individual inadequacy was hardly relevant in such circumstances.

It could be said that the Poor Law guardians were the first State social workers in that they were responsible for providing very basic welfare. Professional care, however, was a long way off!

Alongside State provision there existed various voluntary and charitable societies, the foremost of which was the charity organisation society (COS) founded in 1869. Toynbee Hall, in London's East End, saw the establishment of the first university settlement in 1884; this provided scholars with the opportunity of living and working with poor people so that they would understand their needs better. Together with these organisations, Octavia Hill and other socially aware people helped shape early social work – they introduced group and community work and developed casework as a method of helping families.

Despite this practical and theoretical foundation, much of the early social work was viewed as being of the 'Lady Bountiful' variety where wealthy women of independent means distributed monies to less fortunate people. There was a strong moral blame levelled at those who were destitute, so charity was mainly granted to the 'deserving poor'.

From 1900 to 1945

Early social work was inexorably bound up with poverty as to a large extent it is today, and it was from Toynbee Hall that Charles Booth's enquiry into 'the conditions of the labouring poor of London' was conducted. So too was William Beveridge's early work on unemployment, which shifted the blame from the worker to the organisation of industry. Another late nineteenth century social investigation, carried out by Seebohm Rowntree in York, helped to further expose the extent of poverty and some of its social causes.

At the beginning of the twentieth century, the results of this research caused pressure to be put on the Government to take collective responsibility for social problems. Reforms and innovations in the field of pensions, employment and health insurance followed despite objections made by the COS who, in response to the proposals of the minority report of the Royal Commission on the Poor Laws 1905–1909, argued that increased support for families would encourage dependence and discourage individuals from taking responsibility for themselves.

Social work was developing in other areas in the early part of the twentieth century. In hospitals, social workers – or *almoners* as they were known – were being employed in the London region. Initially, their main concern was with the financial assessment of patients, since there was not yet any universal free medical service. Charges were made unless it could be established that a person was 'without means'. The Institute of Almoners was formed in 1920, although training courses had been started shortly before. The first *Child Guidance Clinic* was founded in 1927, but it was not until the 1930s that the *Psychiatric Social Work* service began in this country. The *Probation Service*, never to be a part of the local authority set-up in England and Wales, had also become established, having its roots in the work carried out by the police court missionaries of the Church of England Temperance Society.

For the local authorities, the statutory obligations regarding welfare were few but they began to increase from the time when they took over the administration of the Poor Law in 1929. However, most social workers at this time, whether trained or untrained, were working with voluntary organisations outside the local authority. It was not until the years immediately following the Second World War, with the further development of the *Welfare State*, that the local authorities were called upon to provide more extensive social services.

From 1945 to 1970

Following many of the recommendations of the *Beveridge Report* of 1942, the Welfare State aimed to eliminate what were described as 'the five giants of **want, squalor, ignorance, ill health** and **unemployment**' and to provide basic security 'from the cradle to the grave' instead. In support of this, local authorities were to establish a range of personal and caring services. The opening words of the National Assistance Act 1948 stated that 'The existing Poor Law shall cease to have effect'. The Poor Law was officially at an end!

Under the Poor Law, older people had been neglected and humiliated, but now appropriate accommodation was to be made available in cases where individuals could not look after themselves or be looked after by their families.

The sad experiences of deprived children kept in huge institutions, including some children who had been evacuated during the war, had been observed. A series of letters published by *The Times* newspaper brought their plight to public attention and in 1948 *children's departments* were set up, following the death of a child (Denis O'Neill) who was left unsupervised in local authority care.

The emphasis was now on professional care in smaller and more personal establishments. *Welfare departments* were set up to take responsibility for the care of disabled people and to provide social training and day centres for them to attend. Families made homeless by unforeseen circumstances now had a right to be accommodated by the local authority. Initiatives in community work were taking place and mental health services and services for people with learning disabilities were developing under the new National Health Service.

Despite the wider social provisions introduced after the war, it was clear by the late 1960s and early 1970s that the Welfare State had failed to eradicate poverty and its related social problems. The work of the Child Poverty Action Group (CPAG), MIND and Shelter all pointed to the continued vulnerability of certain social groups such as disabled people, older people, families in poverty, people with mental illness and those people who were homeless and stressed, and the urgent need for greater equality in the distribution of limited resources. Social work provision was rightly seen as being cumbersome and disjointed. The children's department was the most professional and resourceful; other clients needs were not being met. Rises in the juvenile crime rate, increasing numbers of older people, more frequent breakdown of marriage and a growing awareness of poverty and family problems called for the creation of a unified social services department.

In 1970, following the report of the *Seebohm Committee* two years earlier, the new local authority social services departments (SSDs) were created in England, Wales and Northern Ireland. In Scotland, the social work departments (SWDs) were formed in 1969, following the Social Work (Scotland) Act 1968. The aim of the new social service authorities was to provide an 'effective, family-oriented, community service, available and accessible to all'. This new expanded service would need a larger and more professional personnel. Social workers were to be 'generically' trained in order to avoid the narrow specialisms of the past and were to work with clients within a family and community framework. The new social services departments were formed from the former childrens departments, welfare departments and parts of the health service and began operation in 1971 following the Social Services Act 1970. In Scotland, the newly created social work departments incorporated the work of the Probation Service in addition to their general social welfare duties.

At last a universal and integrated service had been set up with the opportunity of providing standard professional practice and care. The intention was for this to be 'a supportive service for individuals and their families within a community setting'.

From 1970 to the present day

Initially, not all the authorities had the buildings or resources to provide localised social services so they were somewhat restricted by having to operate from a centralised point. Other authorities established *area offices*, which made the services more accessible to everyone and enhanced the departments' community involvement. Eventually most authorities had area offices from which social services were delivered. Some went further and operated an even more localised *patch system*, largely owing to the encouragement expressed by the Barclay Committee. However, we seem to have gone almost full circle as the trend now is towards reducing the number of offices open to the public. Owing to the need to save money some authorities offer access to service users at selected offices only and in some cases this public access is available only at certain specified times in the day.

The Barclay Report

In November 1980, a working party set up at the request of the Government by the National Institute for Social Work, chaired by Peter Barclay, reviewed the 'role and tasks of social workers in (LA) SSDs and related voluntary agencies in England and Wales'. Although no legislation followed its publication in 1982, this report made several recommendations, some of which certain authorities began to put into practice. In recommending a *community approach*, the Barclay Report repeated the message of the Seebohm Committee, adding that this development had not gone far enough.

According to the Barclay working party, most social care is provided not by statutory and voluntary social services but by ordinary people (i.e. relatives and neighbours) and it was recommended that this informal caring network should be supported and strengthened. In order to do this, and to make social work departments even more accessible to the community, the Report recommended that area divisions be divided still further. This has led to the creation of patch or neighbourhood teams within some authorities. Where this situation exists, social workers operate from smaller offices established within the community. Each office is responsible for working in a defined neighbourhood and has the aim of developing local initiative and providing a service to that 'patch'.

Some advantages of the patch/neighbourhood approach

The essential benefit of a patch-based service is that it increases accessibility to those people who use the service. If site offices are within walking distance or a short bus ride from clients' homes then people are more inclined to use the service. Where offices are established within the community they are likely to become a focal point and, indeed, where they have been established referrals have largely increased.

Workers operating from within patch-based offices are able to become familiar with and can more accurately gauge the needs of the local community than, say, their counterparts based in area offices. Accessibility is fundamental to social work. As the Barclay Report points out '. . . professional services carry a moral obligation to be fully accessible to people they wish to serve'; it adds, 'They must avoid both physical and psychological barriers which deter potential clients from seeking help'. The Report further adds that social workers clients' 'are often particularly disadvantaged, suffering as they often do from the effects of poverty. They often lack the confidence which is needed to seek help . . . A community approach offers ways of making social workers more readily available to people who may need help' (Barclay Report, p203). Increased accessibility often meant the opportunity of earlier contact with social services agencies and correspondingly more preventative intervention.

Not everyone favoured the idea of the patch. Indeed there was dissention within the Report itself. There was a fear that neighbourhood services may lead to 'bombardment' of scarce resources. The main objection to the practicality of neighbourhood services was that smaller teams would not be able to offer the expertise of specialised staff currently being provided by area-based teams.

Consequently not every local authority adopted a patch system (in the more rural areas such a system was in practice more difficult to establish.) Some decentralised for a short while only to revert to the more conventional form of service delivery in response to the increasingly specialised nature of social work. However, those authorities who developed a patch/neighbourhood system often did so not only for their SSDs but also for other services such as housing and environmental health. Where this has taken place not only have local services been made more available but the likelihood of interagency co-operation has also increased. But, as mentioned above, the need to make financial savings has led many authorities to operate from fewer public access points and centralise their service delivery so, in many cases, the very spirit of patch has been thwarted.

Child protection

Throughout the 1970s and 1980s there were a number of child abuse enquiries, most notably those concerning the cases of Maria Colwell (1973), Jasmine Beckford (1986) and Kimberley Carlile (1987). These and others were cases where young children died of abuse whilst in the care of the local authority or where the child was known to the authority and there was some active involvement.

Social services departments and social workers themselves came under severe censure from the courts and press who criticised them variously for lack of proper vigilance, failure to carry out their duties, poor decision making and the absence of co-operation with other caring organisations involved in the cases.

In some situations SSDs were justifiably castigated for poor practice. In others they were exonerated from blame, were shown to have acted professionally and it was agreed that they could not have reasonably been expected to have foreseen the tragic events that followed. Social work involves making informed judgements about human beings and this inevitably involves an element of uncertainty.

Just as social workers were criticised for their failure to act swiftly enough, so too were they blamed in cases where they were considered to have acted too hastily.

Heavy censure followed the actions of local authority social workers in Cleveland in 1989 when 125 children were taken into care, suspected of having been sexually abused. Social workers, and the hospital staff responsible for providing a controversial medical diagnosis, were pilloried by the press for over-riding the rights of the parents in their determination to carry out statutory duties to protect the children. Similarly, social workers who suspected ritual child abuse in Orkney in 1991 were criticised for their zealous actions in removing children in the early hours of the morning, once again, seemingly in flagrant infringement of parental rights. In both these complicated cases social workers had some grounds for their actions but subsequent public inquiries criticised the heavyhanded way social workers went about their actions.

By the early 1990s child protection practices of local authorities and related caring organisations had become more sophisticated and effective; consultation and co-operation had increased, flexibility and openness were stressed and named persons within the various organisations were given specific respnsibilities. Clear guidelines were drawn up and there was an emphasis on in-service training for social workers and other caring personnel. However, the events within the field of child protection greatly influenced the introduction of two pieces of legislation which, in turn, are expected to profoundly alter the role of social work for the remainder of this century and beyond. These two acts are the Children Act 1989 (implemented in October 1991) and the NHS and Community Care Act 1990 (implemented in full in April 1993).

The Children Act 1989 in England and Wales, and the NHS and Community Care Act 1991 throughout Britain, represent a radical restructuring of social work. According to the Government White Paper *Caring for People* (1989): 'The two programmes are consistent and complementary and, taken together, set a fresh agenda and challenges for social services for the new decade.' The underlying philosophy for both Acts is one of providing services within the community or family home according to individual need. Common principles embodied in the Acts are: user or parental involvement; 'needs-led' services; a multidisciplinary, inter-agency approach; public accountability; awareness and consideration of race, religion, culture and language; and cost effectiveness and value for money. In a sense these principles are not entirely new; they had already been, to some extent, incorporated into the work of the most committed social service authorities. Now, however, legislation has made them targets for all local authority SSDs and SWDs. (*Note*: the Children Act 1989 does not apply to Scotland.)

A note on anti-discriminatory/anti-oppressive practice

Towards the end of the 1980s plenty of evidence had accumulated that clearly demonstrated that the needs of black and ethnic minority people were not being met by SSDs and SWDs despite the claims of many of those departments of their being 'equal opportunity' employers. Nearly all local authority staffing levels showed a low proportion of black and other minority groups represented at social work level and an even lower representation within the ranks of managers and policy makers. There was evidence, too, that minority needs were being ignored, indicated by the low take-up of services and the fact that many practices lacked a cultural awareness. In such cases the identities of black children in care were rarely affirmed and black elders stayed away from local authority day centres that provided only typically English fare and traditional English passtimes.

In addition to the work of others, the work of black academics, black professional social workers and black community organisations helped bring this matter to the attention of local authorities and social work training bodies. The result was that by the early 1990s many more LAs were actively implementing equal opportunity policies by various methods, for example recruiting more black staff, monitoring services, consulting minority communities and genuinely attempting to make their services culturally sensitive and appropriate. In addition, the principle of antiracism became more firmly enshrined in all social care/social work professional training.

The late 1980s and early 1990s marked a time of greater awareness of issues related to equality and antidiscrimination, not just for black people but for women, people with learning disabilities, physically disabled people and gay men and women. Antidiscriminatory practice formed the backdrop to the developing standards of social care and social work training and was alluded to in legislation. For example, the Children Act 1989 places LAs under a duty to '. . . give due consideration to the child's religious persuasion, racial origin, and cultural and linguistic background'. This was the first piece of legislation to specifically address the significance of a child's 'race'. However, there has been some criticism of the Act because the duty is not mandatory.

Despite the heightened awareness and distinct progress made towards antidiscriminatory practice the struggle for equality continues and will need to do so until such time as Seebohm's vision of social services departments being 'accessible and available to all' is closer to being realised. There is by no means widespread acceptance about the need for social workers to be vigorously antidiscriminatory in their work. Opposition to CCETSW's Paper 30 (which lays down the curriculum universities and colleges must teach for the Diploma in Social Work), particularly annexe 5, a statement on antiracism, has been expressed by the incoming Director of CCETSW, Jeffrey Greenwood. He is concerned that 'politically correct nonsense should be rooted out.' (*Independent*, 23.8.93, p1).

The work of local authority social services authorities

General administrative responsibilities

Every local authority in Britain is obliged by law to provide a social services department or, in Scotland, a social work department. Under the present two-tier structure of local government, the population size of an area determines whether services are organised at county or district level. Thus a densely populated area such as Brent, in London, in common with many inner city areas, runs its own social services department at the district level, whereas social services for geographically larger yet less highly populated areas such as, say, Thetford or Kings Lynn are provided at county level by Norfolk County Council. In Scotland all social work departments are administered by the regional authorities. In Northern Ireland social services departments are administered by the Regional Health and Social Service Boards.

Throughout England and Wales there are 107 councils with responsibility for administering social services, a further nine regional authorities and three island authorities in Scotland and health and social services boards with 16 management units for personal social services in Northern Ireland.

Each council has a social services committee made up of local councillors. This committee appoints a director of social services from outside the council to run the service on its behalf. The director in turn selects and appoints staff to carry out the workings of the department; however, it is the councillors who are ultimately responsible for the actions of social workers.

As each local authority runs its SSD independently, according to its own priorities, there exists a variance in the standard of provision. There are two main elements which determine the quality and range of service provision: the commitment of councils and the availability of adequate funding. This, in turn, is further affected by the specific composition of the population: in other words, the number of people who are living on low incomes and the proportion of the population who are vulnerable and dependent on local authority services.

A council's commitment to the provision of social services is very closely related to its political persuasion. For example, generally speaking, Labour councils have been more prepared to spend on developing their social services than Conservative controlled authorities. Not all provision is statutory, i.e. required by law (Government statute), so local authorities have a good deal of choice about the range and quality of services they wish to offer. However, provision is ultimately determined by the amount of money available.

Local authority social services funding

Local taxation

Local authority SSDs and SWDs derive their finances from two main sources: central Government grant and local taxation. Prior to 1989 in Scotland and 1990 in England LAs obtained their local funding through the long established rating system whereby all property owners were required to pay rates, calculated according to the size and characteristics of their homes or business premises. Thus a householder living in a large house with all basic amenities would pay proportionately more than a householder who lived in a smaller property. Business properties would be rated similarly in accordance to size and amenities. Each local building was accorded a ratable value upon which the rates were calculated. People who lived in council accommodation paid a contribution towards the rates within their rent payments.

In addition to the income generated from the rates, which was the main source of revenue, local authorities also received a rate support grant from central Government.

Today the basis of local authority finance is very similar except that the rating system for households no longer exists. In April 1989 in Scotland and in 1990 in England, it was repaced by the *community charge* (or poll tax, as it became known). Under this system all residents of the borough were required to make an individual financial contribution to local authority expenditure regardless of whether they owned property. People with restricted incomes such as students and pensioners were not expected to pay the full community charge. However, under the system the owner of a mansion paid exactly the same as a person living in a terraced house or council flat and it was considered by many to be iniquitous. There were a substantial number of people who initially refused to pay the charge, collection costs mounted and it was eventually withdrawn. It was phased out in April 1993 when it was replaced by the *council tax*. The council tax focuses on buildings and dwellings and takes into account such variables as the status and number of people who live in them.

Cuts in local authority expenditure

Since the mid 1970s all local authorities have been forced to make periodic cuts in expenditure (some more than others) as their role as providers of services has gradually reduced. During this period there has been an expansion of the influence of central Government at the expense of the LAs generally because central Government has sought to more directly control council expenditure. It has been able to do this by financially penalising those LAs which have 'overspent'. In other words, by withholding or threatening to withhold the revenue support grant, central Government has been able to deter LAs from spending what the government regards as too much on the provision of public services.

In the days of the rating system central Government proportionately reduced the amount of its rate support grant to an overspending local authority in order to deter that local authority's current and future spending: those LAs affected were said to have been *ratecapped*. Similarly during the years of the Community Charge those LAs whose spending exceeded its standard spending assessment (the amount fixed by central Government that a local authority should spend on providing services) were 'poll tax capped' or 'Community Charge capped'. It is anticipated that a similar penalty will exist with regard to the Council Tax which was introduced in April 1993.

Charges for services

The 1980s and early 1990s saw a growing awareness in the potential income to be retrieved from providing services. Social services departments and social work departments developed ways of generating income in order to continue to provide services to vulnerable clients. Depending on their circumstances and commitment, SSDs or SWDs may have developed any of the following strategies: make small (income related) charges for services such as home care; sell off capital assets such as residential homes; reduce or, in extreme cases, cease to provide some or all non-statutory duties in order to concentrate on providing a restrictive service based on the minimum legal requirements. All local authorities have had to make cuts in their service provision. The extent to which they have done so is indicated by the increased variance in social service provision throughout Britain.

The need to generate income from services is likely to grow. Indeed, in March 1993 the Department of Health was developing plans to *force* local authorities to charge for services. This would mean local authorities having to put many more of its services out to tender in order that they may be undertaken and provided by the most competitive bidders from the voluntary and private sector.

Field social workers

Field social workers receive a generic training and have done so since the early 1970s following the recommendations of the Seebohm Report in 1968. This means that they study all aspects of social work, including the needs of many different client groups. Until recently it was common practice for newly qualified social workers to work with a wide range of people initially, before eventually deciding to specialise in an area of their own interest, still viewing their client within a family and community perspective. Nowadays social workers can expect to specialise as soon as they complete their professional training. There are a number of reasons for this:

1. The volume of complex legislation – for example; the Mental Health Act 1983, the Children Act 1989, the NHS and Community Care Act 1990 – and the increasing expertise required to do the job properly have meant a certain degree of specialisation has become necessary. Indeed, only approved social workers (those social workers who have successfully undergone additional professional training in the area of mental health) are permitted to carry out the local authority's duties under mental health legislation. In the field of child protection, social workers, ideally would have already received a substantial amount of postqualification training and it is anticipated that additional qualifications may be developed in the future.
2. The need for local authorities to save money has resulted in their cutting costs in some training; for example, the cost of training only a specific number of social workers in current developments in practice, as opposed to providing training for all those who would be interested in it, is obviously cheaper. In the past social workers were encouraged to undertake a wide range of in service training courses and to attend conferences as part of their personal development and in order to remain informed on aspects of their work. Today they are more likely to attend courses directly related to their specialism.
3. External factors, such as the critical media attention following on from isolated incidents of malpractice and abuse, have helped generate an atmosphere of mistrust and uncertainty around some social work operations. Consequently social service authorities, with less money at their disposal, have been concerned to concentrate their energies on their statutory responsibilities.

Some people argue that the move towards specialisation has been accompanied by an increasing emphasis on work done with children and that this has been achieved at the expense of other groups, notably older people and disabled people. Furthermore, it is claimed that the approach towards families in need has changed, with less emphasis now being laid on preventative social work. To quote a former SSD director, John Rea Price: 'Throughout the seventies we used to do quite a lot to support parents. That preventative work was undermined. Social service departments have been putting all their resources into child abuse' (quoted in Bob Holman's Tawney Lecture, 'Reconstructing the Common Good').

Broadly, the aim of field social workers is to clarify problems for service users and assist them to develop ways of coping. They have access to a wide range of resources, which include the provision of a place in a day nursery or nursery centre. In addition to obtaining day care or residential places, social workers may enlist the support of a whole range of domiciliary services which are aimed at helping people function better in their own homes. Increasingly these services are being provided by the private and voluntary sectors.

Legislation has extended the role of field social workers, and has granted them additional statutory duties with regard to all client groups – for example, the duty to 'have regard to the racial origin of a child in need when encouraging foster care applications and arranging day care' (Children Act, 1989, Sch 2(1)). Among other statutory duties, social workers have the right in certain circumstances to remove a child from her or his home, even if this action is against the wishes of the parent(s).

Most social workers operate from area offices or neighbourhood offices, but some are based in other settings including day centres and hospitals or, less frequently, they may be attached to general practitioners' (GPs) practices.

Fieldworker levels of responsibility

Generally, field social workers are paid at three different rates – level one, level two and level three – according to the responsibility they carry, the complexity of their caseloads and the decisions they are expected to make. The Barclay Report defined these levels as follows:

Level one   Social workers under close and regular supervision are expected to manage a caseload which may include all client groups and all but the more vulnerable individuals or those with complex problems. Such social workers are not expected to make decisions affecting the liberty of clients or in relation to place of safety orders (these have now been replaced by emergency protection orders under the Children Act 1989).

Level two   With supervision and advice, social workers are expected to manage a caseload that may include the more vulnerable clients or those with complex problems and may be expected to accept responsibility for action in relation to the liberty of clients in emergency situations. They may be expected to concentrate on specific areas of work where such concentration arises primarily from organisational needs and to supervise trainees or staff other than social workers.

Level three   With access to advice, and within normal arrangements for professional accountability, social workers are expected to accept full responsibility for managing a caseload which will include the more vulnerable clients or those with particularly complex problems in situations where personal liberty or safety is at stake. Such officers are expected to concentrate on specific areas of work which require more developed skills. They may be expected to contribute to the development of new forms of work or service.

More recently some local authorities have introduced a fourth tier, in an attempt to provide a *career grade* for those social workers who seek professional advancement yet do not want to move into management, who prefer instead to continue working directly with service users. Field workers at this level will usually be senior social work practitioners with many years social work experience, who are able to share their expertise and develop skills within the rest of the team. They will normally have a supervisory function but no managerial responsibility.

Care managers

Following the NHS and Community Care Act 1990 the traditional role of local authority field workers is likely to change in a radical fashion. Since the act was fully implimented in 1993 many social workers have become involved in the new role of *care manager*.

The White Paper *Caring for People* which followed the publication of the Griffiths Report on Community Care stated that social authorities should be responsable for designing care packages to meet individual needs. The NHS and Community Care Act recommends that where an individual's needs are 'particularly complex' or where 'significant resources are allocated to them' then a care manager should be appointed to ensure that the care package is well co-ordinated and remains appropriate. Not all field social workers will act as care managers; instead they will continue to be engaged in the more traditional social work role with service users.

The care manager does not necessarily have to be someone from the local authority social services or social work department; they could, in fact, be a person's career or even the service user. In practice, owing to the centrality of the role of social services, the care manager is likely to be a local authority worker. Their role will be to 'take responsibility for ensuring that the individual's needs are regularly reviewed, resources are managed effectively and that each service user has an individual point of contact' (Hammersmith and Fulham SSD Community Care Plan 1991/92, p96).

Under the NHS and Community Care legislation the local authority's general duties concerning the care management task are fairly broad. Essentially the local authority is involved in the following:

1. Defining need;
2. Devising forms of assessment;
3. Planning care;
4. Securing appropriate resources;
5. Monitoring;
6. Controlling the delivery of the care plan;
7. Reviewing the progress of the care plan with a view to reassessing needs.

At the same time it is important that the views of carers and service users are sought and that adequate information is made available to the public about the care management process.

Social work assistants (SWAs)

Several Social services authorities employ social work assistants to carry out the more routine social work tasks such as escorting, processing applications and registering people for basic services. Social work assistants are supervised by a qualified social worker and usually go on to undertake professional training themselves when they have gained sufficient experience. Similarly some LAs give their team clerks minor social work responsibilities in order that the incumbent can gain social work experience at a basic level. More formalised training is offered by those LAs who provide trainee social worker posts or take on unqualified social workers. Both types of inchoate social worker will have a restricted caseload and professional supervision and will be encouraged to develop a width of experience before eventually going on to apply for full professional training, if they can afford to do so.

Residential social workers (RSWs)

As the title implies, residential social workers (RSWs) are employed by social services authorities specifically to work in one of the authority's homes. Their chief function is to provide day-to-day care for the residents of the home, whether the service users are older people, people with a physical disability, people with a learning disability or children.

In the past, RSWs were concerned only with what happened in their particular establishments but nowadays they are becoming increasingly involved with the community. This is particularly true for, say, a RSW of a children's home preparing children for adoption or fostering. The worker not only needs to establish a trusting relationship with the children with whom she or he is working but also needs to get to know the prospective substitute parent(s). This will obviously require visits away from the establishment and so the role of the RSW overlaps with that of the fieldworker. Closer parental involvement and increased community liaison have been further encouraged by the Children Act 1989 and the NHS and Community Care Act 1990.

Care officers/care assistants

Care officers, also known as care assistants, provide basic social care for a whole range of client groups in different care settings, which may be residential, day care or now increasingly in the client's own home. They form the majority of the personnel within social service authorities. Some social services authorities have abandoned the distinction between COs and RSWs owing to the similarity of their roles, although it is generally true to say that where they are both employed within the same authority, COs focus on carrying out basic care whilst RSWs are involved in planning as well as providing care. However, there is often an overlap depending on how much additional responsibility a CO is allowed or encouraged to take. Significantly, in most boroughs care officers are usually paid weekly whilst RSWs receive a salary. This arrangement reflects their comparative status.

It is widely recognised that the role of CO has been undervalued and that their developmental and training needs have been largely ignored. Research shows the majority of care officers to be 'mature, committed, long-serving and willing to take on responsibilities and training' (*The Lost Potential*, SCA/Help the Aged, 1992). The fact remains they are comprised predominantly of women, a disproportionate number of whom are from black and ethnic communities, and they are in the main unqualified. The recent development of NVQs and SVQs in social care has the potential to redress some of the limitations of the care officer's role.

Types of difficulties presented to SSDs and SWDs

Social work authorities are faced with a wide range of emotional and social difficulties presented to them by individuals and their families. As several studies have indicated these difficulties are overwhelmingly related to the low income of the client. However, poverty is not always the main component of the presenting problem; it may be one of or a combination of the following:

a) *Relationships* – Difficulties between partners or between children and their parent(s).
b) *Drugs and alcohol* – Problems related to the misuse of alcohol and or illegal or prescribed drugs.
c) *Housing* – Inadequate housing, overcrowding or isolation.
d) *Absence of parent* – Single parent families are prone to poverty. Additional difficulties may occur if the parent is temporarily absent (in prison, for example).
e) *Children* – Behaviour problems, offences against the law, non-attendance at school or theft.
f) *Parents unable to cope* – Pressures stemming from several children of the same age or difficulties in managing.
g) *Financial* – Individuals or families may have rent arrears, debts and/or a basic lack of amenities.
h) *Illness* – One parent may be permanently or temporarily ill and be unable to care for the children.
i) *Mental ill health* – A family member may suffer from periods of various forms of mental illness (depression, for example).
j) *Older age* – Difficulties tend to increase with age particularly for those who are living by themselves.
k) *Physical or learning disability* – Of any family member may involve difficulties for the whole family.
l) *HIV positive and people with AIDS* – People who are infected affected by HIV and may need the support of the various services.
m) *Violence* – A person may be the subject of physical, emotional or sexual abuse.

The above examples by no means exhaust the range of difficulties presented to the SSDs or SWDs. Further, many of those listed are inter-related and are experienced by some individuals or families at the same time. In some cases it may be that social services authorities will not have the resources to resolve the situation and will need therefore to engage the co-operation of another caring organisation. In other instances they may refer the case in its entirely to a more appropriate agency, for example if the matter is essentially a 'housing allocation issue'.

Assessment

Before any action can be taken the client's situation needs to be assessed. Most referrals are received by the *duty officer* of a general social work team, who collates the information about the individual or family. This may have been gleaned directly in a

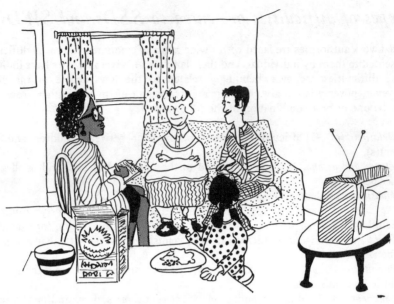

A Social Worker will visit people in their homes

face-to-face interview; the subject of a letter to the department; the result of a telephone call; or a combination of all three. Referrals may also come direct to the home care organiser as head of the home care service or straight to the head of the occupational therapy section, where there is one. The first task of the duty officer or home care organiser is to check whether the client is known to the department and is already in receipt of services. If, say, a social worker or a home carer has been allocated, then the information is merely fed to that person.

In social services authorities and SWDs which have adopted a specialist structure, a specialist *intake team* or assessment and investigation team, made up of social workers and social work assistants, may deal exclusively with new referrals. There are advantages to this arrangement: intake workers can develop an expertise in both diagnostic work and short-term intervention.

It is well known that a good deal of social work referrals are for short term practical assistance only and that this can be provided without recourse to long term resourcing or formal assessment. More straight forward issues may be rectified relatively simply: for example, the provision of a bus pass for someone who qualifies through disability or age; referral to a local women's refuge in instances of domestic violence; or sucessful negotiation with another agency, say the Gas Board or the Department of Social Security. Intake workers may deal with all new cases for a maximum period of about three months, by which stage, if more intensive and specialised intervention is deemed necessary, then the case will be reallocated to the appropriate specialist (long term) team (see below).

A more recent development has been the creation of *access teams* made up of specially trained administrative workers whose task it is to deal with straightforward matters, decide whether an initial appointment with a social worker is necessary and if so, which specialist team is appropriate for the client to be referred on to. The main advantage of this system is that it saves social workers spending time on routine matters and allows them to concentrate on their more specialised work.

There have been misgivings about the introduction of access teams from both social workers and their unions. It is claimed that clients may be put off by having to outline their difficulties first to an access team member and later again to a social worker. 'People who come to the office bursting with problems will be told to come back in a few days and go through the whole story yet again with someone else.' Furthermore, it is argued that experienced social work duty officers are able to detect and probe beyond the presenting problem and gain a more holistic view of the client's situation. Where access teams have been introduced this expertise has been lost: '(Now), if someone is making a nursery application he or she is given an application form. In the past, a social worker might have spotted other issues' (Community Care 19.3.92). Another concern is that it is not always apparent which specialist team should take a case and cases that are not attached to a specialist team may not receive a service. For example, a single adult who is not classified as physically disabled, mentally ill, elderly or has not got a learning difficulty, yet is in distress, may not receive social work support.

Within a political climate where the clear trend of Government initiatives has been to encourage LAs to distinguish between, and concentrate on, those members of society who are most obviously in need, it seems likely that access teams will be more widely adopted. Furthermore, in addition to the initial assessment arrangements carried out by access teams, LAs will need to develop secondary assessment for those people whose needs are more complex and full assessment systems for those people who require care management, to develop, oversee and implement a care plan in order to comply with the requirements of the Community Care legislation.

Prioritisation

It is important to remember that social services authorities have statutory rights and duties to provide a service in specific circumstances. For example, they are obliged to pursue any allegation of child abuse, since under the Children Act 1989 (and before, under a succession of acts since 1948) (in Scotland the 1980 Children Act applies), they have a duty to protect children from harm. Social service authorities are empowered by law to intervene, with or without the parents' permission, and to remain involved until they are satisfied as to the child's safety. On the other hand they have no specific statutory duty to assist, say, a middle-aged man who has an artificial leg and has no bus fare home or even a mother of an adult with learning difficulties who refuses to attend a day centre and is becoming depressed at home. Of course, provided they have the resources, SSDs and SWDs will do all they can to assist the people in both sets of circumstances towards a resolution of their difficulties, either directly themselves or with the co-operation of another agency. However the first duty of social services authorities is to meet their statutory requirements. In a time of economic cutbacks and decreasing resources SSDs and SWDs are forced to prioritise accordingly.

In recent years many social services authorities have been accused of delivering a crisis-based service only. It is claimed that in concentrating their resources on statutory work as it arrives, focusing particularly on child care and serious mental health cases, SSDs and SWDs have done so at the expense of delivering a more

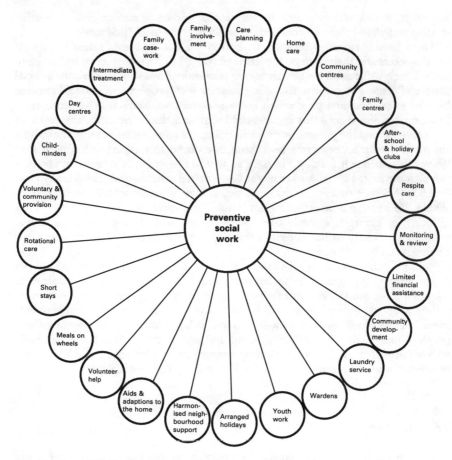

Fig 2.1   Preventive social work

generally preventive service. Whilst there is a good deal of truth in this accusation, particularly so far as the more financially restricted authorities are concerned, preventive work is still being carried out wherever possible. After all, to enable somebody to cope before she or he experiences insurmountable difficulties, to assist someone to manage by themselves in their own home or to facilitate community support for a person in their own neighbourhood remains the essence of good social work practice. Moreover, in view of its long term impact, such a policy is not only more humane, it is ultimately cost-effective.

Preventive social work

Preventive social work is aimed at enabling individuals or families to manage their lives more easily and avoid the occurrence of a breakdown or crisis. However, it is often the very experience of a crisis itself which leads a family to first seek help from the social service authority. In such a case, it is the task of the social worker to help resolve the immediate situation and thereafter to employ the various preventive resources at the disposal of the department.

Figure 2.1 illustrates the different services which can be described as preventive. They will be discussed more fully throughout this chapter. 'Community care' is one philosophy of social care/social work practice which is incorporated within the broader concept of preventive social work.

Recording

Once a person becomes known to the SSD or SWD and that person is allocated a worker, whether a social worker, a social work assistant, a home carer or an occupational therapist, a file is allocated to them and the workings of the case are recorded by the worker as they occur. Since 1987 under the Access to Personal Files Act, all service users have the right of access to what is written about them and are entitled, subject to certain specific conditions, to read and inspect their own files. Clients may apply in writing for access but will not be allowed to see third party records (i.e. those written by a doctor or a psychologist). This move was generally welcomed by social workers and clients alike. Indeed, it is considered good social work practice to use the substance of the files to emphasise agreements, responsibilities and mutual commitments and to show progress, so that recordings can be used in an enabling way. Essentially the file provides a summary of the department's ongoing involvement with an individual or family. It needs to be kept up to date and contain accurate information, including the precise times and dates of visits and the substance of discussions and agreements, as well as the social worker's summary of progress made. In the event of court proccedings taking place, written records may form the basis of evidence. The actual physical process of recording may help the worker reflect on their actions and direction and the file may be used for reference by senior managers, particularly in formal supervision sessions.

Recording is also an important function of the social care/social work task in both day and residential care settings. Most establishments will have a 'day book' where information about service users, such as changes in medication, sickness or significant events which may have occurred during the day, are entered in order that this may be made known to the whole staff group.

Some settings will hold a changeover meeting in order to give carers finishing their shift an opportunity to pass on relevant information to the oncoming shift of care officers. Where no changeover meeting takes place a senior member of staff will be responsible for verbally informing incoming staff of necessary information. Such practice will be reinforced by the expectation that all workers will familiarise themselves with what has been written in the day book at the beginning of their shift. Any serious occurrences happening during the day or night will be recorded in more detail in the incident book. Information which is of a particularly sensitive and confidential nature may need to be passed on verbally to appropriate staff.

It is important that recording is clear, concise and accurate in order to succinctly convey the essential details and to prevent any misunderstanding occurring. Many establishments are now using word processors for the storage and transfer of information. Where this has been set up a potentially more effective communication system exists, providing the staff are 'keyboard competent'. Naturally, there is the same need to guard against any breach of confidentiality as there is with handwritten records.

Supervision

A common practice throughout social care/social work in fieldwork, day and residential settings is that of professional supervision, where a designated person, usually the worker's own line manager, is responsible for providing one-to-one support and guidance. To be effective this needs to be practised regularly, carried out in a quiet and comfortable space and, so far as is possible, be uninterrupted. It is a two-way process with benefits to the practitioner and manager alike.

Some benefits for the practitioner

Supervision enables the worker to discuss any difficulties they are having working with any of the clients on their caseload and to seek advice and guidance on this. The worker is also able to outline the planned intervention strategies they intend to use with individuals or families and to report on the up-to-date progress being made with other service users. A field social worker may request resources for a client or discuss where these might otherwise be obtained. The supervision process allows for the exploration of a worker's feelings and attitudes towards their work and the people with whom they are working, in order to ensure that this does not prejudice successful intervention.

Supervision is just as important for residential and day care staff but it is generally less available for care officers. Most residential social workers can expect regular supervision. This gives them a chance to explore their relationship with service users, consider ways of working, any progress being made and action which needs to be taken. They may want to look in detail at their involvement with a particular client or even the difficulties in their own relationship with another member of staff. Once again, there should be the opportunity for self-examination and purposeful exploration in order that the worker might gain insight and work more effectively and assertively in the future.

Some benefits for the supervisor

Supervision should be an honest and open exchange allowing the supervisor to in some way evaluate the effectiveness of the worker and gain some reassurance that planned action is being carried out. The supervisor can identify training needs or may use the occasion of supervision to admonish the worker where this is necessary. Generally the process is supportive. On the strength of decisions reached during supervision sessions, a worker may decide that it is time to close a case, to try an alternative approach or to intervene more directly in the life of an individual or family. It may turn out to be necessary for a number of reasons to take a worker off a particular case and replace them with someone more appropriate.

In residential and day care settings supervision can similarly be used to monitor the work being carried out by staff. Generally it should be used as an occasion to praise

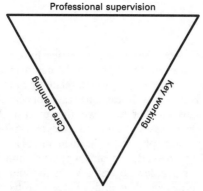

Fig 2.2   Interrelated activities in residential social work. (Diagram devised by Richard Johnstone.)

and reward workers for the contribution they make although there is room too for constructive criticism.

Team meetings

Teamwork is at the core of all good social care and social work practice and this can be fostered in some way by the provision of regular team meetings. At meetings staff can learn of any proposed policy changes, share ideas, comment on the progress made by individual service users, discuss any innovations in practice and consider practical ways of introducing new forms of good practice. Team members can also offer support for one another and use their combined strength, as a group, to challenge management on matters of concern to them and so help to shape policy.

Accurate recording, quality supervision and open team meetings all contribute to the development of teamwork which in turn contributes towards the establishment of good practice.

Figure 2.2 shows the interrelatedness of professional supervision, care planning and key working. *Care planning* is concerned with stating jointly agreed aims and objectives between the agency and service user and supporting that agreement with a regular review. (Young people in residential care can expect a review at six monthly intervals, after the initial reviews have been held. The Wagner Report recommended that this practice become mandatory for all client groups but this has not been universally adopted.) It is therefore up to agencies to decide on the regularity of reviews. Those people who have been admitted to residential care since April 1993 are entitled to a review every six months following the National Health Service and Community Care Act 1990. *Key working* is concerned with accountability where a named person is principally responsible for the delivery of service to specific individuals on behalf of the agency. Key working, care planning and professional supervision are the tools of the trade for residential social work.

Specialist services

As we have already said, social services authorities have a number of statutory responsibilities and to some extent these govern the deployment of resources within the department. Most of these legal obligations relate to children and their families and for this reason there is normally at least one team concentrating on working with this group. There is usually another team working exclusively with older people, reflecting the high number of cases within this category. Separate specialist teams may similarly exist to work with physically disabled adults and people with learning difficulties; in less populated areas these teams may be combined. Most areas have a specialist team working with people who are HIV positive and another serving people with mental health difficulties which includes those who have problems related to alcohol or drug misuse. Within these teams there are individual specialists such as an interpreter for people who are deaf or who have hearing impairment; a visual handicap specialist; an under-8s co-ordinator and approved social workers (ASWs) (mental health). Some other specialists who may or may not be team based are welfare rights officers, intermediate treatment officers, fostering officers, after-care social workers and language interpreters. In addition to this social work support each department has a home care team led by a home care organiser. This service usually provides care in the service user's own home. Finally, an occupational therapist may well be based in an area office or in social services authorities day centres.

The children and families team

The work with children and their families may be divided between a team specialising in serving younger children (i.e. those under eight) and a team working with older children (i.e. mainly teenagers). Of course many families include children in both age categories and the social workers concerned will be working with the whole family. However, working with families with very small children requires different skills from working with teenagers and their families, hence the need for social workers to specialise.

As part of a team, a social worker may well work with a family on a regular basis to help overcome difficulties that may be of long standing. They will have a number of families or young people on their caseload and will apportion time according to the urgency and importance of the case. Experienced social workers may have a caseload made up almost entirely of clients who are on the child protection register. Employing whichever form of intervention is considered appropriate, the social worker may be able to assist in a number of ways ranging from the provision of practical help, such as arranging transport or liaising with the school welfare department, to giving sustained emotional support and offering direction.

A fulltime place in a day nursery for one of the children in the family may help alleviate family stress and provide the child with the care and attention she or he requires; this may be arranged by the social worker. They will not allocate the place personally; rather, the social worker will recommend the family to the under-eight specialist who, in liaison with the officer in charge of the local day nursery, will consider the case in the light of those already waiting. Sometimes it is possible for social workers to arrange holidays for families with the help of voluntary organisations or to obtain financial help, say, for a family with a child with special needs, again through the voluntary bodies concerned (the Rowntree Trust, for example).

Financial aid

Ever since the Children and Young Persons Act 1963, SSDs have been allowed to distribute a certain amount of money to families with children, but only in special circumstances. Originally this money was used 'to diminish the need to receive a child into care' (section 1, Children and Young Persons Act 1963, retained as section 1 Child Care Act 1980). (*Note*: Since the Children Act 1989 the term 'children in care' is not applicable to all children being 'looked after' by the local authority: some children and young people are admitted through accommodation orders and others through the courts, following care proceedings. Strictly speaking, then, only those children who are cared for as a result of a care order, i.e. via the courts, can be said to be 'in care' – the others are said to be *accommodated* when they are removed from their family homes. The term 'being looked after' refers to *all* children who are cared for by the local authority) i.e. those 'in care' and those who are 'being accommodated'.)

This money, formerly known as 'section one money' and now known as 'section 17 money' (Children Act 1989, section 17), continues to be available but owing to restrictions on expenditure, it is less widely applied by social services authorities than it was in the past. It may still be used to help a family forestall the cut-off of gas or electricity supplies, for example, or to part finance a holiday in order to help the family take a needed break. This limited budget remains the only legal means by which the department may financially assist its clients. Other families in need of financial support are referred to the DSS and in some circumstances social workers may help a family to contact a charitable organisation or voluntary body to try to obtain additional funds, provided their circumstances are appropriate.

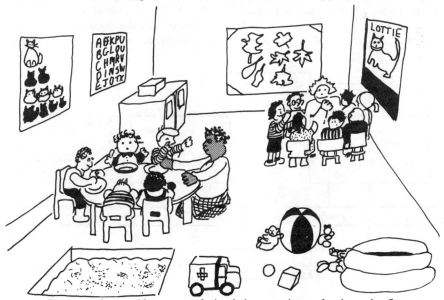

Day nurseries provide a range of stimulating experiences for the under-fives.

Services for families with young children (under eight's)

Day care

An overwhelming requirement of many families is the provision of adequate day care for their children. This may be sought in order to allow the parent(s) to take up paid work or to allow the parent(s) some time away from the demands of young children and so relieve family stress. Nationally there are LA day care places available for less than one percent of children age 0–4: England 0.81 percent, Wales 0.11 percent and Scotland 1.61 percent (1991 statistics, Great Britain, National Children's Bureau) so social services authorities are forced to prioritise their allocation of day care places and, in most cases, establish a waiting list. Traditionally SSDs have initially offered places to children considered to be at risk; that is, those children already on the child protection register and, in some instances, their sisters and brothers; other children who are suspected of being abused and children who are not felt to be developing, who would benefit from the structured love and care provided in the stimulating surroundings of a LA day nursery. The Children Act 1989 reinforced this emphasis and directed that services to children should be centred on children in need a category which automatically includes children with disabilities.

In a society with a general paucity of adequate day care provision the value of fulltime day care in a LA day centre with its professional staffing, long day and its high level of support is recognised by many families, including those who are able to afford the full cost of day care and whose children are not 'deprived'. Some LAs, mindful of the need to generate income, have decided to allocate a set number of nursery places to children of full fee paying families. This has meant a political compromise for the authorities concerned in that such a policy effectively reduces the amount of places available for the more disavantaged children. However this policy does yield one major advantage in that it lessens the stigma attached to children who attend LA day nurseries and provides a wider social mix within which the children can develop.

Family centres, a relatively new form of provision, are aimed at serving the needs of the family and the child. They originated in the 1970s and are usually run by

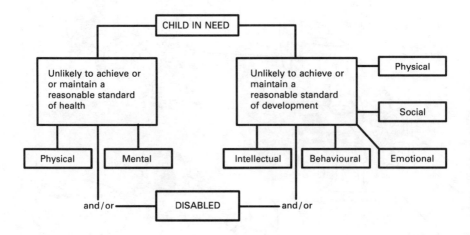

Fig 2.3   A child in need.

voluntary organisations, either in conjunction with social work authorities or independently. In 1989, of the 352 family centres in England and Wales only 57 were exclusively in the statutory sector (Community Care 30.7.92). There exists a wide diversity of provision from centre to centre, ranging from recreational, cultural, occupational or social activities to the provision of advice, guidance, counselling and family therapy. According to Bob Holman, family centres can be broadly catogorised into three types:

> The first is the client-focused model, which concentrates mainly on families referred for child abuse, with professionals in charge of running the centre. The second is the neighbourhood model, which has an open door to the community and so draws residents in as users and helpers; and the third is the community development model, rarely found, which encourages residents to initiate and run the services.
>
> (Community Care 30.7.92)

It has been noted that there is a danger of the client-focused model becoming the dominant mode of family centre provision, mainly owing to many social services authorities' need to meet the demands of existing child abuse cases, so they concentrate their resources on a few, very needy clients. Where either of the community models have been established, a wide range of service users continue to give and gain support in a friendly, non-stigmatised way. By facilitating community contacts and helping to develop skills and confidence these types of family centre are often able to equip families with the ability to cope and ultimately

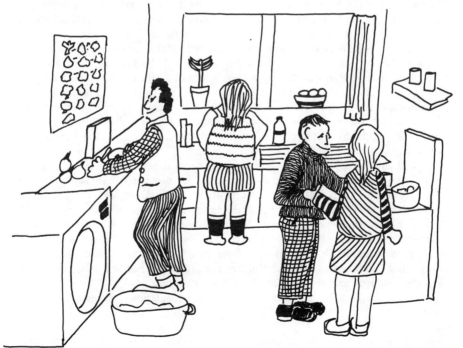

In family centres, parents come together to share and enhance their skills in a group setting.

avert the potential family crisis that usually heralds the need for more intensive social work intervention.

Childminders offer a personalised form of day care for young children but they are not provided directly by the local authority. LAs have a duty to register childminders according to strict criteria including the number and size of rooms, toilet and washing facilities and the maximum number of children allowed to be looked after during the day. Childminders work in their own homes, usually on their own, although some may work with an assistant or in partnership with another childminder. Whatever the arrangement, specified ratios of carers to children have to be adhered to. The standard recommended ratios are:

1:3 children aged under five
1:5 children aged between five and seven
1:6 children aged under eight of whom no more than three are under five.

Basically their homes need to be free of hazards and to be welcoming to children. The premises are subjected to periodic local authority inspection and childminders are encouraged to maintain records of the children they care for.

The main advantages offered by childminders to young children and their families are their local accessibility, flexibility and the intimacy of care provided by the same adult to a small number of children. This is offset against the relatively high cost to parents who use such a service particularly when it is compared to an allocated day nursery place which is generally subsidised or charged at an income-related fee. In situations where a child has been assessed as qualifying for a fulltime day nursery place and there is no vacancy, she or he may be offered a sponsored place with a childminder. Under this arrangement the LA will pay the whole childminder's fee, until such time as a day nursery place becomes available.

It remains illegal for parents to pay unregistered childminders although many still do owing to the convenience of the arrangement and the fact that they are often cheaper than registered minders, but the standard of care is not guaranteed. Low incomes are a factor behind the continued use of unregistered childminders and partly account for the fact that most preschool age children are cared for by members of the child's family or by friends or neighbours. As stated earlier only a very small proportion of children are provided with a fulltime day care place by the local authority.

As well as having to register childminders the local authority also has a duty to register play groups and other forms of sessional day care where care is provided for mornings or afternoons only. Furthermore, under the Children Act 1989, all services to children should 'have regard to the different racial groups to which children within their area, who are in need, belong'. 'Local authorities have the power to cancel a group or an individual caregiver's registration on the grounds of "inadequate care" to have regard to the child's religious persuasion, racial origin and cultural and linguistic background.' So now all services to children need to be planned and delivered to meet the racial, cultural and religious needs of those children.

Volume 2 of the 'Children Act: Guidance and Regulations' makes the following point:

People working with young children should value and respect the different origins, religions, cultures and languages in a multiracial society so that each child is valued as an individual without racial or gender stereotyping. Children from a very young age learn about different races and cultures, including religion and languages, and will be capable of assigning different values to them. (It goes on to add) The same applies to gender and making distinctions between male and female roles. It is important that people working with young children are aware of this, so that their practice enables the children to develop positive attitudes to differences of race, culture and language and differences of gender.

(Children Act 1989; Guidance and Regulations Vol. 2, 6.10)

Playgroups offer part-time care to children and have the advantage of being local, flexible and usually relatively cheap. They give parents a break, freeing them for part-time paid work or to do tasks best done without young children around. Some playgroups will encourage the active involvement of parents for some of the sessions. Children benefit from interacting with other children, learning to play and share and having new experiences in a caring setting outside the home.

Some local playgroups have been successful in obtaining partial funding from the LA in which they operate. This helps to reduce the direct cost to users and to extend the provision to more children within the community.

Services outside school hours
The Children Act 1989 extended the duty of LAs to regulate day care for children under five to children in need under eight. This includes day care services which provide play opportunities for school age children outside school hours and in the school holidays: summer play schemes, out-of-school clubs and various drop-in centres, for example. For this type of care strict regulations need to be complied with; for instance, the ratio of staff to children needs to be 1:8 for children under eight. The Act requires registered providers of out of school hours care to make observations and keep records on the children in order to contribute to future planning. There is enormous value in the provision of both after-school and holiday day care service to families with young children whether it is for allocated places only or is of an open access, drop-in variety. Often the resource is flexible and informal and enables the children more scope to develop confidence and social skills.

The advantages of day care
There are several studies of day care settings which reveal the positive developmental benefits for the children who attend them in terms of improved cognitive and language development; skill in interaction with other children; and the increased ability to form secure attachment relationships with adults. This last point is closely related to the stability of care: it is argued that the greater the stability of care, as measured by the continuity of the placement and by a low staff turnover, the greater the potential for the child's development.

Many people advocate the provision of fulltime preschool day care for all young children because of the obvious social, educational and psychological advantages it offers particularly to those children who are disadvantaged in some way. It is felt that the provision of quality day care can go some way towards mitigating the social and emotional disadvantages experienced by many children in our society. Whilst the value to ordinary children of day care has been widely acknowledged, until recently less has been said about its appropriateness for children with disabilities, who would appear to have even more to gain.

Children with disabilities

The Children Act 1989 provided a framework for incorporating children with disabilities into mainstream service provision and so both physically disabled children and those with learning difficulties are now placed in ordinary day care settings wherever possible. This move towards integration can be seen as a positive step forward for the estimated 360 000 children with disabilities living in England and Wales. It may improve a child's chances of being seen as a whole person, rather than having her or his disability viewed as the main focus to the exclusion of important aspects of her or his personality and identity.

Children with disabilities are automatically included in the 'in need' category of the Children Act 1989 and therefore quality for service provision. The Children Act 1989 reiterated the principle of the earlier Education Act 1980 in stressing that the development of young children with disabilities is more likely to be promoted if they attended ordinary day care and nursery establishments. 'Generally the development of young children with disabilities or special educational needs is more likely to be enhanced through attending day care services for under-eights or educational services for under-fives used by all children' (Children Act 1989, Guidance and Regulations Vol. 2, p 34). Prior to the Act some of the more enlightened local authorities had already moved towards integrating children with disabilities with ordinary children in their day care provision, but the Children Act 1989 now offers specific direction to all local authorities. LAs are encouraged to liaise with other organisations such as the health authority and relevant voluntary bodies in making arrangements for integrating children and to pay particular attention to 'the physical environment, staff/child ratios and training (e.g. in sign language)' (ibid). However, owing to the speciality or profundity of some children's disabilities it is necessary to provide separate services in some instances. Where possible it is recommended that such provision 'be attached to a service used by all children so that joint activities can be arranged from time to time' (ibid).

Children being looked after by the local authority

The aim of social work intervention with families with young children is to provide guidance and support and, where possible, practical resources to enable the family to help themselves. Ultimately the goal is to dispense with any social work involvement and to rely on the inner strengths and resilience of all families to meet and deal with their own difficulties.

Unfortunately it is not always possible to prevent breakdown, which may occur for a number of reasons. When this happens it is sometimes necessary to remove a child from home in order that she or he may be looked after by the local authority. It must be remembered that this step is only taken as a last resort when all other alternatives have been explored. For example, the feasibility of placing the child with relatives or of supporting the family through the allocation of a home carer will need to be considered.

Once a child is accommodated by the authority the aim of the social service department, following a brief period of assessment, is to work towards one of two aims, both of which embody the *permanency principle*: either reunification with the child's own family, i.e. a permanent return home, or finding a substitute family, i.e. establishing a permanent home with foster carers or adoptive parents. In most cases where children are removed from their homes they return before the end of a six month period, the crisis having been resolved with the possibility that the very action of temporary separation may have in itself contributed to the resolution of the family's difficulties. In other cases where a return home is neither sought nor deemed desirable, for instance in circumstances of danger or complete rejection of the child or in cases where the child is totally beyond the control of the parents, long term alternative accommodation is required.

Although practices and policies vary throughout the country the general trend, accelerated over recent years, has been away from providing residential accommodation for children in the care of the local authority in favour of providing a comprehensive *fostering service*. It is felt that the needs of children, especially in the lower age group under ten, are better catered for in a foster home because the care is provided in a family-based setting more typical of society in general than any institutional provision. In 1992, of the 55 000 'children in care' in England, 32 100 were in foster homes (*Hansard*, 18.5.93, pp 147–50).

Fostering services

Fostering is the bringing up of a child in a local authority or a registered voluntary organisation's care by substitute parents. It is one of the oldest services provided by the LA and was formerly referred to as 'boarding out'. The 1980s saw an overall decline in the number of children in care, the closure of many children's homes and a growth in the proportion of children placed with foster carers. In 1981, 92 270 children were in the care of local authorities in England, of whom, 35 749 were placed with foster carers. In 1991, 59 834 children were in the care of local authorities in England, of whom, 34 766 were placed with foster carers (*Children in Care of Local Authorities, Year ended 31 March 1991*).

There are two main reasons for the increased use of foster carers firstly, the drive towards improvement in child care practice; it is recognised that the fostering arrangement incorporates better practice since it is more personal, does not have the problems of staff turnover which characterise some residential establishments and takes place within a family setting, however this is composed. Secondly, there is the financial factor; the increased popularity of fostering has coincided with the reduction of local authority finances. Fostering has a superficial attraction to local authorities because it may be provided at a lower cost than residential care. However, good quality fostering, where carers are paid an appropriate allowance for their skills and are provided with an adequate support system, may cost as much as the average residential provision.

The fostering service has been greatly influenced by the implementation of the Children Act 1989, in particular the emphasis of the Act on the importance of the family and the continued responsibility of the child's parents, even when they are not physically looking after their children. As has already been said, the Act stresses the need of care agencies 'to work in partnership with parents' and insists that parents are involved in planning for their children's care. The LA must promote 'contact' between parents and children and work towards reunification of the family wherever possible. Even where it is felt that children are unlikely to return home permanently there should still be provisional arrangements for contact between children and their families.

Any adult can become a foster carer, but first they need to be approved by the local authority. Foster carers do not have to be married (indeed, many carers are single) or in a long term relationship with another person; if they are then the local authority would want to be satisfied that the relationship is a settled and stable one. Neither do foster carers need to have children of their own. Some children who need to be fostered find it much easier to settle in homes where there are no other children although others find it easier if there are children because they relate more readily to another child than to an adult. The important requirement of potential foster carers is that they have had some experience with children and that they are committed to providing loving care and support to a child or young person within their home.

Before children may be placed, the foster carer(s) needs to be approved either by the LA or an authorised voluntary organisation, e.g. Banardos or Catholic Children's Society, except for emergency placements. In carrying out an assessment of prospective foster carers and their households, all other children, adults and any lodgers are taken into consideration because they will have an influence on any child placed in the home. Police records on all adults in the household and health records on the foster carers are checked with the appropriate authorities and the two personal referees submitted are interviewed by the social worker undertaking the assessment.

Potential foster carers may be assessed on matters such as age, race, sexual orientation, personality, occupation, experience with children, culture and religion and views on HIV and AIDS. A confidential written report will be produced which is normally shared with the carers being assessed. The social worker will discuss with the carers the age range of children they would feel comfortable caring for. Some foster carers will state a preference to look after physically disabled children or children with special needs. When they are approved, carers are given a written agreement and are informed about the number of children and the age range they have been approved to foster and the kind of foster care approved of, e.g. short term or long term (permanency). In return foster carers broadly agree to 'comply with the terms of the foster agreement: to care for the foster child as if she or he were a member of the family and to safeguard and promote the child's welfare' (*Foster Care Placements: Regulations and Guidance*, National Foster Care Association, 1992, p 6).

Placement agreement meetings

According to the recent Foster Placement (Children) Regulations the local authority is obliged to hold a placement agreement meeting within 14 days of a child being placed with a foster carer. The broad aim of this meeting is to get all parties together in order to give the placement a firm direction. The people who will be invited to attend are the child or young person being fostered; her or his birth parents; the foster carer(s); the foster carer's social worker and the child's social worker. During the meeting issues such as the child's schooling, her or his cultural and religious requirements and the 'house rules' of the carer's home will be discussed and an agreement drawn up between the parties outlining the specified tasks of all concerned. If this meeting follows a planned admission then it would have been preceded by a preplacement meeting, made up of the same personnel who would have already been involved in a similar planning process; nevertheless a statutory placement agreement meeting would still have taken place. For an emergency admission the placement agreement meeting would be the first time that all the interested parties have been brought together. These initial planning meetings will be followed up by statutory reviews which are required to take place (after one month) after three months and at six-monthly intervals thereafter.

Training for foster carers

Apart from having responsibility to 'match' children to foster carers, a LA fostering officer has a duty to recruit and support foster carers. The fostering officer will normally be a qualified social worker who will carry out assessments on people who are willing to become foster carers. Once they have been assessed and are considered appropriate, they are invited to join ongoing groups of experienced foster carers. Groups are run to promote an understanding of the requirements of the work and to allow foster carers to share their experiences, express their views and provide mutual support. The local authority will outline what is expected of carers. Foster carers will talk about what they expect from the arrangement and receive and contribute to general practical advice for the age group they are fostering.

Fostering is a demanding job and requires a wide range of skills from foster carers who, in turn, need regular support. In addition to visits from the field social workers working with the child, carers will also receive visits from the foster carers' link worker whose role it is to support them and help sort out any difficulties they may be having. The local authority or local branch of the National Foster Care Association (NFCA) may encourage the development of foster carers' support groups. The Children Act 1989 requires that children being looked after are reviewed at regular intervals and foster carers will be invited to attend these reviews and to contribute to the local authority's plans for the child's future.

Local authorities pay foster carers an allowance to cover the cost of keeping the child but they do not usually pay a salary as such (although this arrangement would appear to be changing in some authorities). The payment of a basic allowance stems from the older thinking that people ought not to make a profit from looking after children. Nowadays, however, since the service has expanded to include provision for children of all ages and with a wide range of disabilities, allowances are being increased in relation to the degree of difficulty and responsibility involved. In some areas of the country, with regard to 'hard to place children' (for example, children who have displayed severe behaviour difficulties), fostering is recognised as being

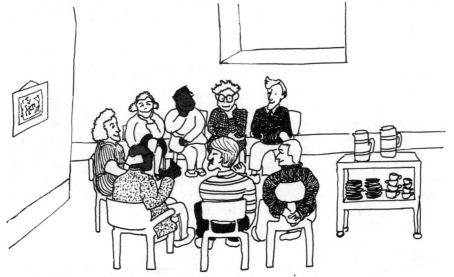

Regular group meetings enable foster parents to be supportive to each other.

equivalent to a fulltime job and is paid accordingly; in other areas only the basic recommended allowances are paid.

It may be that foster carers will seek to adopt the child they have been fostering and under the Children Act 1989 there is provision for them to do so provided they have been caring for the child for a certain number of years although in some instances carers may make the application sooner. Not all foster carers want to adopt; they may wish to continue long term involvement and carry on receiving the fostering allowance or, under certain circumstances, they may apply for a *residence order* which will automatically give them parental responsibility. This may be simpler and quicker to achieve than adoption and has some security benefits for the children concerned. It must be remembered that whilst a child is being accommodated by a local authority, birth parents have a right to remove their child at any time, except in extreme cases when foster carers can refuse to hand back a child if they feel they are 'reasonably safeguarding or promoting the child's welfare'. This might apply when a foster carer refuses to hand over a child to parents who are clearly under the influence of alcohol or drugs.

Types of fostering

There are three main types of fostering:

1. Short term fostering;
2. Long term (permanency) fostering;
3. Teenage (task centred) fostering.

Short term or temporary fostering   Young children who are being looked after by the local authority may first go to a short term foster carer who would have been especially prepared to take children on a temporary basis. While the child is with the foster carer the social worker will be working towards reunification with the family or a subsequent placement with a more permanent foster carer. In extreme cases, where a return home or permanent fostering is not considered to be viable, a place may be sought within a therapeutic community. Here the child may benefit from living in a structured caring environment with other children. As has already been stated, contact with the child's parents will be facilitated and actively encouraged throughout the placement. For many children this short period of being looked after by the local authority will be their total experience of care, since most children return home within a six month period. Figures suggest that children who remain in care beyond six months are unlikely to be reunited with their family. In their study 'child care now – a survey of placement patterns', the authors, using a sample of 20 local authorities showed that 35 percent of children left care within the first month, 11 percent of children left care within two months and 15 percent of children left care within six months. During the next 18 months only 8 percent of children returned home, leaving the authors to conclude, 'if children do not leave care quickly they may well remain in care for a very long time'. *Child care now – A Survey of Placement Patterns*, Jane Rowe, Marion Hundleby and Louise Garnett, BAAF, 1989, p 50).

If the child is heading for permanency care then it may be necessary to place the child in a 'bridging' placement with foster carers to help the child to adjust to moving to a permanent placement.

Children will have mixed feelings about being permanently cared for away from their own home, regardless of their family experience. There may be feelings of relief, fear, distress, shame or anger, but if these can be worked through in the temporary setting then the chances of long term foster placement breakdown can be reduced.

Emergency foster carers   Emergency foster carers specialise in receiving children at any time of the day or night, often at very short notice. They are contacted in emergencies by social workers who have had occasion to remove children from their homes and need immediate accommodation for them. Unplanned reception into care can be very traumatic for children and so foster carers need to be particularly sensitive and welcoming. Out of hours duty social workers, who operate in the evenings and at weekends and bank holidays, will have a list of emergency foster carers who are available at all times. This list should be updated at least once a week.

Respite care   Respite care initially developed because of the need for parents with children with learning difficulties to have some respite from the continuous care of their children. Foster carers were recruited so that a child with learning difficulties could stay with the same foster carer at regular intervals while her or his parent(s) have a break to take part in activities that are either denied to them or are not easily performed while they are caring for children. Sometimes the child will stay over night and on other occasions for the weekend. In addition to providing a break for the parent(s), the child also has the opportunity of developing a relationship with the respite carer and her or his friends and family. This arrangement has proved successful with children who have learning difficulties and it has now been extended to ordinary children.

Long term (permanency) fostering   Permanency foster carers are concerned to provide children with a loving and caring permanent home. The children may have already experienced a placement with a task centred foster carer or they may have come from 'permanent' placements that have broken down or they may have been placed directly with a permanency foster carer as a result of being 'matched'. The latter involves the selection of an appropriate foster carer for the child in relation to such factors as similarity of social background, common interests and proxmity to present school. The placement would have been planned and have included a series of meetings, visits and overnight or weekend stays before it became a fulltime arrangement. The child's wishes would have been continuously sought and taken into account. Some foster carers may eventually seek adoption of the child. Here again, the child's wishes and needs, where age permits, will be considered. As with all matters concerning the child, the child has a right to determine her or his own future.

Teenage fostering   Teenagers may be 'accommodated' in the same way as young children but because of the difference in age and related experience there may be more obstacles to overcome before a suitable placement is found. Some teenagers are placed in the usual way but there are now specialist foster carers who offer places to youngsters whose behaviour makes them unsuitable for traditional fostering. Many such carers are in fulltime work outside the home and are only available for the young person whom they are fostering in the evenings, at weekends and during holidays, in just the same way as many ordinary parents of teenagers. It is only where small children, are being fostered that the Local Authority generally insists on a carer being full time.

Specialist teenage foster carers, over a set period of time, seek to actively reduce the difficulties that youngsters have and help them to return to their families or to move on to more independent forms of living. For example, a gay teenager would benefit from the love, understanding and support of a gay foster carer at a time in her or his life when positively coming to terms with one's sexuality is profoundly important. It should be noted that gay teenagers are not always automatically placed with gay carers, nor are gay foster carers restricted to looking after gay teenagers. Sexual orientation is one factor which would be taken into account when seeking to match the young person to the carer. Some kinds of specialised fostering are recognised as being particularly demanding and the carers therefore need greater expertise and professionalism. In some cases, local authorities acknowledge this by paying a higher allowance to foster carers of teenagers.

Although considered here as a distinct type of fostering it needs to be remembered that foster carers specialising in caring for teenagers may also undertake emergency care, bridging or respite care.

Fostering and adoption panels

Following the Children Act 1989 some LAs have established fostering and adoption panels similar to the ones already set up by the more proactive authorities. One panel is concerned with fostering and the other is concerned with adoption.

Fostering panel   This panel is responsible for recommending to the authority the suitability of potential foster carers and to consider whether the proposed foster placement(s) is suitable for a particular child(ren). The composition of the panel will be different in each authority but, may be made up of the divisional manager, experienced members of the foster care team and the children and families team and at least two registered foster carers and related professionals. It will meet regularly in order to minimise the delay in approving carers or placing children. The panel is also responsible for periodically reviewing existing foster carers.

Adoption panel   The panel's primary responsibilities are to consider whether certain foster carers could eventually become adoptive parents of a particular child and whether a child's interests are best served by a permanent placement in a foster home or by being adopted. The panel is also responsible for recommending the approval of prospective adopters and considering the suitability of particular children to the prospective adopters with whom they have been matched. This panel will have a similar membership to the foster care panel but in addition it may have members of the council's social services committee and other independent persons.

Same race placements

Before a child is placed with a foster carer it has to be established that fostering is the best service for the child and that the particular foster carer is the best carer in the circumstances. It needs to be remembered that following the Children Act 1989, all agencies now have a responsibility to ensure that the child's needs, related to racial origin and cultural and linguistic background, will be met as far as practicable and that the child will be brought up in her or his religion.

Immediately prior to the passing of the Children Act 1989 there was considerable controversy concerning a child's right to a same race placement and to some extent this controversy still exists. It is generally argued that only carers of the same 'race' as the child can properly look after a child or prepare her or him for later life. This argument applies particularly to 'black' children who will face racism throughout their lives and will need to be prepared and helped with regards to this. Like all children they also need to express and have their cultural identity affirmed. The controversy came to a head in isolated instances when local authorities removed children from their existing foster carers in order to place them with other foster carers of the same race as the child. This practice was viewed by some as being disruptive and unkind to the child. For instance, in response to an Appeal Court ruling by Lord Justice Balcome and Lord Justice Glidewell in August 1989 that a 17½ month old child be transferred from a white foster carer who had cared for the child since shortly after birth to a black foster carer, in accordance with the local authority's child care policy, MP Marion Roe said it was, 'Absolute cruelty'. She added, 'If a mother loves, cares for and nurtures a child, that child does not care what colour her skin is. Human beings relate to one another whatever their colour'. (*Daily Mail*, 24.8.89).

This view ignores the negative experiences of many black children in care who were brought up by white foster carers and the fact that children from a young age learn about different races and cultures and are capable of assigning different values to them. It is felt that they are likely to value themselves more positively with foster carers of the 'same race.'

According to one anonymous social worker: 'It is wrong to pretend to colour blindness. The melting pot ideal of the coffee-coloured children of the seventies, where everyone was seen as the same, could never have succeeded. People should be proud of their differences. There is so much evidence of the benefits of same race placements. I have seen children who were performing badly at school, were unable to concentrate, and were experiencing racism who, after moving to a black family, become confident and outgoing. They began to perform to their full potential' (*Independent*, 13.1.93).

Even though the Children Act 1989 stresses the right of children to an environment which facilitates their whole development, which tends to support the idea of same race placements, the issue remains controversial and local authorities vary on how they interpret the guidance of the law.

The issue is less clear for children with parents of distinctly different racial origins; for example, the child who is 'part Sri-Lankan, part French, part Jewish and a large part British'. 'How', the authors of *The Colour of Love* ask, 'can that cultural amalgam which is part of a multiple identity be described just by the work 'black'? (*New Statesman & Society*, 7.2 1992). All aspects of the child's cultural identity need to be acknowledged. Sue Norris, a white mother interviewed in *The Colour of Love*, says: 'I have three children. They are all shades and colours. They say my children are black – well, where does that put me? Where is that side of me? I am their mother, for God's sake – not their maid . . . When they call them black they take away my genes, my motherhood, with that word. I have no problem with the word black, I am not racist. I love their father and I fight very hard against racism, but I am not black and my children are not just black, but black and white.'

Anne Wilson, author of *Mixed Race Children – A Study of Identity*, believes it is important for children to 'accept both sides of their dual heritage, provided that they do not lose sight of the fact that white society sees them as black and metes out to them the same degree of disadvantage that it does to all black people'.

One reason for the development of the controversy was that in the past local authorities failed, for a number of reasons, to attract in sufficient numbers foster carers from black and ethnic communities. This was owing partly to negligent and discriminatory foster care recruitment procedures, partly to ignorance of service provision and partly to a general mistrust of social services departments within black and ethnic minority communities. Some of the more enlightened local authorities have already begun to redress this imbalance, but now the Children Act 1989 has instructed local authorities to follow the directive that, 'in recruiting foster carers the local authority must have regard to the different racial groups to which children within their area who are "in need" belong and recruit appropriate foster carers'.

The strength of fostering is that it is carried out in a variety of ordinary family situations that are broadly cross-representative of society. However, it is not an arrangement which suits all children; not all children are 'fosterable'. Some have behavioural or emotional difficulties that require more intense help. Others have physical or learning difficulties that cannot be accommodated in a carer's home. There are also children who have too strong a relationship with their own parents to want to form a new one with a foster carer and there are those children who have had enough of family life of any kind. These children may be better placed in a children's home or a therapeutic community.

Adult fostering

Foster services are also available for older people although this service is nowhere near as extensive as it is for youngsters. There are over 21 schemes throughout the country. Coventry SSD has the widest ranging service; it provides for 200 adults between the ages of 18 and 102 who are fostered by a total of about 130 carers, (Community Care 13.2.92). The client group includes people with learning difficulties, people with physical disabilities, older people and those who are recovering from mental illness or alcoholism. All carers are vetted in a similar way to those who undertake fostering of children and young people.

Fulltime and respite care is available and the foster carers are provided with support and are encouraged to share their experiences with one another. They may be invited to attend inservice training sessions along with social workers on relevant issues such as sexuality, new legislation and advocacy. Adult fostering has particular relevance for the continuity of care for adults with learning difficulties who have been fostered as children but need continued care beyond the age when they should officially leave care. Clearly, it has an equivalent application to all other adult groups because it enables them to be cared for within the community instead of inside an institution.

Adoption

Adoptions take place when the courts transfer all the legal responsibilities for children from either the legal parent(s) or the local authority to the adopter(s). In rare circumstances, because a child can be adopted more than once, the transfer of parental authority may be from an adoptive parent. Where a court makes a care order on a child or young person and that person is looked after by foster carers, then the local authority will have parental responsibility as well as the child's parents. Adoption is different because when a child is adopted the previous parents and the local authority will lose any parental responsibility they had prior to the adoption order being made. However, once an adoption order is made a LA still has a duty to provide post-adoption support where it is required by the adoptive family.

'Natural parent' is a term still found in adoption law. Practitioners vary in the use of the terms 'parent', 'birth parent' and 'natural parent'. 'Birth parent' is generally favoured because 'natural parent' implies that others are unnatural. It is important, before adoptions, to identify who has parental responsibility. Those who do have parental responsibility must either give their consent to an adoption or have their consent dispensed with by a court before an adoption order can be made. Unlike the mother, the father will not always have parental responsibility: if he was not married to the mother when the child was born then he will not have parental responsibility unless he obtained it at a later date, for example, after the mother has obtained a 'parental responsibility agreement' in order to share responsibility for the child.

Only an adoption agency can legitimately place a child with adopters. Most local authorities do this through SSDs (or SWDs) that are organised as an adoption agency and have an adoption panel to make decisions. However, social services authorities can delegate their role to one of the private voluntary adoption agencies which exist locally (e.g. the Catholic Child Service (CCS)).

The nature of adoption work has changed over the years and fewer babies have become available for adoption. This trend reflects a growing social acceptance of single parenthood, developments in contraception and, to a lesser extent, the availability of abortion. At the same time, the service has been extended to include older children and children with special needs. Children with learning difficulties were formerly considered to be 'inappropriate for adoption' but nowadays the right of any child to family life is increasingly being recognised.

Adoption work is complex because it is carried out within a legal framework. Once an adoption order has been made, the responsibilities of the previous parents are transferred permanently so, because of the irrevocability of adoption, the situation requires sensitive and careful handling. Giving up a child voluntarily so that she or he will benefit from the care of another family takes strength and the person(s) concerned needs time and support from an experienced, emphathetic social worker or independent counsellor, so that this important step can be fully considered, understood and valued.

There has been increased recognition of the value of openness in adoption, of maintaining significant links between the adopted child and her or his birth family if this is appropriate. Arrangements for contact can vary greatly from an exchange of information about a child's well-being from adopters to birth parents via the agency, to actual meetings between the child and the birth parents. Arrangements for contact may be informal agreements or by order of the court.

Since 1975 adopted adults over 18 years of age have been able to apply for access to their original birth record. If people were adopted prior to 12 November 1975 they are required to see a counsellor first in order to discuss the implications of learning about their birth parents and the reasons for their adoption. This change in law acknowledged the need and right for adopted people to have access to information about their identity and birth families. This is now integrated into adoption work practice by the provision of information to all adopters and children.

Adoption panels

Preparatory work for an adoption is normally carried out by specialist family placement social workers, some of whom will serve on the adoption panel made up of other social work personnel from the local authority and specialists from other agencies (for example the probation service and voluntary organisations). Meeting regularly, the panel makes recommendations on the appropriateness of adoption for particular children and the suitability of prospective adopters and agrees matches of children to parents. Frequent meetings of the panel are essential because undue delay can be harmful to the family and children whose circumstances are being considered.

The process of 'freeing' a child for adoption was introduced to allow parents to give up their parental responsibility to an adoption agency if they did not want to be involved any further or did not want to have responsibility handed over by the courts to the adoption agency despite the parents' wishes to retain it. Delays in this process have meant it is rarely used in practice.

After an application to adopt has been made to the court the local authority must produce a report covering the areas included in schedule 2 of the Adoption Act 1976. The court will expect this to include the child's wishes and feelings in relation to the adoption depending on her or his age and understanding. In adoption cases the court will appoint either a *guardian ad litem* or a *reporting officer*. The guardian ad litem is an independent guardian for the child, appointed either when the case is particularly complex or when the parents have not given their consent to the adoption. The guardian will meet with everyone concerned and eventually make a recommendation to the court. The reporting officer is appointed if the parents are consenting to the adoption; their principal duty is to witness the birth parents' written consent to the adoption having first ensured that they do so freely and fully understand what adoption involves.

Step-parents

Some of the work of the local authority adoption agency involves applications made by step-parents wanting to formally adopt the children they are already caring for. This applies in cases where one of the child's parents remarries (or marries for the first time) and the couple want to formalise their joint parental commitment. If such applications are granted, the birth parents surrender their natural parental rights in regard to the child and an adoption order grants both partners equal status as adopted parents.

The court must be satisfied that adoption is in the best interests of the child and is better than any alternative to adoption, including making no order at all. One step-parent cannot make a parental responsibility agreement with the child's birth parent because this option is currently only available to two birth parents.

As has already been stated adoption work is necessarily complex because of the legal framework, which includes the Children Act 1975, The Adoption Act 1976 and the Children Act 1989. These have all increased the statutory definitions of what must be done. The Adoption Act 1976 remains the dominant piece of legislation in adoption but is currently being reviewed in the light of changing attitudes and practices. The Children Act 1989 introduced a number of changes and requires local authorities 'to give due consideration to a child's religious persuasion, racial origin and cultural and linguistic background' when a local authority looks after a child. This applies equally to adoption placements.

Children who are accommodated

The notion of voluntary care was replaced in the Children Act 1989 by the provision of 'accommodation'. Children are no longer said to be in voluntary care; instead they are said to be 'accommodated' by the LA. The relationship, however, is still a

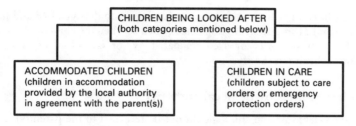

Fig 2.4   Children being looked after by the local authority.

voluntary one, so children can be removed at any time by the person with parental responsibility for them (or the child may leave, if old enough) except in certain circumstances.

A child must be provided with accommodation if:

(a) There is no person with parental responsibility for him or her;
(b) If he or she is lost or abandoned;
(c) The person who has been caring for him or her is prevented from providing suitable accommodation or care, whether or not permanently, and for whatever reason.

The following are examples of circumstances when a child could be accommodated by the LA:

1. When the child's parents die suddenly, say in a traffic accident, and there are no relatives willing or able to look after the child. Or when a refugee child arrives in this country and she or he has no contacts. Such children would be accommodated under condition (a).
2. When a baby is found abandoned in a public space or when a young child is lost and is unable to provide information about his or her parents or home address. Such children would be accommodated, usually only as a temporary measure, under condition (b).
3. When a parent is admitted to hospital and the other parent is either absent or unable to provide proper care and there is nobody else available. Or when a parent or child feels 'at the end of her or his tether' and is concerned that the situation is going to deteriorate and harm may occur, such a child would be accommodated under condition (c).

Condition (c) is the one most used since it broadly incorporates 'family breakdown' which is the main reason children are accommodated. 'Disrupted family relationships are a contributory factor in over half of admissions' *Patterns and Outcomes in Child Placement – messages from Current Research and Their Implications*, HMSO; 1991, p15). It must be remembered that accommodation is only resorted to (other than in emergencies) when all other appropriate forms of intervention have been explored; and when it is used, it is used in a positive way to help families stay together wherever possible.

Accommodation is provided when the LA considers that it will safeguard or promote the child's welfare. Even if the child or young person is not technically 'in need' the LA has a duty to provide accommodation up to the age of 18 and between the ages of 18 and 21 in certain circumstances, such as when the child has been looked after by the local authority or accommodated by, or on behalf of, a voluntary organisation or health authority.

Children looked after by the local authority

If the LA considers that the child should not be returned to the parent(s) it can no longer apply for 'assumption of parental rights', as it could for a child who was in voluntary care prior to the Children Act 1989. Now in order to obtain parental rights the local authority has to apply for a care order or, in exceptional circumstances for the sake of speed and expediency, and emergency protection order (EPO). This order is often used in cases of child abuse.

The Children Act 1989 introduced the concept of looking after a child. Children are classed as being looked after by the LA if they are in care on a care order, if they are being accommodated or if they are on remand, or away from home following emergency protection orders or child assessment orders or in certain other circumstances.

When a child is looked after by the local authority, the child should where it is reasonably practicable be placed with a person(s) who is connected with him or her; be accommodated near home; and remain with sisters and brothers. If a child has a disability then the accommodation should be suitable for that disability. So children may be looked after by the local authority but placed with relatives or a family friend so long as that person is regarded as being suitable by the local authority. In certain circumstances children may be placed, under a protection order, with their own parent(s) in their own home.

Before the Children Act 1989 there were several different routes into compulsory care. Now this is achieved solely by means of an application made by a local authority either under care proceedings or under other family proceedings. The Act sought to simplify the procedure and integrate private law with public law (for example, with regard to divorce law and reception into care).

In order to ensure that the child's welfare is paramount the court must use the following checklist before deciding which action to take (once again, it must be remembered that the court will only make an order if it considers that to do so would be better than making no order):

1. The wishes and feelings of the child as far as the court can find these out.
2. The physical, emotional and educational needs of the child.
3. The likely effect on the child of any change in her or his circumstances.
4. His or her age, background and any other characteristics which the court considers to be relevant.
5. Any harm the child has suffered or is at risk of suffering.
6. How capable each parent, or any relevant person, is of meeting the child's needs.
7. The range and powers available to the court under the Children Act. The court can make a care order or a supervision order if it is satisfied that:

    a) the child has suffered significant harm or is likely to suffer such harm; and
    b) the harm or likelihood of harm is attributable to:
      i) the care given to the child, or the care likely to be given to the child if an

order were not made, not being of a standard that would be reasonable to expect a parent to give him or her, or:

ii) the child's being beyond parental control.

Harm is defined as: 'ill treatment or impairment of health and development'. It is now possible for a local authority to receive a child into care before any actual harm occurs to the child in cases where potential abuse is strongly suspected.

Care orders and supervision orders
A care order or supervision order can only be made after an application has been made by a qualified social worker, who works either for the local authority or the NSPCC. However, such orders can be discharged or ended on the application of the local authority, the child or any person with parental responsibility. Education supervision orders can be initiated by local authority education departments (Children Act 1989, Section 36). When an application is made, the court may decide to make an interim supervision or care order until the court hearing takes place. These orders can take effect for up to eight weeks initially and can be renewed for up to another four weeks if necessary.

Care orders There is very little difference between the old care order of 1969 (Children and Young Persons Act) and the new care order of 1989 (Children Act). The main difference is that now parental responsibility is shared between the local authority and the parents of the child. Care orders operate until a child's 18th birthday, unless they are discharged earlier (and 19 if the child is made the subject of a care order after she or he is 16).

Supervision orders These last for six months in the first instance but the supervisor can apply for it to be extended, but it must be for no more than three years in all. Under the supervision order the child is placed under the supervision of a local authority social worker whose duty it is to 'advise, assist and befriend the child'. (This is the same guidance, incidentally, under which probation officers are encouraged to relate to their clients.) Supervision orders may be used in conjunction with one or more of the following section 8 orders.

Section 8 orders
In addition to the care order and supervision order, the court can make section 8 orders. These cover residence, contact, specific issue and prohibited steps orders. The court can also make family assistance orders under section 16.

1. *Residence orders* – Settle the arrangements to be made with the person with whom the child is to live. The person in whose name the residence order is made has parental responsibility for the child and can, in instances of disagreement with others who have parental responsibility, over-rule the other parties.
2. *Contact orders* – Are orders requiring the person with whom a child lives to allow the child to stay with the person named in the order or for that person and the child to have contact with each other. (This order replaces access orders.) Normally this would be used for the father of the child but it can be used for 'any person to whom the court considers the question to be relevent'. It cannot be made if a child is subject to a care order. In such an instance a care contact order can be made.

3. *Specific issue orders* – Means giving directions with the purpose of determining a specific question which has arisen or may arise in connection with any aspect of parental involvement with a child. For example, a 15 year old girl wants to have an abortion but her parents refuse. The court may make a specific issue order allowing the young woman to have an abortion.
4. *Prohibited steps orders* – Can be used to decide on a specific issue relating to a child or young person. For example, the court may issue an order prohibiting a father from removing a child from the country when this is seen not to be in the child's paramount interest.
5. *Family assistance orders* – Enable a social worker to 'advise and befriend' any person named in the order and can last up to six months.

The Children Act 1989 sought to offer sufficient safeguards to children at risk and to protect families against children being removed without their being given the opportunity to contest the order. There was a good deal of dissatisfaction with the old place of safety order (Children and Young Persons Act 1969) which had a duration of up to 28 days and the parents were unable to challenge this order while it remained in force. The place of safety order was replaced by the *emergency protection order*. This is a short term order which anybody can apply for if they feel the child is suffering, or is like to suffer, harm if the child remains where they are or if the child is removed from where they are. For example, a child may be considered to be at risk in their own home and may need to be removed for their own safety or a child may need to remain in a hospital ward or a children's home, again for their own safety.

The initial order can be for up to eight days with a possible extension for a further seven. The parent or person with parental responsibility can apply for the order to be ended 72 hours after it has been granted unless they had notice of the application and were present when the order was made. Parental responsibility is acquired by the person who obtains the EPO (e.g. the SSD) for the duration of the order, but contact with the family must be allowed unless the court says otherwise. The court may give instructions for a medical or psychological assessment of a child, although this can be refused by a child who has 'sufficient understanding to do so' regardless of his or her chronological age.

Guardian ad litem   Since May 1984 courts have been required to appoint a *guardian ad litem* in care and supervision proceedings and since the Children Act 1989 they have also been required to do so for an emergency protection order. The guardian ad litem's duty is to provide the court with an independent investigation into the child's circumstances. They may be appointed when there is a clear conflict between the interests of the child and the parents or between the family and the LA. The guardian ad litem must represent the views of the child and put these before the court. In addition the child is likely to be represented by a legal expert, usually a solicitor. In all other proceedings the court may request a report from the court welfare officer, either a probation officer or a social worker, depending on the age of the child. In most areas social services will tend to take responsibility for younger children, say those aged 14 and below. This report will outline the child's background and will include the child's views and a recommendation to the court concerning any action(s) that should be taken.

Children's homes or units

Children are said to be being *looked after* if they are being *accommodated* or they are the subject of a care order. As has already been stated, children are only accommodated as a last resort. Once it is decided that a child needs to leave the family home the first stage is to find a placement within the child's extended family. This might only be a temporary measure but it is likely to be less traumatic for a child to be placed with relatives than to be accommodated either with foster carers or in a children's home.

When it becomes clear that the child is liable to need accommodation the LA will hold a planning meeting which will be attended by all the relevant personnel. If the decision reached is that the child needs to be looked after, the social worker will contact the fostering team and request a place. If an appropriate foster carer cannot be found then a place in a children's home will be arranged. As a general rule, it is considered undesirable to place children under the age of 12 in a children's home; they will only be offered a place if a reliable relative cannot be found or an appropriate foster carer is not available.

Not all children are accommodated with such careful planning and forethought; some admissions are of an emergency nature that follow a family crisis that may have occurred that day, during the night, over the weekend or on a bank holiday. Each local authority will have a set number of 'emergency beds' reserved to accommodate children and young people at very short notice. The field social worker effecting the emergency admission will be expected to outline the immediate circumstances and the factors that precipitated the move. The social worker will also be expected to provide all the basic personal details of the child with regard to their schooling, medical or health needs and any particular cultural and religious needs, in order that the residential staff are not hampered in their work and that planning can begin straight away.

There are several types of children's homes; they are differentiated by the functions in which they specialise; that is to say, they may operate as an assessment unit; an emergency unit; a short stay (or task centred unit; a long stay home; a prefostering or preadoption unit; a home preparing youngsters for independence; or, in rare instances, a home caring predominantly for black or ethnic minority children. In practice, homes normally have more than one function. They will cater for different age groups and the establishments will vary in size.

Short stay/task centred children's homes or units

A typical short stay/task centred children's home will also act as an emergency unit and carry out assessment. It may cater for a maximum of six to eight children, say between the ages of 14 and 16, and may limit the length of any child's stay to a period of three months before she or he is returned home or to foster carers or, if the young person is unlikely to fostered, then to a hostel or bedsit accommodation. A place in the home could be refused by the head of home or unit manager if it was felt the child would be joining a disturbed group and would not benefit from a placement at that particular time. Conversely, if it was felt that the incoming young person would adversely affect the balance of the existing group a place could, again, be refused.

Within 48–72 hours of a child or young person being admitted, even in an emergency, a planning meeting will be held. This would have been discussed with the field social worker who brought the child or young person to the home. The people likely to attend this planning meeting are as follows:

1. The unit manager or the deputy;
2. The key worker (the care worker who will work closest with the new entrant and who will be 'responsible' for the child or young person). The key worker is allocated to the youngster as soon as they are admitted to the home or unit, in recognition of the young person's right to have individual support from the point of entry into the process of accommodation. Where a planned admission takes place an attempt is usually made to match the youngster and careworker along such grounds as interests, age closeness, gender or race;
3. The field social worker;
4. The field social work team leader (only if the case is particularly complex, otherwise they will rely on the field social worker's contribution);
5. The parents (or the person with parental responsibility);
6. Any other person who is significant to the young person (for example, an older friend);
7. The young person.

Care is taken to balance the meeting in its composition so that even representation is achieved and to ensure that the meeting is not too big or intimidating. It may be preceded by a short separate meeting of the 'professionals' involved to enable them to clarify the issues of concern. These issues will then be shared with the young person and the family in the main meeting.

The first question that the unit manager will address to the three main parties – the child or young person, the parents and the social worker – is, 'What can we do for you?'. This is to establish the objectives that need to be made. It may be possible to return the child or young person home almost immediately. If not, then during the meeting everyone will be given tasks and a contract will be drawn up. If the child has not been attending school the social worker may undertake to contact the school and see what help is available. The key worker may offer to accompany the young person to school or to assist with getting up in the morning. In turn the young person will also make a commitment, say, to attend school, to be in for an agreed time at night, to manage their pocket money and to abide by the rules of the home. The parents will also agree to appropriate tasks, perhaps to visit the children's home regularly or to make an appointment to see the social worker. Arrangements for bus passes and spending money will be settled, taking good care that the parents are in no way undermined. The parents are still responsible of course but are acting in partnership with the LA.

Two weeks later the first fortnightly contracts meeting will take place. A smaller number of people will be present; perhaps only the young person, the parents, the social worker and the key-worker who will chair the meeting. The focus will be on how well people have kept to their tasks and the overall contract and any developments will be noted. By the eighth week it should be clear whether or not the youngster is to return home. If not then a fostering officer or a placements officer will be invited to attend the contract meeting in order to begin procedures to obtain an appropriate placement.

The placements officer will be aware of all the children's homes within the borough, including those run by voluntary and private organisations, as well as those outside the borough that the local authority use. If the child is not going to be fostered, then the placement officer will discuss the alternatives available.

Semi-independent living units

A child of 15 or over is likely to be placed in a hostel or a unit which offers semi-independent living. Here the young person will normally have their own room but will share kitchen, bathroom and toilet and, perhaps, a common recreational room. There will be a few care staff around, mainly during the day, who will offer support. They will provide help with obtaining grants, dealing with the DSS and may assist the young person to look for a job in addition to offering support in more personal matters.

The staff may also be involved in the training of social and life skills, such as budgeting, cooking and self-care. The transfer from one establishment to another should never be abrupt; there should be some continued involvement in the form of outreach from the previous home for a short period, until the person is settled. With good quality continuity of care young people are more able to wean themselves off any dependency over a period.

Longer term childrens' homes

Although the fashion is undoubtedly towards the provision of smaller units, the larger, older style, long term children's homes continue to exist within some authorities. Once again it is possible for a young person to be admitted as an 'emergency' or, more usually, after careful planning has taken place. It is now not uncommon for one establishment to be the only children's home in the borough. Planning will be integral to its purpose so it should no longer be possible for children to 'drift through care' as many were allowed to do in the past.

The initial aim for long term homes is towards reunification of the child with their own family. In some cases this goal is not feasible because of the child's family circumstances and therefore a decision to try and find appropriate permanent accommodation will already have been taken by the social worker involved with the child and their family. If 're-unification' is still viable then the staff of the children's home will work towards this in much the same way as they would in a short stay home.

If a substitute home is sought then the child needs to be prepared to be fostered or adopted by another family. A useful aid in this process is known as *life story work*, an ongoing exercise in which the child and the residential social worker are engaged in the process of reaffirming and establishing the child's identity, by tracing the child's past and representing it in an album. Materials such as photographs, letters and drawings are used to illustrate events and landmarks. Some children who are looked after by the LA, particularly if they have been looked after for a long time and perhaps have moved from one children's home to another, may not have a clear sense of their own history. The task of life story work is to restore this history for the child. The worker and the child may decide to revisit homes where the child has lived or visit significant places and take photographs. The youngster may not have any photographs of themselves as a baby or a small child and may wish to choose from pictures in magazines close approximations to how they felt they looked at that age. Sometimes this process can be upsetting for the child because painful memories are revived, but carried out gently and supportively, life story work can provide a young person with a stronger sense of themselves and make them feel less different from other children. When the child moves on they will take the life story book with them so that it can be continually updated.

Children preparing for a move to a substitute family may spend some weekends in the homes of willing staff so that they get used to living in ordinary homes with generally smaller rooms. This practice, however, depends on the co-operation and commitment of individual care staff. Children may also stay in the homes of approved volunteers for the same reason. These arrangements will be carried out over a trial period. If an appropriate foster carer is found then the young person will, after initial meetings at the children's home, go and stay with the prospective foster carers. Early visits will be for the day only, progressing to overnight or weekend stays until all concerned are willing to try out the arrangement on a fulltime basis.

Therapeutic communities

Therapeutic communities may offer places to children and young people who have displayed behavioural difficulties and need the intimate care provided by a structured environment, away from the immediate influence of their own family and neighbourhood. The chief value of such communities lies in the availability of qualified staff and the focused nature of the regime. The community aims to give young people time, space and support to work through their needs and develop awareness, confidence and a belief in themselves as valued members of society. They are confronted with their own behaviour and its consequences and encouraged to develop positive changes. Each young person will work with their key worker to devise and carry out a programme appropriate to their needs. The programme may include work and task centred activities and offer the young person an opportunity to engage in new experiences, such as weekends away, crafts and sports. Young people of school age will be offered education on the premises and be able to follow the National Curriculum in the same way as in ordinary schools. The following example may serve as an illustration of a young person referred to a therapeutic community.

Keri was 14 when she was first placed in the community. Prior to this she spent three months in an assessment centre. She was accommodated by the local authority at the request of her parents after she had been disruptive at school, been in trouble with the police, had been stealing from her mother and staying out overnight without informing her parents. Of particular concern was her increasingly violent behaviour, both verbal and physical, towards anyone who prevented her doing what she liked. This behaviour had been going on for over 12 months and both working parents felt Keri was beyond their control; they also felt that she was vulnerable.

Keri spent two years at the therapeutic community during which time both her parents visited regularly and Keri herself went home some weekends. The visits home were closely monitored and built up gradually, an hour one weekend, two hours the next and so on. This helped rebuild Keri's relationship with her parents which had been severely strained over the preceding 12 months. She also periodically ran away from the community home and stayed away for some days before returning, only to leave again, sometimes the same day. She now lives in her own bedsit, near to her parents whom she sees quite regularly.

During her time at the community Keri displayed evidence of her educational potential and was entered for relevant examinations. She had not previously shown any interest in her schooling. Significantly, after a prolonged one-to-one session with her key worker, following her return from a period of absconding, Keri disclosed that she had been sexually abused by a regular babysitter over a number of years. The careworker was the first person she had been able to tell and so the painful process of acceptance and growth could now begin. The disclosure would almost certainly not have happened had Keri remained at home, since the atmosphere of constant friction was not conducive.

Therapeutic communities recognise that young people are ready to leave at different ages and offer help with finding appropriate accommodation. They may continue to offer support through a structure of after-care, tailored to the needs of the individual.

After-care

There has been a good deal of criticism about the lack of provision offered to youngsters leaving local authority care. In the main young people leaving care constitute a vulnerable group of people. Many have had disruptive home lives and therefore cannot return to their families; they may have spent much of their lives in a variety of care establishments, some of which may not have proved suitable and they may have generally experienced a range of unsettling events. By contrast other care leavers have gained from being looked after by the local authority in situations where they have met with consistency, love, understanding and security, either in children's homes or with the foster carers with whom they were placed. They have grown sufficiently mature to feel confident of facing the outside world and living independently.

However, a sad picture emerges of the young people who leave local authority care, ill equipped to face life on their own, once their eighteenth birthday has arrived and they are no longer the responsibility of the local authority. Two reports published by the National Children's Bureau in June 1992, *Leaving Care and After* and *Prepared for Living*, conclude that a comprehensive planning of support services is needed. Figures show that young people who have been looked after by the local authority are disadvantaged in a number of ways. As has been stated earlier, young people leave care on their 18th birthday, or before in many cases, and therefore leave 'home' at an earlier age than the majority of the population where the average for both men and women is in the early twenties (*Child Facts*, NCB 1992). Furthermore, leaving home for most young people is a gradual and reversable process unlike the experience of young people leaving local authority care. The report also showed that 80 per cent of young care leavers were still unemployed 2½ years after leaving care and 75 per cent had no educational qualifications. It was further estimated that over one third of all homeless young people had at some time been looked after by the local authority, as had 23 per cent of adult prisoners and 38 per cent of young prisoners. Two other reports showed that nearly half of the young people found begging in London had in the past been looked after by the local authority and that two out of three male prostitutes had a care background (ibid).

The implementation of the Children Act (1989) in 1991 was welcomed by those concerned with care leavers because of its emphasis on the value of maintaining links between a child and their family and because it gave local authorities wider powers to help teenagers leaving care. Under the Act, LAs are required to help all young people aged 16–21 years who have been looked after for at least three months by a LA, a voluntary organisation, a health authority, an education authority or private foster carers. Not only are LAs required to assist those who have been looked after by the LA or other organisation, they are enabled to help other young people who have lived away from home.

The LA must 'advise, assist and befriend' young people who have left care 'with a view to promoting their welfare'. This duty includes preparing young people to leave care and to provide financial assistance in certain circumstances. They are also obliged to support a care leaver in their education and training even after the age of 21.

Some LAs have already gone beyond their statutory duty to offer support to their care leavers but there is a variation in provision nationally. How positively each LA interprets its responsibilities under the Children Act will determine its commitment to its young people and the standard of service it will provide.

Services to children and young people

Some authorities have created specialist teams to deal with particular aspects of recent legislation, namely the Children Act 1989 and the Criminal Justice Act 1991. Such *youth justice teams* will work with young people, up to the age of 17, who are considered to be 'at risk of custody'. In some parts of the country the probation service will undertake responsibility for young people, sometimes from as early as 15.

The YJT will write reports, such as pre-sentence reports (PSRs), for the court. These reports will provide information about the young person which is related to the offence and will be used by the court when deciding what action to take. The social worker is likely to offer community based options to the court and to have carried out preliminary investigations in order to establish feasibility. The team will also implement any court orders on young people, such as a supervision order or a specified activity order.

Intermediate treatment (IT)
IT grew out of the recognition that children and young people from deprived backgrounds, lacking proper parental support and without any formal educational achievements, become bored and experience life in a negative way. These are the very children and young people who are most likely to appear before the court or be received into care. The IT worker, whether a social worker or a probation officer, seeks to prevent this happening.

Some LASSDs still have an IT centre where young people can go for group meetings or activities. 'Latch-key' provision in the form of rooms and meeting places may be available in the morning and early evening for those whose parents are out at work and indeed the centre may offer 'drop-in' facilities throughout the day. During group meetings, children and young people are encouraged to discuss and share their feelings about matters that are important to them. Meetings are held on a regular basis with the aim of developing trust and friendship. Other activities, including outward bound courses organised from the centres, will aim to strengthen a person's self-worth and sense of achievement. However, the main emphasis is on offence-based groupwork.

There was a fashion for IT to be offered away from the locality of a young person's home, at a residential IT centre. This physical separation from their usual surroundings was intended to enable young people to distance themselves from previous patterns of behaviour and to learn new skills in a more therapeutic setting. This form of IT is rarely provided nowadays because it is thought to only have a short term benefit and the current focus is on helping young people cope with the difficulties of living in their own communities. Furthermore, residential IT is an expensive provision. Today's interventions are more directly geared to confronting and encouraging young people to alter their offending behaviour.

The members of the youth justice team will be called upon to attend police stations in order to act as an 'appropriate adult' under the requirements of the Police and Criminal Evidence Act (PACE). The social worker will be present whilst the young person is interviewed by the police. They will stand in for the parents who may be unable or unwilling to attend the police station. In the evening and at weekends and on bank holidays a member of the out of hours emergency duty team will perform this task and refer the information to the youth justice team on the next working day.

The team will also ensure that people adhere to bail requirements and that they attend specified places according to the conditions set out by the court. They will visit the homes of people on their caseloads and may adopt a range of social work interventions.

The YJT is a provider service and will only have care management responsibility for the young people referred to them who are not known to the district or area social workers. If a child or young person is already known to a child protection team or a children and families team then an area social worker will be the young person's case manager.

Services to adults

Community care

Just as the Children Act 1989 has greatly influenced the provision of services to children in England and Wales, so the National Health Service and Community Care Act 1990 has shaped the provision and delivery of services to adults throughout the whole of Great Britain. Other pieces of legislation such as the Education Act 1980 and the Disabled Persons Act 1986 have effected changes in service delivery and provision but nowhere as profoundly as the NHS and Community Care Act. Both the Children Act 1989 and the NHS and Community Care Act 1990 have stressed similar principles: for example, service users have:

1. the right to be made aware of services and to be informed of them in all 'living languages' presently spoken in Britain;
2. the right to complain through a standardised and accessible complaints procedure;
3. the right to 'choose' and determine as far as possible the services they receive.

The intention of providing a 'needs led service' and for there to be increased co-operation between the various caring organisations was stressed in both acts, as was the need to extend the principle of partnership to parents of children who are accommodated or to relatives who care for people in their own homes.

Essentially the NHS and Community Care Act 1990 sought to radically alter the primary role of the LA from that of main care provider to that of an assessor and manager of care with a responsibility to co-ordinate and purchase care services. Although it was envisaged that the LA would continue to provide some services, other agencies, be they statutory, voluntary, 'not-for-profit' or private, would submit their services for tender to the LA. In other words, LAs would help stimulate the creation of a mixed economy of care from which they would purchase services whilst they relinquished their historical role of being the major service providers. It was further envisaged that local authorities would still provide some services, particularly to very dependent people or those with challenging behaviour or where there are no other suitable forms of provision.

The NHS and Community Care ACT 1990 was staggered in its implementation. The Government timetable for implementing Community Care was as follows:

April 1991   LAs to publish complaints procedure.
              LAs to establish an 'arms length registration and inspection unit'.
              Specific grant available to begin community care services for mentally distressed people.
April 1992   LAs to publish their community care plans (this becomes an annual duty).
April 1993   LAs to implement assessment and care management.

Local authorities had some difficulty meeting these targets because they had initially to plan for community care services without knowing exactly how much money would be available. Resourcing remains a key issue concerning community care: plans may be far-reaching and imaginative, they may embody all the essential elements of good care practice but without adequate funding they are mere statements of intent. The following extract from a local authority's community care plan points to a number of factors beyond the LA's control which will ultimately determine the effectiveness or planned service provision:

> Realistically, the extent of local control of these processes is already quite limited by the impact of wider social and economic change on generating social need and people's ability to pay for it, and by Government financial and social policies. Our plans can be critically affected by national or regional decisions to set priorities, service standards and resource levels.
> (*Community Living*, Islington's plan for Community Care, 1991, p 13)

Community care is not a new concept. Its earliest official mention was in the Percy Report which preceded the Mental Health Act 1959. While community care has only recently become official policy it has effectively been practised, albeit under a different guise, for quite some time by the more committed and enlightened local authorities. Preventive social work such as the provision of a holiday for a young family to help reduce the pressures of everyday living; the provision of respite care for a child with learning difficulties to lessen the strain on the parent(s); or the provision of a laundry service or a day care place for an older person in order to enable that person to remain living in their own home are all examples of the spirit of community care practice.

Community care basically has two meanings: firstly it refers to the policy of decanting large scale institutions such as hospitals of long stay patients, in order that they may be cared for in the community either by relatives in their own homes or in group homes or on their own with social work support. This practice has been going on since the early 1970s, particularly with adults with learning difficulties and mentally distressed people.

The second and more recent use of the term Community Care refers to the policy enshrined in the NHS and Community Care Act 1990 of maintaining people in the community with a holistic range of services in order that they may avoid being placed permanently in residential accommodation and live instead in their own communities in the same way as ordinary people who are not so dependent on the care of others.

The NHS and Community Care Act 1990 outlined the main functions for the LA with regard to assessment, care management and service provision.

Assessment

In contrast to assessment in the past, assessment now has to be needs led and not service led. In other words, instead of merely fitting a client into existing services the assessor is required to start by establishing exactly what the client needs and then to go about trying to find a service, or range of services, which will meet that person's needs within the context of their community. Crucially this service provision must be allocated within the framework of 'available resources'.

The assessor is required to look at the client's services not only from the point of view of whether the person qualifies for services but to look at ways in which the client's daily living can be enhanced. So, for example, instead of simply providing a place in a nearby local authority day centre for an isolated housebound man, it may be better to vary provision and arrange attendance at, and transportation to, a former social club, chess club, bowls club or community luncheon centre and so maintain the client's interests. It is important that in carrying out an assessment the assessor is governed by the wishes of the client or their carer. Essentially the assessor acts in partnership with the client.

In addition the local authorities have a responsibility of targeting those services available to those in need: in other words, to prioritise services to the more vulnerable members of the community.

Care management

Some people's requirements will be fairly straightforward but in more complex cases a care manager will be appointed to oversee the delivery and review of services. In most instances this person will be the local authority social worker but it need not be so. The role could be performed by the client or their carer who, many argue, are in the best position to evaluate service provision. But not all clients would want to take on the responsibility involved in trying to co-ordinate services from different agencies; they may not be physically or mentally able to carry out the necessary negotiations or they may lack the confidence required. However, the service user, or their carer, remains central to the process of community care; they must be consulted and be involved in the decision making process as far as possible.

Service provision

The care manager need not rely upon the local authority for the provision of services. It will no longer be acceptable, for example, to say to a client that there is no community care service available over the weekend simply because the local authority does not employ home carers on Saturday or Sunday. If the client has been assessed to be in need of a visit from a home carer over the weekend, the care manager may buy in that service from any other organisation, statutory, voluntary or private. Needless to say, the care manager, in buying in the service, will endeavour to obtain 'value for money' so that the maximum service provision is available to all clients for whom a 'specific budget' is allocated within which services may be purchased. The purchaser of the services need not turn, in the first instance, to the local authority to provide a service such as, say meals on wheels: they may go direct to a cheaper provider although the purchaser should accept no deterioration in quality.

The NHS and Community Care Act 1990 stipulated the provision of a clear *complaints procedure* to enable service users, or their representatives, to complain about the quality or nature of the services and to bring about a resolution of the difficulties identified. In addition all local authorities are required to have inspection units. Local authorities are responsible for the registration of private and voluntary homes and for inspection of all residential establishments in the area, including, for the first time, their own. The inspection units have to be set up so that they are independent of the day-to-day management of local authority homes. This has led to their being known as the 'arms length' inspectorate. In addition to ensuring that residential homes meet statutory requirements the inspection units must work towards the development of good care practice by recommending training or necessary changes in practice. Ultimately they have the power to close a care home.

The NHS and Community Care Act 1990 represents a new direction in social policy. It stresses the importance of service users' needs, rights, choices and control over the services they receive. The Act further emphasises the need for additional co-operation between all the agencies involved in assessment, management, and provision of care. The next few years will show how the caring services respond to this new challenge and how they manage the changes within the context of available resources.

Services to older people

Older people form a relatively high proportion of our population. There were 3.1 million people over the age of 75 in 1981 and over half a million were over 85. These numbers are increasing and it is forecast that by the year 2000 there will be 4.3 million people over 75 and more than 1 million over 85.

Many older people continue to make an important contribution to their communities. Not all elders will need social services. Some are capable of looking after their own needs well into their eighties or even nineties and others are cared for by relatives and do not require much additional support. However there are many older people who have become increasingly frail or disabled or have reduced mental abilities or a declining income, who experience poverty and loneliness and who need support if they are to remain in their own homes. Even when they are in receipt of help from a member of their own family or neighbours they may still require additional support from the social services.

Elders are of course eligible for a whole range of services and can expect to receive counselling, information and advice in the same way that this is made available to younger people. However, many local authorities have tended to neglect the ordinary needs of older clients because they have concentrated resources on meeting their statutory responsibilities for children and those adults who are seriously mentally ill. This ageist attitude towards service provision has also been observed with regard to the health service, where older people are rarely offered therapeutic counselling, for example, and are often faced with long delays for simple operations.

There are two main kinds of social services provision for older people: domiciliary and day care services and residential services.

Domiciliary and day care services

As the name 'domiciliary' suggests, these services are generally provided in the service user's own home. Their aim is to improve the quality of the client's life and enable them to continue to live independently in the community. The range of provision varies throughout the country but the main services are as follows.

Home care
Formerly this was referred to as 'home help' and is granted to people who are either too frail or disabled to manage daily living tasks by themselves. A home carer may do the shopping, and collect pensions or cash prescriptions. They may also, if required, clean the home, change the curtains or perform those tasks that the service user needs to do but cannot. In some local authorities the name home help or home carer has been disregarded in favour of the term community carer and the role too has been widened. In addition to performing the tasks already described, the carer may also provide personal care such as taking a person to the toilet, helping the client in and out of bed, preparing meals and even, if necessary, administering pills. Doubtless many home helps and home carers of the past performed some of these tasks although it was not strictly their brief to do so. The strength of this kind of help lies in the personal contact and the potential for a relationship to develop between the care giver and service user. The home carer is in an ideal position to monitor the client's condition and to advise if additional services are required.

Under certain circumstances LAs provide home carers during the night to sit with someone who is ill, either because the person is waiting to go into hospital or because the person has been discharged and is still seriously, or terminally, ill. Such night sisters, as they are called, are used to give relief to an informal carer who would otherwise have to stay up with their partner or relative, so that the carer may get some rest. Night sitters do not carry out medical duties; they help with routine care tasks such as providing a drink or assisting someone to the toilet.

Meals on wheels
This is a more straightforward provision and is allocated to people who cannot manage to prepare a hot meal for themselves and are unlikely to obtain one otherwise. They may receive meals on wheels on a certain number of days of the week depending on need. Service users have a choice of menu and it is important that their cultural and dietary needs are acknowledged and catered for. This service may be provided alongside others including 'neighbourly help,' which is usually only made available to support people living alone.

Neighbourly help money
This money, often only a nominal amount, is made available by some LAs in acknowledgement of the support and help that a neighbour may give to an elderly or housebound person. It may be paid to the neighbour who calls in on the days when the community carer does not visit or to the person who provides something hot to eat for their neighbour on the days when there are no meals on wheels delivered. It is anticipated that under the community care legislation this kind of informal arrangement will be encouraged. Local authorities will have some difficulty in establishing a

fee that on the one hand does not exploit a neighbour's willingness to help and on the other does not jeopardise the natural development of community spirit.

Aids and adaptations

Major structural alterations to a service user's home may be made in order to keep a person at home. In some special instances a lift may even be installed in order that a disabled person may independently, or with minimal assistance, get up and downstairs freely. Smaller adaptations include the fixing of hand rails beside steps or alongside stairs and the provision of non-slip mats, domestic gadgets and adapted cutlery. The decision about what aids or adaptations are needed will be made following an 'aids to daily living assessment' which is carried out by an occupational therapist.

Day care

Day care is available for elders to ensure that, at least, they have the opportunity to meet with others, receive a hot meal and have access to professional care so that their condition may be continuously monitored. In addition, various services may be available such as a regular visit from the doctor or health visitor, a chance to have a bath or to have one's hair done, to see the chiropodist or physiotherapist. In one day centre the local greengrocer sets up a stall inside the establishment on one morning each week so that elders are able to purchase their own fruit and vegetables. At the end of the day these service users take their shopping home with them and are assisted, where necessary, by staff and the driver.

Centre users' interests are various; they may include painting, card playing, dominoes, music and sewing and these are often catered for. Even opera appreciation meetings have been organised where demand, facilities and expertise are at hand. It is important for older people to feel close to their roots at this time in their lives so it is vital that day centres reflect all the cultures of the community in their service delivery. Food needs to be culturally appropriate for all service users; staff and day centre membership has to be representative of the community and the music and pastimes need to reflect the interests of the cultural groups of the neighbourhood.

Confused older people

In some authorities the care of confused elderly people may be integrated with the care of other older people, whereas in other authorities those with a diagnosis of dementia may receive separate provision. This specialised care is made available because of the extra needs of those people with dementia. It has long been recognised that stimulation staves off further mental deterioration, so activities are devised especially for confused elders to help to maintain their level of functioning and to improve their orientation. The staff: client ratio is usually high in centres that specialise in providing care for elders who are thought to have some dementia to allow for small varied groupwork and one-to-one work to take place.

Reality orientation strategies will be relied upon throughout the day, beginning with the initial 'Welcome' activity when staff remind the centre users where they are, where the centre is situated, and familiarise users with the daily programme and enable them to make choices about their meals and what activities they want to be involved in. The staff may start a session by looking at the newspapers for an interesting story upon which a discussion may be based, or draw from the group a topical issue to discuss. Later there may be small group activities aimed to increase confidence, such as completing simple cooking tasks, or activities centered around self-care, or for example, making decorations for Christmas or other festivals or a card for someone's birthday. Creative activities are likely to be many, short and varied, separated by frequent breaks to accommodate the low concentration span of older people with senility. During a sedentary activity staff may attend each of the members administering personal care such as grooming their hair or cutting or filing their finger nails. Such individual physical attention can create a feeling of well-being in the service user and may serve further to orient them into the 'here and now'. It needs to be remembered that touch is a powerful way of communicating, particularly when one is trying to connect with someone who has dementia.

Transport
Transportation may be available to take an older person or disabled person to day care. The service can be used more imaginatively as well, say, to take a number of local elders on an outing to a place of interest or on a shopping expedition.

Telephones
Under the provision of the Chronically Sick and Disabled Persons' Act 1970 all disabled older people are entitled to help with the installation of a telephone in their own home. The potential cost of delivering this service has inhibited SSDs from fully implementing the Act. Instead many authorities have allocated help only in a limited number of cases operating on a priority basis.

Residential Care

Only a small proportion of elders are cared for fulltime in a residential home. As mentioned earlier, the majority of older people live in their own homes and are supported mainly by families or neighbours. Indeed many older people manage entirely by themselves. However, there are others who, for various reasons, are no longer able to live in their own homes and need fulltime care. Residential care should not be seen as being distinctly separate from community care: a residential care establishment is, after all, a home within the community. Furthermore, care homes have many different functions, including a rehabilitative one to enable residents to return to their own home, when this is possible. Care homes need to be viewed as a community resource and an integral aspect of community care provision.

Respite care
Respite care may be offered to an older person mainly to allow the carer, often the spouse or younger relative, who is invariably female, to take a break from the strain of providing continuous care. When respite care is planned and taken up at regular intervals it enables the care relationship to be more easily maintained. This kind of care is also sometimes referred to as rotational care. Carers may find it easier to manage if they know that they will obtain a break for, say, a week or two, every two or three months. The length and regularity of the respite break will of course vary according to need and individual circumstances.

Short Stay care
Short stay care is also offered to elders when it is felt that they may benefit from a sort period of residential care. The person may be self-neglecting or they may have been

observed to be deteriorating. A short stay may check deterioration and restore an older person's equilibrium. Alternatively a few days or weeks in care may be offered as a strategic resource for an older person whose home is unsafe because it is undergoing repair, for example, rewiring; or to cover the period when the principal care giver is temporarily unavailable. A short stay can also be used to familiarise an older person, for whom permanent residential care is eventually planned.

Fulltime residential care

Residential care was formerly provided mainly by local authorities and some voluntary organisations but in recent years there has been a growth in the number of privately owned establishments offering permanent care. The NHS and Community Care Act 1990 and continued restrictions on local authority expenditure have tended to reinforce the trend towards private and voluntary sector provision.

Standards of care may vary from establishment to establishment although today there is much greater awareness of what constitutes good practice. *Home Life: A Code of Practice for Residential Care* (Centre for Policy on Ageing, 1984) was produced prior to the passing of the Registered Homes Act 1984 and was considered an 'integral part' of the Government's measures to regulate and control care establishments; In 1988 the Wagner Report, *Residential Care: A Positive Choice* (HMSO, 1988), outlined minimum standards of good practice in residential care and more recently, the National Integrated NVQ/SVQ Standards in Health and Social Care (August 1992) have enshrined the principles of good practice in the 'value base' and all the units of competence which make up their care awards. These standards need to be met by care establishments otherwise their workers will not be able to be assessed as being competent.

Allocation of places in local authority residential establishments is usually carried out by a panel and decisions are reached on a priority basis. This is because of the widespread and high level of demand. Although more and more older people are being cared for in the community, the number of elders needing fulltime care is still rising, in accordance with the increased proportion of older people in the population. The allocation panel is generally made up of a senior social worker, the care manager, the team leader of the elders section and the head of home. Together they will assess the various applications presented to them by the social workers concerned. The panel will also consider any emergency admissions that have taken place and view these as potential fulltime admissions. Fulltime care is also often referred to as 'part three' care. This stems from the local authority's duty to provide care for older people under part three of the National Assistance Act 1948. In arriving at a decision about an application for fulltime care the panel must be certain that the older person is 'part three fit'; that is, that they are suitable for residential care and would not be more appropriately placed in a nursing home where medical attention can be given.

Nowadays the residents of care establishments increasingly tend to be less able and more dependent. There is a higher proportion of residents suffering a degree of dementia to be found in local authority homes than at any time previously. However, homes still have their rehabilitative function; some residents do eventually return home or move on to live with relatives. It remains vitally important that the care environment provides stimulation and an opportunity for the maximum involvement of all the residents and provides for their differing levels of ability.

Reality orientation therapy (ROT)

Reality orientation therapy is a practice used to encourage the maximum involvement of residents in their care setting. It has a number of purposes: to help residents to become accustomed to their new surroundings; to enable them to have an understanding of things going on around them; and to give residents opportunities to take more control over their lives. Its main aim is to orientate people in time, place and their present surroundings in order to lessen confusion and to make sure that residents feel safe so that progress can be made.

Residents, particularly those classified as EMI (elderly mentally infirm), may become very disorientated when first admitted to care owing to the new surroundings and new people. For residents to be orientated in time, clocks need to be big, bold and visible. Day recognition can be achieved in serveral different ways; for example, residents may have calendars in their rooms and should be encouraged to routinely check the day. Newspapers are a good means of orientating people, not only by the date but by using the topical information provided; residents should also be encouraged to have their own newspapers for personal use. Display boards can be used to provide information; they can state the day, date and name any activities that are due to take place.

It is sometimes argued that signs and notices are not part of good practice since they go against the spirit of *normalisation*; that they would not be found in ordinary homes but serve only to institutionalise an establishment. This objection misses the point. There are, of course, 'official signs' erected for the sake of the organisation, such as 'private', 'out of bounds', 'manager's office' and 'staff only' but use of such signs should be kept to a minimum in order to reduce the institutional nature of the establishment. However, signs that help to clarify the environment, such as 'bathroom', 'toilet', 'bedroom', help people to orientate themselves, so that they can manoeuvre more freely, and are essential to a client's dignity. Signs can be used in conjunction with particular colours; all toilet doors, for example, could be painted green. Inability to find the toilet is one of the main causes of incontinence and to have to continually ask is both embarassing and undignifying.

Not all residents have the same level or type of dementia and some, of course, are very mentally alert, so not all ideas are appropriate for all residents. Photographs and possibly other small, familiar objects, can be used to enable residents to feel at home as well as to assist them in orientating themselves in time and place. A key worker can set up an album with a resident, labelling photographs with their name and age when the picture was taken. Photographs of places where the resident has lived or pictures of favourite places the resident has visited might also be included in the album. Residents who are less confused can be encouraged to keep diaries in order to record information or plan for the future. Residents' meetings, too, can be regarded as a part of reality orientation therapy since they take place regularly, concern themselves with day-to-day issues and prescribe roles and responsibilities.

Compulsory admission to residential care

Under section 47 of the National Assistance Act 1948, local authority social workers have a duty to compulsorily admit to residential accommodation any elderly person who is unable to cope for themselves and is considered to be in need of care and attention because of their infirmity and who is, as a consequence, living in insanitary conditions. If this is the opinion of the specially appointed doctor – the medical officer of environmental health – and the social worker concerned, then a compulsory admission will be carried out. Before this can be implemented, the elderly person will have to have refused all domiciliary services offered. This rarely used provision is a safeguard to protect an individual whose confused mental state is life-threatening. (The medical officer of environmental health is appointed by the local authority after being nominated by the district health authority. A deputy will also be appointed and, depending on the size of the area covered, may take geographical responsibility for some of the area. In Scotland there is no formal title for this post, but a community physician will be designated and approved in the same way, to undertake duties under section 47 of the Act.)

Services to people with learning difficulties/disabilities

The term learning difficulties is very broad and is used to describe a range of learning problems experienced by a diverse group of people. Those designated as having severe learning difficulties may need considerable support throughout their lives. Severe learning disabilities is often associated with brain damage, before or after birth, various illnesses and genetic abnormalities, for example, Down's syndrome. People with moderate learning disabilities often have problems learning basic skills but usually manage to lead fairly independent adult lives.

Although there is a tendency to think of people with learning difficulties as having below average ability, it should be noted that there is another group of people who have specific learning difficulties, for example, dyslexia, who may well be of average or above average ability but have a major problem with some aspects of literacy or numeracy. The terms learning difficulties or learning disabilities are therefore used as umbrella terms to cover a wide range of needs.

The range and level of services offered to each person with a disability will depend on the extent of their need and the service provision available locally. For people with severe learning difficulties, services are provided by local authority SSDs, the health authority, voluntary organisations and private bodies, including those who are 'not for profit'. Nowadays the emphasis is on helping people with severe learning difficulties to live in the community. Admission to hospital is now only usual for the purpose of specialist treatment, not for long term residence. Indeed the larger hospitals are still engaged in the process of transferring residents to care homes within the community.

Social work support

Social workers from the team dealing with people with learning disabilities and their families will attempt to support families soon after the birth of a disabled child, or at least from the time when it becomes clear that the child has a learning difficulty. It is often a distressing time for the parent(s) as they learn to handle disappointments, change their plans for the future and begin to appreciate the added responsibilities they face. Emotional difficulties are common; they are related to the strain of providing continuous care, of being avoided by relatives or friends who are uncertain how to react, of being shunned by those who associate stigma with disability. Social workers may provide counselling support in addition to giving practical advice on such matters as pointing out any benefits the family may be entitled to; giving names and addresses of voluntary organisations who provide funding; and drawing attention to the existence of any local support group. This kind of help may first be provided by the hospital social work team, then followed through once the child leaves hospital.

All children with learning difficulties are entitled to fulltime educational provision between the ages of two and 19. Once a person with learning difficulties reaches the age of 19 they are no longer the responsibility of the local authority education department. In common with other young people, unless they have a profound disability, the young person will want to find some form of paid employment outside the home. During times of high unemployment finding paid work suitable for someone who needs attendant support is often very difficult. There are successes, however, as firms become more mindful of their obligation to meet the needs of a wider section of the community. Not everyone, of course, is ready for or capable of obtaining work. Some still require support and further training to enable them to live as independently as possible in the community.

Local authority day centres

These were formerly known as adult training centres (ATCs) but are now more commonly called social education centres (SECs). At the SEC there will be a similar emphasis on developing the service user's life and social skills with the object of helping each student to be as self-reliant and independent as their abilities will allow. The staff will try to educate the public about people with learning difficulties and they will provide every opportunity for the public to become aware of the potential that exists in all people with learning difficulties. They will also endeavour to assist families with practical advice and guidance; to understand the nature of services available; and to involve families in *individual programme planning* (IPP) for their son or daughter. The link between parent(s) and the establishment is important to the overall aim of encouraging maximum development for the service user.

At the centre each student will have their own timetable and will take part in a variety of both individual and group-based activities. Before the timetable can be worked out students need to be assessed. This is done provisionally while the student is gradually being introduced to the centre – say, for one day per week – over a period of five or six weeks, in order to arrive at an approximation of the student's needs and abilities. A more sophisticated form of assessment based on the Copewell Assessment devised at Manchester University then follows; it assesses a whole range of skills including dressing skills, personal care skills and skills in arts, drama and gardening.

Social education in domestic skills may take place in a training flat that has a fitted kitchen, bathroom and laundry facilities. In a community context the social education will be centred on using public services such as transport, libraries, sports centres, shops, cafes and restaurants. As part of their social and personal education students will learn about sex education and responsible relationships with friends and families. For some, prework training will be offered and work experience will be organised locally and links will be established with job clubs. Some people with learning difficulties may attend as part-time or fulltime students at colleges of further education. This is a growing trend in service provision.

Normalisation

It is argued that the existence of special day centres for client groups, such as those for people with learning difficulties, conflicts with the principle of *Normalisation*. This principle underlines the entitlement of all people, including those with learning difficulties, to live a life as close to that of an ordinary citizen as possible: in other words, they have a right to make decisions and choices and to participate as fully as possible in everyday life and not to be dependent upon segregated provision.

Social education centres (SECs) have done much in the past few years to strengthen their students' links with the outside world by encouraging their participation in community settings and their use of community resources and facilities. A few service users eventually move on to live more fully independent lives. Some may find paid work. Others, who have more severe learning difficulties, who are unable to function without support outside the centre, need to continue with the secure, structured, specialised care that is provided by the day centres. The service is aimed at maximising involvement and developing independence, but this needs to be provided in a segregated setting because of the specialised nature of the care and support that is required. LASECs are in general enlightened and progressive institutions; they have come a long way from the days when service users used to spend every day performing repetitive mechanical tasks for a small weekly allowance. This was the practice in some adult day centres of the past.

Advocacy

The last decade has seen the growth of a variety of forms of advocacy in connection with people with learning difficulties. Advocacy means 'to speak and act, persuasively or forcefully, on behalf of someone's rights and interests, whether these are your own or someone else's' (*Developing Self-Advocacy Skills with People with Learning Difficulties*, Mariette Clare, 1990). Three forms of advocacy have been identified:

1. *Citizen advocacy* is the voluntary involvement of a member of the public in the life of the disabled person; the latter is usually someone who is institutionalised and has no other contact with the 'outside' world. Citizen advocates undertake to become the resident's friend. Their role is to find out what her or his wishes are, to speak to members of staff on the resident's behalf and to represent her or him on such occasions as case conferences. At the minimum they try to ensure that the person is treated in such a way as citizen advocates would accept for themselves (ibid, p9).

2. *Legal advocacy* does not necessarily involve a personal relationship. 'Volunteers who become advocates are independent members of the public, who are therefore able to monitor the legal and financial affairs of disabled people who are unable to do so for themselves. This is a check against their exploitation by institutions or, indeed, other members of their family' (ibid, p9).

3. *Self-advocacy* is more simply defined as 'a process whereby users are encouraged to speak out directly for themselves' (Staff Practice Handbook – a Guide to Practice in Services for People with Learning Difficulties, David and Althea Brandon, University College Salford, 1991, p31) or 'speaking up for yourself so that your life goes the way you want it' (*Developing Self-Advovcacy Skills with People with Learning Disabilities*, Mariette Clare, Further Education Unit, 1990). The idea of self-advocacy encouragement was first developed in Sweden and the United States when people who had lived in long stay hospitals were returned to live in the community. Nowadays self-advocacy groups are to be found in social education centres, adult training centres, hostels and some hospitals. Commu-

nication may take place orally, by signing or writing, or through a tape recording. As a group, individuals may rehearse ways of speaking up for themselves, familiarise themselves with their rights and choices, and contribute towards combatting the, often negative, ideas that exist about people with learning difficulties. A well-known self-advocacy group, People First, has done much to educate the public about the range of abilities people with learning difficulties have, as well as their needs. Some people with learning difficulties have given an input on training courses for doctors, nurses and social workers. Others have been involved in making educational videos.

Residential care

As we have already said, the trend nowadays is to care for people in the community. However, a number of people with learning disabilities are so profoundly handicapped they require 24-hour attention and therefore need to be cared for in hospital or a residential home. But there are a number of former residents of long stay hospitals now living in a variety of establishments within the community. A few live with their families; others live in group homes with or without live-in social work support; and some are able to live on their own. Group homes are situated in ordinary housing. Usually a terraced or semidetached house has been specially adapted to accommodate a set number of adults. There may be room provided for a social worker to live in, depending on the degree of support required. The residents will be involved in making choices about their home so they will decide on such matters as colour of curtains, style of seating and choice of furniture in the same way as ordinary people. And they will be involved as much as possible in the decisions and practices of daily life.

Residents of the establishments may attend day centres during the week and will use the resources of the local community when they are appropriate. Some of the larger establishments will offer respite care to those people with learning difficulties living in the community. As well as offering a stimulating experience for the service user this periodic short term care provides the person normally responsible for care with an opportunity to take a break. Respite care may be provided over a weekend or for a week depending on the needs or requirements of the person with learning disabilities. When respite care is provided at regular intervals it is often referred to as rotational care. Nowadays respite care is provided not only by establishments but by approved families who act as foster carers.

Services to people with mental ill health

Mental distress is a common human experience. It includes anxiety, depression and a fear of not being able to control strong feelings. It may be triggered off by such everyday events as separation, loss or bereavement; child birth; being made redundant or being long term unemployed; the strain of the responsibility of caring for a large family, or a number of children, without support and living on an inadequate income for a continuous period. People may feel unable to cope with such stresses and may experience sleeplessness, irritability or withdrawal and then may become overdependent on drugs, food or alcohol in an attempt to establish a sense of control over their lives.

While physical illness is generally regarded sympathetically by society, mental ill health is often looked upon less than supportively by people who may fear it who are confused about the reality of being mentally ill. There is often a powerful stigma associated with mental distress and blame may be attributed to the person for their condition. Negative attitudes of others can hamper the recovery of a mentally distressed person; such a person needs a supportive and understanding environment to help them regain strength. Adverse or stressful social conditions reduce a person's chances of reintegrating into society after they have experienced mental ill health and increase their chances of suffering a relapse and further hospitalisation. However, unlike a mental handicap which is permanent, most forms of mental illness are self-limiting and the majority of people who experience mental distress make a full recovery just as people overcome various physical illnesses.

Services are provided through social services authorities, the National Health Service and the voluntary sector; in particular through the work of MIND which has made an important contribution over the last 20 years. The NHS and Community Care Act 1990 encouraged local authority social services departments to continue the practice of working collaboratively with other agencies so services now tend to be jointly planned and funded. However, not everyone who needs support receives it: lack of funds and cutbacks in expenditure have limited provision for those who are not 'dangerously mentally ill'. As a consequence the burden of care falls on relatives and families who are themselves often in need of support.

Community care

The thrust of the work of both the SSD and the NHS over the past 15 years has been concerned with the movement away from institutional care in large hospitals towards the development of local community-based services. While a few large psychiatric hospitals have that yet closed completely, resources and bed spaces within them have been gradually run down over the years. Former residents have been settled in the community, either with relatives or in group homes, with or without live-in social work support.

Community mental health teams

Community mental health teams are made up of representatives of the SSDs and the NHS and include such personnel as an approved social worker, and senior social worker, an occupational therapist, a community psychiatric nurse and a GP. The team may also have access to the services of a clinical psychologist. Together the team will normally prepare a multidisciplinary assessment on an individual in order to plan for the appropriate support and resourcing. For example, it may be decided that a long stay hospital resident is now ready to live in supported accommodation within the community. The social worker may plan to help with the development of life and social skills and provide emotional support; the occupational therapist will focus on developing practical living skills; the community psychiatric nurse (CPN) will visit frequently to ensure that medication is taken or to administer injections; at the same time they will provide continuity of contact to help facilitate the client's adjustment to a new way of living. The CPN and the GP will together monitor the client's medical condition. Even though their contributions may overlap all the members of the team will try to ensure that the care provision will be comprehensive and they will encourage the service user to make decisions about their own life so that they may live as independently as possible. The community team may also undertake the assessment function required by the NHS and Community Care Act 1990.

Drug and alcohol services

Since the NHS and Community Care Act 1990 specific grant funding for mental health services has been available (annually) in order to improve the quality of social care provision in the community. An additional smaller grant was intended to be made available exclusively for the expansion or improvement of drug and alcohol services within the voluntary sector but the government reversed their decision to 'ring fence' this money. Drug and alcohol services have traditionally been provided by voluntary organisations *mainly* because local authorities have had no statutory obligation to provide a service. The grant from the Government for drug and alcohol services first awarded in April 1991, has ensured that the service will continue to be provided almost exclusively by specialist voluntary organisations.

Social services authorities have a central role in assessment and have been encouraged to develop joint planning initiatives with the relevant agencies such as the NHS, voluntary organisations and, in some instances, the police. Specific issues dealt with by drug and alcohol services include supporting people who misuse drugs, both illegal drugs and those which have been prescribed; supporting the families of drug misusers and providing support for people and relatives of people who misuse alcohol. In addition workers are concerned with HIV prevention. Service provision is centred around education, counselling, groupwork and day centre provision, both the drop-in and structured type of settings. Residential care is also offered.

Day centres for people with mental distress

Day centres are open to people suffering from mental distress who live in the community either in their own homes, on their own or with their families, or to people who are living in group homes, with or without support. In every case the centre provides a valuable source of social contact for people who may otherwise be quite isolated. For some day centres social services authorities may set an upper age limit of around 25 in order to tailor a service to suit the special needs of young people. (Alternatively the LA may fund a voluntary organisation to provide this service.) Most day centres do not have an age limit; they aim to offer a range of services directed at supporting a wide range of people.

Day centres vary in the way provision is organised. Some offer informal drop-in care: a relaxed warm environment; advice and guidance for those who request it; the provision of light refreshments; subsidised hot meals and general recreation activities. Other day centres are more structured and hold group sessions on assertiveness, basic life skills, self-advocacy, art therapy and group or individual counselling. Of course, centres may combine the provision of both informal and structured support. One important value of day care is that it allows the well-being of service users to be monitored and thus provides some form of safety net for vulnerable people living in the community.

Residential care

As has already been mentioned, the late 1970s, 1980s and the early 1990s have seen a large scale transfer from hospital to the community for people with long term mental ill health. This movement is continuing. Some people have been able to sucessfully live by themselves others have needed differing degrees of support, so various forms of accommodation have been made available. Group homes where former hospital patients live together in the community, are a common form of provision: In some, 24-hour live-in care is available; in others it is not necessary for a social worker to be always on the premises.

Institutionalisation

People who have been in hospital for a long time have become accustomed to having things done for them and therefore may be resistant to doing things for themselves. They may be reluctant to take decisions, make choices or take on responsibility because they have never been asked to do this in the past. They may not have been treated as individuals and because of their illness and the medication they have to take they may operate at a low energy level, not caring greatly about themselves or others. They may be prone to self-neglect, withdrawal, violence or other forms of antisocial behaviour. Such people, whose individual needs have been made subservient to those of the establishment and who have systematically become less able to function independently, are described as being the victims of the process of *Institutionalisation*. It is important therefore that group homes in the community address these matters and are structured in such a way as to maximise an individual's potential for independence.

A residential group home needs to strike the balance between providing a safe structured care environment that encourages personal development and one that functions as much as possible like an 'ordinary' house. Homes will seek to provide a programme of care which will include opportunities for *experiential learning* (i.e. learning by doing) and *formal learning* (i.e. teaching or training individuals to develop skills) that will enable them to grow in confidence and become more fulfilled. Counselling, therapies, possibilites for relationship building and medical supervision are offered to residents with the view to facilitating their development within the home and perhaps leading them towards a more self-sufficient lifesyle elsewhere in the future. So complete has been some people's rehabilitation into the community that they have decided to get married or to live on their own. Others have graduated from a group home with support to a home with less support, to a semi-independent unit and progressed eventually to full independence. With others, however, the arrangement broke down and they had to return to hospital. Some people need sanctuary from the stress and strain of the outside world and it is one function of the hospital to provide *asylum*.

Compulsory admission to hospital

Some people with mental ill health have no insight into their condition and may display threatening behaviour. Such people are unlikely to voluntarily accept help from a doctor and may need to be compulsorily admitted to a psychiatric hospital.

Under section 2 of the Mental Health Act 1983, any person suffering mental illness who is considered to be either a danger to himself or a danger to other people can be compulsorily admitted to hospital (or *sectioned*, as it is known) for assessment or assessment and treatment for a maximum period of 28 days.

For a compulsory admission to take place, the hospital administrators require three forms. Two of these are medical recommendations – one is signed by the person's GP and the other by an approved doctor (usually the hospital consultant). The third form, requesting admission, is supplied by either an approved social worker or the distressed person's 'nearest relative'. Often it is the approved social worker who completes the 'section' form, since compulsory admission can be personally distressing to the nearest relative, who may prefer to leave matters to the detached professionalism of the social worker.

In emergency situations, section 4 of the Mental Health Act 1983 can be used to compulsorily admit somebody suffering mental illness, under the same grounds as section 2. This order needs to be signed by only one approved doctor and an approved social worker or nearest relative, but the person can only be legally detained for up to 48 hours. A 'Section 4' order is carried out only when it is impossible to contact the person's own GP and to avoid 'undesirable delay'.

Where the nearest relative has signed a 'section' form, the social worker has a responsibility to visit the home of the person admitted to hospital and to provide a report on the family circumstances.

An approved social worker's consent is also required under 'section 3' of the 1983 Act before compulsory treatment may be given. This 'section', of six months' duration, is usually passed on somebody already in hospital. Today only approved social workers (ASWs) who have successfully undergone extra training are allowed to sign 'section' orders, but before 1983 any social worker could do this.

The role of the approved social worker in a compulsory admission

The role of the ASW with regard to compulsory admission is basically to safeguard the rights of the person to be 'sectioned'. Before signing the order, they must be sure that such action is necessary and that the person is unwilling to go into hospital voluntarily, otherwise the social worker can refuse to sign and the section becomes invalid. The ASW is also responsible for transporting the committed person to the hospital and this often requires patience and understanding. Sometimes resistance and violence occur and the ASW may need to call upon the assistance of the ambulance service or, in extreme cases, the police. It is also important for the social worker to spend time with the person's relatives who may feel devastated that a family member's illness has developed to such an extent that they to be forcibly taken to hospital.

In accordance with the Mental Health Act Code of Practice (SSD Policies and Procedures) 1990, ASWs are currently expected to take account of several specific factors before making a decision about a compulsory admission. These include the client's wishes and views of their own needs; information received from friends, relatives and professionals; and the impact that compulsory admission would have on the person's life after discharge from hospital (code 2.6). In addition the client should be informed by the ASW that they are able to have another person, such as a friend or advocate present with them while they are being assessed (code 2.12).

Mental health in a cultural context

There is a good deal of evidence that black people have been discriminated against by mental health professionals particularly with regard to compulsory admission. It is estimated that 'black patients are nearly four times more likely to be sectioned under the Mental Health Act 1983 than their white counterparts' (Community Care 27.2.92). Racism, language difficulties and an absence of appropriate cultural understanding amongst mental health professionals are seen as the main reasons behind this disproportionate representation. At the same time there is concern that other minority groups are not receiving sufficient support from mental health services. In Tower Hamlets, an impoverished area of East London, where Bengalis make up between a quarter and one third of the population, only between 10–12 percent of hospital admissions are Bengalis. This is surprisingly low because proportionately mental illness should be more prevalent because of the stresses and difficulties such a disadvantaged community faces. According to Manowara Ahmed, a member of the social services team in that borough, Asian communities may not be receiving help because of the attitudes of mental health authorities. She believes Asians are expected to tolerate more strain than other groups: 'We have to fight to get people into hospital because families are expected to take care of themselves' (Community Care 27.2.92). This view, that minorities are expected to 'look after their own', has been commonly expressed.

More is now known about the need to develop services that are culturally sensitive and of the dangers of being influenced by racist or sexist assumptions. Improvements in publicity concerning service provision, more emphasis on understanding mental health in its cultural context and increased recruitment from minority communities are some of the ways forward for social services authorities.

Services for people with physical and sensory disabilities and people with HIV

This section deals with non–elderly adults with physical and sensory impairments and people with HIV who have particular service needs. The majority of people with physical disabilities, those who have sensory impairments and people with HIV live in the community. Only a minority live in residential units.

Services for people with physical disabilities

People may experience a whole range of disabilities which may or may not result in their becoming wheelchair users. Disabling conditions include the progressive illnesses of muscular dystrophy and multiple sclerosis; strokes and thromboses which may result in reduced levels of limb function; and other accidents and illnesses which lead to permanent disability. Some people, for example those suffering from cerebral palsy, were born with their disability; others acquired it. Sensory disabilities mainly include visual and hearing impairments. Some people experience a combination of disabilities.

Needs for services will differ according to each individual; some individuals are able to manage entirely by themselves, others will require up to 24 hours' care, depending on their condition.

Assessment

Under the Disabled Persons (Services, Consultation and Representation) Act 1986, all physically disabled and sensory impaired people are entitled to a *community living assessment*. This is normally a jointly funded service and will be carried out by a multidisciplinary team made up of the following personnel: a social worker; a home care organiser; an occupational therapist; a physiotherapist; a district nurse and a housing advisory person. Members of the team will assess the environmental, social, treatment and rehabilitation needs of people with disabilities. The overall assessment will take account of a person's medical history and current medical needs and is likely to be carried out in the service user's own home. The Act requires the local authority to take into account the ability of a carer, that is anybody who is providing a 'substantial ammount of care', to continue to provide care on a regular basis.

Note: Not all sections of the Disabled Persons Act 1986 have so far been implemented. Every local authority is currently providing community living assessments for people leaving fulltime special education but they have not all yet extended this service to all adults. And the provision for each disabled person to have an authorised representative to act on their behalf, where incapacity makes this necessary, also awaits full implementation.

Domiciliary services

Occupational therapists will carry out an aids to daily living assessment on the service user. The assessment is aimed at establishing a person's needs and considers ways in which they can be assisted to manage more independently. Various aids and adaptations to the home may be provided, ranging from non-slip bath mats and specially adapted furniture to the installation of a stair lift. Home care may be allocated for a certain number of hours per week. A laundry service is available to all disabled people provided they meet the provision criteria. In some instances financial help will be provided towards the installation costs of a telephone.

Day centres

Day centres are used by older people with a disability or a sensory impairment as well as by younger disabled people. It is argued that having a disability itself is not a sufficient reason to attend a centre if this is all the members have in common; the needs of older disabled people and younger disabled people can vary substantially. Nevertheless day centres do provide a constructive and imaginative service and cater for different disabilities across a wide age range. Centres usually employ occupational therapists who will work towards the service users' rehabilitation: assisting them with practical help, with skills acquisition and confidence building, to help people to adjust to a new lifestyle, particularly those who have recently been disabled. Day centres provide a link for otherwise isolated people and continuity of care for those who have recently been discharged from hospital. Other professionals, for example physiotherapists, may be employed on a sessional basis to attend to the service users' physiological needs: to stimulate limb movement, to demonstrate exercise and to encourage maximum use of muscles and joints to prevent unnecessary deterioration and loss of usage. These sessions may be held for individuals or for groups and although they may be hard work, they are often relaxing and enjoyable. Art therapists, music therapists and speech therapists may also make a contribution to a person's care.

The main emphasis of day centres is on rehabilitation, therefore places will be made available to each person on specific days of the week only. Factors such as age, degree of disability, home environment, job prospects, support and social network will be taken into consideration so that an individual care programme will be devised for each service user with the ultimate aim that they will be able to move on.

Sheltered workshops and homemaker schemes

These have become less popular with service users in recent years. The institutionalised character of workshops and the repetitive nature of their routinely carried out tasks are now generally thought to be unstimulating and dignity depriving. Instead sheltered placements in ordinary work settings are sought, where possible.

Transport

Transport should be the concern of mainstream transport providers, not social services authorities, but much public transport remains inaccessible to people with disabilities. Local authorities may provide travel passes, taxi card schemes or 'dial-a ride' services.

Services to people with sensory disabilities

Some social workers work exclusively with people who have one, or more than one, sensory impairment and their families. They may specialise in working with people who are hard of hearing or profoundly deaf; with people who are visually impaired; and people who have severe speech difficulties.

Social workers for people with hearing disabilities will need to be skilled in lip reading, be familiar with Makaton (a visual, sign-based aid to non-verbal communication) and be a British sign language user if they are to be able to communicate with all people who have a hearing disability. They will offer the full generic service to users and will specialise in providing advice and assistance in matters relating to the implications of hearing loss. Many profoundly deaf people need no social work support at all; they either manage by themselves or are supported by their families and friends. People with hearing impairments experience difficulties in just the same way as ordinary people; they experience mental ill health, have difficulties with their children and have domestic or financial difficulties, but these problems are compounded by the added difficulty of coping in a hearing environment.

Access has become a significant issue for people with physical disabilities generally so over the last few years more has been done to make public buildings accessible for disabled people. Similarly deaf people need to be received and understood in the public domain. It is important, for example, that receptionists of social services departments are acquainted with a basic sign language. Some authorities have assisted hearing impaired people by providing them with Minicom systems in their own homes. These visual communication systems allow typed messages to be transmitted to places where other Minicom systems have been installed. In this way a deaf person is able to communicate with organisations such as social services authorities, hospitals and police stations, where similar devices have been installed.

Social workers may work with visually handicapped people and those who are blind. Once again it needs to be stressed that many visually impaired people do not need or request support from social services authorities. People are more likely to need support at the onset of visual disability particularly if it was sudden and unexpected. Social workers will know about the services of voluntary organisations; for example, they will be aware of the special support and residential training provided by the Royal National Institute for the Blind for people who become blind.

Mobility rehabilitation workers, who are not qualified social workers, may provide practical help: for example, assistance in the use of a cane or in planning safe routes to community resources, in supplying equipment and demonstrating its use. They will also contribute to the person's needs assessment.

Services to people with HIV and AIDS

In response to the development of HIV and AIDS in the population over the past decade, social services authorities have needed to make service provision available in order to assist both those infected with the virus and those whose lives are affected (i.e. friends or other family members). Specialist social workers who provide services to people living with HIV and their families are usually located within the disability team. The team might typically include two social workers, three support workers and an occupational therapist. Recent legislation, namely the Children Act 1989 and the NHS and Community Care Act 1990, requires local authorities to work in partnership with parents of children or families of adults and to work alongside voluntary, not-for-profit and private organisations in assessment and service delivery.

HIV is a recent condition. The earliest recorded case in Britain of somebody being diagnosed as HIV positive was in 1982. It is expected that everybody who is HIV positive will eventually develop AIDS, an illness for which there is no known cure (although there can be no certainty of this). One fact already known is that HIV is preventable and that by avoiding direct contact with other people's blood and seminal fluids, infection can be averted.

People who are HIV positive may experience considerable rejection and disapproval from others because of the widespread ignorance and myths that surround the condition. Originally, gay people and black people were blamed for the cause and spread of AIDS despite the fact that the World Health Organisation is still unable to identify the origin of the disease. People living with HIV have been physically attacked, ostracised and discriminated against by individuals and organisations. Many have lost their jobs been forced to move from their homes and have been denied access to services available to other members of the community, all as a result of society's intolerance.

However, there are signs of more enlightened attitudes developing towards people living with HIV; this in marked contrast to the initial hysteria that characterised early public responses to the spread of the virus. Work carried out by leading voluntary organisations such as the Terrence Higgins Trust, London Lighthouse and Body Positive has helped to break down myths and stimulate a more dignified and human response. The recognition that everyone is vulnerable to HIV and AIDS is becoming more apparent as the increased incidence of people who are infected through heterosexual relations has become known.

Because of the public hostility and the subsequent stigma felt by many people who are HIV positive, not everyone with the virus is willing to seek help and receive services. It is now incumbent upon every local authority to provide or co-ordinate a discreet and sensitive service founded upon confidentially. Where services have been developed people with the virus and their families are offered advice about benefits and allowances and community care grants where appropriate. In common with people with other disabilities, people who have HIV are often unable to work and are therefore more likely to experience poverty.

Referrals to and liaison with housing specialists will take place and occupational therapists will advise on the home environment. Practical help is also available: for example, assistance with transport to and from hospital or medical appointments and assistance with applications to voluntary groups and charities for financial support.

Meals on wheels can be provided. These need not be delivered just for the service user but for the whole family or for friends: eating is a social activity, from which the service user should not be excluded because of incapacity. Foodchain, for example, is a voluntary organisation which specialises in such a service, providing wholesome, tasty meals. The meals may be deliberately high in calories in order to encourage weight gain and imaginatively presented in order to stimulate appetite loss. Because they are delivered in ordinary unmarked vehicles confidentiality is maintained (Neighbours may otherwise wonder why a young man or young woman is receiving meals on wheels).

An evening or night sitting service may be available to provide non-medical assistance to people with HIV and AIDS, perhaps to provide an opportunity for informal carers to have a break from caring or to give additional support to someone with the HIV virus living at home.

For families with children, the social worker will need to co-ordinate through voluntary organisations such as Body Positive or Positive Partners, babysitters, play schemes, child-centred outings or respite care to help lessen the strain on infected parents whose condition is often draining of energy. Black people with HIV or AIDS who may be distrustful of local authority social services departments may need to be put in touch with local black organisations, where they exist, such as Black Liners where they can expect a sensitive service.

The social worker may need to provide considerable emotional support for people living with HIV or AIDS and to their carers, partners, families or friends. They may put them in touch with carers' support groups who help with establishing support networks. Some parents will need help in deciding when to inform children of their (the parent's) HIV status – there are no rules about when or whether a child should be informed of their parent's HIV status, or of their own infection or the infection of siblings. Parents may need help to explore the options available.

Working with people with HIV and their families is recognised as being particularly stressful because of the nature of the virus and the distress which so often accompanies it; consequently, it is recognised that all people working with people with HIV need support. Group support meetings can help workers deal with issues and feelings raised. Indeed, the Terrence Higgins Trust insist that all those who act as 'Buddies' to people with HIV and AIDS should attend support meetings as a condition of their continuing to work for the organisation.

Occupational therapists (OTs)

Each social services authority normally employs a team of occupational therapists, or OTs as they are more commonly referred to. They may work with a wide range of client groups, including children, physically disabled adults and people with learning difficulties as well as elders. To some extent their role inevitably overlaps with that of social workers, nurses, physiotherapists and even psychologists, since the focus of their work is on how individuals use their time: that is, their occupational behaviour. The broad aim of the OT is to restore, reinforce and enhance performance in order to maximise a person's level of functioning so that clients can, as far as possible, take control over their own lives. In their work, OTs are encouraged to view the service user *holistically* – that is, to see the person in terms of their physical, emotional, psychological, cultural and social needs. The practice of occupational therapy draws on the theories of the social, medical and biological sciences and in recent years has been influenced by the work of Gary Kielhofner whose *Human Occupational Model* was published in 1985. An OTs work is chiefly divided thus: making assessments, problem solving and providing rehabilitation.

Assessment

As mentioned earlier in the chapter, OTs may carry out an *activities of daily living assessment* on a client in order to find out what the person is capable of doing by themselves. This process may involve a degree of measurement and testing and will focus on the service user's mobility level and ability to carry out daily tasks independently within the home environment. From this analysis the OT, in conjunction with the client, will be able to arrive at a treatment plan. OTs may also assess, to a degree, a person's level of cognitive functioning: they may carry out perceptual tests on people who are recovering from strokes or head injuries by using shapes or they may check an individual's memory in order to establish the kind of support needed. OTs may also contribute towards the special needs statementing assessment, for young people with learning difficulties.

Rehabilitation

OTs are concerned with the individual's wider rehabilitation so they may spend some time working to improve someone's mobility, standing balance or posture. The therapist may break down a difficult activity into component parts so that, for example, a person undergoing rehabilitation is finally able to make a cup of tea, having sucessfully rehearsed all the stages of the process. The provision of equipment may be necessary in order to support the achievement of a higher level of independence. In such cases it is the responsibility of the OT to select and issue equipment as appropriate. An OT may work with someone who is recovering from mental ill health to help to develop the client's confidence and enable them to become more involved in the community.

Much of the work is carried out on a one-to-one basis although OTs also run groups such as carers' support groups or 'stroke' clubs. Periodically they may undertake family work; that is, working with the whole family in order to assist in a member's rehabilitation at home. OTs may also visit small group homes in the community to assist residents with community integration. The OT may devise a series of purposeful activities such as using various forms of public transport or planning shopping expeditions or regular visits to job clubs or they may accompany a person to an interview.

The work of the emergency duty team

The area offices of most social services authorities open between 8.30 a.m. and 5.30 p.m. Outside these normal hours, the standby team is on duty to deal with any emergencies which may arise. In larger urban areas more than one officer will be on standby duty at a time, whereas in some less populous area only one social worker may be involved and this, among other considerations, limits the time spent with any one client. Some areas of the country have no separate standby service – instead, social workers work on a rota system following a normal day's work.

All kinds of emergencies occur outside office hours and special arrangements have to be made. Designated residential establishments will have beds reserved for emergency admissions and certain foster parents will be available to receive a child into care at short notice. Home helps will be contactable if their sitting services are required and senior management will be available for telephone advice if necessary. Daytime fieldworkers may inform the standby team of family situations which they regard as being potentially difficult and outline the relevant circumstances in case the standby duty officer is forced to intervene during the night or over the weekend.

The existence of a standby team does not prevent the necessity of social workers working in the evening with their own cases, as the role of the standby duty officer is strictly concerned with emergency matters.

Problems that face the emergency social worker are usually precipitated by some kind of crisis and it is part of their duty to resolve the situation as calmly as possible until the normal daytime services come into operation. If people contact the standby duty officer with routine requests which could wait until the following day, they will not be dealt with out of hours but will be referred to the daytime staff.

A standby social worker has to be adaptable in dealing with the range of problems they are presented with. The police may phone to say they have an elderly confused man found wandering in the road who is unable to tell them where he lives. The social worker may respond by checking with the establishments to see if any residents are missing or visit the area office to see whether the name is known to social services and the address is obtainable from the files. If this procedure is likely to take some time, they may arrange for the man to go to the local elderly persons' home and wait there. The social worker's enquiries may yield no information and the man may still have not recalled his address, so a bed would be made available for the night until he is eventually reported missing.

If acute family discord occurs at night when all members of the family are together, the social worker can be contacted to help settle the dispute. A wife may phone from a neighbour's house to seek refuge from her violent husband. Initially a place in a women's aid hostel will be arranged for a mother and children – a rendezvous and transport will have to be provisionally arranged as quickly as possible. However, if a visit by the social worker to the family home is likely to resolve the situation, then this will be made, but there are certain circumstances in which this course of action is plainly not appropriate.

If a child under 16 is held at the police station and the police are unable to obtain the child's parents, or the parents are unwilling to attend, the social worker's presence may be requested so that the child has the support of a 'responsible adult' before any questioning or fingerprinting procedure can legally be carried out. Similarly, the duty social worker has a responsibility to return children who have absconded from children's homes in the area. If the home is too far away, then a temporary placement at a local children's home will have to be arranged.

Since 1983, all standby duty officers have had to undergo extra training in order to become approved social workers able to administer the new regulations contained in the Mental Health Act 1983.

People who have difficulty coping often experience their worst fears when alone at night. They may seek help from the overnight duty officer. Their need to be available in case of other emergencies will limit their involvement, although reassurance over the telephone is often all that is required. The social worker is continually using their judgement to decide upon who should be visited. Sometimes, however, there is no choice.

A visit from a social worker, who will listen to the particular circumstances of the family and outline the support services available, will often resolve a crisis and render immediate action unnecessary. All contacts made with the emergency team are referred to the daytime staff the following day and followed up by the appropriate social workers.

People made homeless through unforeseen circumstances (a house fire or flood, for example) are the responsibility of the SSD 'out of hours' and the social worker may have to obtain places in a local authority housing department hostel if no other arrangements can be made. Married couples with children, elderly and disabled people, pregnant women, all children under 18 and those under threat of violence in their own homes are all entitled to temporary accommodation. Capable single people or couples without children are not the responsibility of the local authority; however, the social worker would advise and direct them to hostels or hotels in the area if they present themselves as homeless.

The emergency duty team consists of experienced fieldworkers who need to be particularly flexible and resourceful, with friendly dispositions. Having to wake residential social workers up at two in the morning to request accommodation requires a little tact! The establishment and maintenance of good relations with other agencies, notably the police and the hospitals, is of course essential.

Conclusion

This chapter has examined the work of local authority social services authorities at a time when they are undergoing great change. This change, as we have pointed out, has been mainly brought about by recent legislation, principally the NHS and Community Care Act 1990 throughout Britain and the Children Act 1989 in England and Wales. The proposals contained in this legislation alter fundamentally the core business of social services departments and social work departments in Scotland. The scale of these changes has been compared with the inception of the Social Work Scotland Act 1968 and the Social Services Act 1970 and 'have even been described as changes akin to those initiated by Beveridge in 1942' (*Community Care in Context* Part 2, 1992, p 1).

Local authority social service authorities are no longer expected to be 'the monopolistic provider of services'; instead they are to have a central assessment and purchasing role. They now have a duty to develop further the 'mixed economy of care' and encourage good quality provision from the private and voluntary sector. So far as residential care is concerned local authorities will have a principal role in carrying out an 'arms length inspection' on homes in the non-statutory sector as well as their own establishments. The standards of other services provided by non-local authority agencies are intended to be protected through contract agreements.

The local authority's historic role of chief provider of care is at an end. Local authorities no longer have any incentive to provide their own care homes for older people except for the most needy and dependent residents. Other services such as day care, domiciliary care, sections of fieldwork and the training division all have the potential to be 'floated off' to operate as independent providers.

These changes are not restricted to local authority social services authorities: much of the public sector has been affected by the introduction of management principles which proclaim efficiency and accountability as a consequence of exposure to market forces. Quality and 'value for money' are expected to emerge. Inefficient practice is expected to disappear because it is ultimately unprofitable.

The pattern of service provision has always varied between different authorities depending on their commitment to care and the resources available. This has not changed. It remains to be seen how well social services authorities act out their central assessment and purchasing role and whether the standard of care improves or deteriorates.

Appendix 1 – an example of short term social work involvement by a social services department (a deliberately oversimplified case study)

Monday – 11.00 a.m.

Mrs Baker arrives at the social services office and sees the duty social worker. She is concerned about her son Arthur (aged nine) who has recently begun to absent himself from school. Mrs Baker shows the duty officer a letter she has received from the school indicating Arthur's absences over a two month period. This is the first time that Arthur has ever stayed away from school, which he has always seemed to enjoy.

The duty social worker takes down some information about the family's history and present home circumstances. She tells Mrs Baker that another social worker will come and visit her and Arthur in their home during the week.

Tuesday morning

The case is allocated to a male social worker from the children and families team. (Not all offices have a special intake team for short term work.)

Wednesday – 5.30 p.m.

The social worker calls on Mrs Baker at her home. The family live in a small terraced house. The social worker is shown into the main living room in which there are two comfortable chairs. Arthur is present, but withdrawn and a little apprehensive.

Arthur tells the social worker and his mother that he has stayed off school for a number of isolated days during the last 2½ months. He has spent the time wandering around the park or 'messing about on the wasteland'. None of his school friends has been with him.

He is unable to say why he stays away from school – he likes the subjects, particularly maths and geography, and has 'two close mates'.

At the suggestion of his mother, Arthur takes the social worker to show him his new bedroom – it is brightly furnished with new unit shelving, a small computer and a small black-and-white television. Arthur says quite proudly that his mother decorated the room for him. The social worker goes downstairs to see Mrs Baker, while Arthur remains upstairs engaged at his computer.

Mrs Baker tells the social worker more of the family history: how Arthur's father left shortly after Arthur was born and how Mrs Baker has brought up Arthur single handed. She met her present husband five months ago, having almost despaired of ever finding anyone with whom she had so much in common. They have been married for three months. Her husband works quite long hours as a sales representative and likes to relax when he comes home in the evening. He sometimes spends Sundays fishing at the local reservoir.

By the end of their discussion, the social worker concludes that Arthur's staying away from school could be a form of attention-seeking behaviour. He points out that, before his mother's recent marriage, Arthur and Mrs Baker spent a good deal of time together. Now that Mr Baker has moved into the home, Arthur may be feeling a little excluded – this is symbolised by the fact that there are only two comfortable chairs in the living room. He recognises that Arthur's material needs are adequately met – the child has, for example, a well-equipped and cheerfully furnished bedroom – however, the social worker feels that, in her enthusiasm to establish her relationship with her new husband, Mrs Baker may have neglected Arthur's emotional needs.

Mrs Baker can see some truth in this appraisal and decides with the social worker that it might be useful if the family could do a few more things together. A third comfortable chair in the living room might encourage Arthur to spend more time with his mother and stepfather. Perhaps Mr Baker could take Arthur fishing one Sunday.

It is further decided that Arthur should not be criticised for his non-attendance at school – rather he should be encouraged to forget about the past few months and start going regularly.

Mrs Baker and the social worker feel that, if Arthur could be made to feel that he is still loved and wanted by his mother and could form a closer relationship with his new stepfather, he would begin to feel more secure. This might result in Arthur resuming his previous readiness to attend school.

Exercise 1 – emergency duty social work

Below are a number of problems presented to an emergency duty social worker working outside normal office hours. Imagine you are the social worker. How would you respond to the telephone calls and what kind of help would you offer? It is important to remember that the social worker would be basically concerned to find a practical short term solution to each problem, which would later be referred for follow-up social work support when the office next opens.

a) Sunday night – 12.05

The social worker receives a phone call from a Mr Dell who, together with his wife and two young children (aged three and five), is stranded just off the motorway but within the local authority boundary, having run out of petrol. They have no money. They are 40 miles away from home and 30 miles from the hotel where they have spent the last week on holiday. Mr Dell is requesting overnight temporary accommodation and is presenting the family as homeless. If no help is offered, he threatens to inform the Sunday newspapers.

Note Under certain circumstances, local authority housing departments have a duty to temporarily rehouse families presenting themselves as homeless in their area. Not many housing departments have overnight duty staff, so housing matters are dealt with by the social work emergency duty team and are referred the following day.

b) Saturday night – 12.30

Mr Cheeseman (44) is known to the social services. He is an unemployed single parent caring for his two sons in poor rented accommodation. He phones the overnight duty officer, saying 'The keys to my house are in the door. The two children are upstairs in bed. I have had enough and am leaving. I am going to walk to the motorway and hitch south. I intend to go abroad.'

c) Saturday – 11.30 a.m.

A neighbour telephones to say that Mrs Reid fell during the night and was taken to hospital only to be discharged and returned home early in the morning. The neighbour feels that Mrs Reid is at risk and could fall again tonight. He says he has done 'all that a neighbour can, but I have my own family to be concerned about'. He would like the social worker to provide some help as, in the neighbour's opinion, Mrs Reid is deteriorating.

d) Bank holiday

Mr Bull telephones. He is angry about the lack of support there has been for his ageing and confused father. Mr Bull has spent three days of the bank holiday caring for his father, who is obstinate and difficult to manage. A request for a full time place in a care home has been refused in the past. Mr Bull is 'fed up with having to make a 50 mile journey every weekend and bank holiday to look after my father'. It has gone on too long, he says, and quite simply, 'I am transferring the responsibility of my father to you.' With this statement he puts the telephone down.

e) Weekday – 7.00 p.m.

Mrs Ettiéne is distressed as she speaks to the social worker over the telephone. Her husband has just been physically violent towards her and her son (14). He has left the home but threatens to return to 'finish the job' later. He has now presumably gone back to the pub. Mrs Ettiéne is using her neighbour's phone, but she is frightened that her husband will return home any minute. She has two other children, aged seven and nine.

f) Weekday – 8.00 p.m.

Gina Houston phones to say she would like a social worker to accompany her to the local psychiatric hospital. She is not prepared to go by herself. Further, she says she has a piece of glass held against her wrist and that if someone doesn't come soon she will inflict an injury on herself. She says she will give the social worker 20 minutes to arrive.

g) Weekday – 11.30 p.m.

Jack Marsh is a 56-year-old disabled man with an artifical leg. He phones from a public call box in the town centre to say he is unable to get back home, four miles away, because he cannot afford the fare. He sounds as if he has been drinking. There is no late night bus service and he would like to be transported home by the social worker.

h) Weekday 9.00 p.m.

The emergency duty officer receives a call from Fanny Baldwin who is a woman in her eighties who lives alone. She is worried because the home help has not arrived to help her bed down for the night. She was due 25 minutes ago and is never late.

i) Weekday 10.15

An anonymous caller informs the emergency duty officer that an eight month old baby is severely bruised facially. The caller gives an address but then hangs up.

j) Saturday 2.30 pm.

A neighbour phones complaining of hearing 'Bloody mayhem next door'. She asks you to visit Mrs Richards, a young mother of two children, aged seven and nine, and adds that the police have also been called.

Exercise 2 – day care allocation for the under-fives

You are the social worker with responsibility for allocating day care places for the under-fives. You have two full-time and two part-time a day nursery places. It would be possible to place two children with registered childminders, although their fees are £3.50 per hour. The social services department would be prepared to help a family meet these fees for one child in the case of hardship. How would you allocate the available places among the families below? What advice would you give to the families you are not able to offer a place?

a) *Mr and Mrs Mathura* are two doctors in their late twenties. Mrs Mathura would like to return to general practice now that their daughter Marion has reached 12 months of age. She would be able to hold surgeries on alternate evenings to her husband.

b) *Mrs Pillai* (31) has recently separated from her husband and has custody of the two children, Dru (seven) and Suriya (two-and-a-half). She has an opportunity of working at her cousin's office and would welcome this for financial reasons and for the social contact a job would bring. She has no friends or relatives near to where she lives. Mrs Pillai would like a day nursery place for her daughter.

c) *Mr and Mrs James* are in their late twenties and have three children Jo (six), Asa (five), and Aileen (three). The family live in rented accommodation of poor quality and, since Mr James was made redundant, have accumulated debt problems. The two school age children both wet the bed and neighbours have complained to the housing department about shouting they hear coming from the house late in the evening. Mr and Mrs James would like Aileen to be offered a place in a day nursery, so that the parents can spend time 'free from the children'.

d) *Mrs Kenrick* (37) is married with two children – Thomas (seven) and Mary (three-and-a-half). Her husband works full time in a well paid job and Mrs Kenrick has spent the last few years looking after the home and the children. Mrs Kenrick has a history of psychiatric illness and, according to her husband, is beginning to display signs of disturbed behaviour. He feels she may need to go into hospital again. Mrs Kenrich requests a day nursery place for Mary.

e) *Miss Starling* (27) would like to return to full time education in order to pursue her interest in a career caring for people. She has two children, one of whom is at primary school. She requests a day nursery place for her two-year-old daughter, Margaret. Miss Starling is a single parent with no relatives or good friends living nearby.

f) *Mr and Mrs Okorafo-Smart* work long hours running a family business and have four children, two of whom – Amy (four) and Fran (three) – are under school age. They would like Amy and Fran to be placed in a day nursery. English is not spoken in the home and the parents would like their children to mix in an English-speaking environment. Previously the children were cared for by their grandmother, who has just died.

g) *Mr Wingate* (30) is a travelling salesman who spends some nights away from home. He is a single parent and until now his daughter Rachael (aged two-and-a-half) has been looked after mostly by Mr Wingate's mother. His mother had a stroke recently and can no longer care for the child. Mr Wingate requests a day nursery place for Rachael. His brother's family, who live nearby, will look after Rachael when Mr Wingate works away from home overnight.

h) *Miss Quinn* is 19 with a young son Daniel (aged two). She lives alone and has become quite depressed recently. The health visitor who calls to see her and the child feels that, although the baby is loved, it is very understimulated. Miss Quinn has never worked but would like to take up the offer of a job as a lunchtime barmaid at a local pub, in order to have the chance to meet more people.

i) *Mr and Mrs Ahmed* are a young couple in their twenties. Their only child Talat (aged three) is physically disabled. Talat has to wear a caliper on his deformed right leg. His parents would like him to mix more with other children and are requesting a nursery place.

Exercise 3 – role-play – a case conference

The following account describes the issues involved concerning Paul, a 15-year-old boy who is attending a community home with education on the premises. At the case conference, Paul's new social worker will recommend that Paul be allowed to return home. Your group will be allocated the various roles of the personnel involved and will have to re-enact the case conference.

Roles

1. Paul's new social worker
2. Head of the home (and chair of the meeting)
3. Motor mechanic teacher
4. History teacher
5. Houseparent
6. Other member of staff (role can be invented)
7. Paul's mother
8. Paul's stepfather

Situation

Paul Yates is 15 years old and has been in care since the age of nine. When he was 13, having previously been returned 'home on trial' to his parents, he appeared in court charged with taking and driving away cars. He was also due to appear for non-attendance at school. Since his court appearance, he has been at a community home with education on the premises (CHE) ten miles outside the city centre. In the last few months his behaviour has deteriorated and he has been disruptive in class. Paul admits that he has been a bit unco-operative but feels that he has been picked on by one member of staff in particular – his history teacher.

Family background

Paul's mother and father are divorced. His mother remarried a friend of her ex-husband and all three – mother, father and stepfather – have a close relationship. Mr Yates and Paul's natural father were themselves in care as children and later experienced Borstal and prison. All three adults are contemptuous of social services. As far as Paul is concerned, they argue that he has already spent 18 months in a community home and has already 'done his time' (equating the time Paul has spent at the community home with a prison sentence). They point out that Paul made good progress during his first 12 months and that his social worker promised that he could return home after the next case conference, three months later. This case conference passed and Paul was not discharged. Since then his behaviour has deteriorated. The parents, who visit Paul every Sunday, feel that Paul is 'not a bad lad' and should be given a chance to return home, where his parents will give him support. They feel that the social worker, Miss Tarrow, let him down by not obtaining his discharge as she previously promised.

Attitudes

1. Paul's new social worker

Paul's new social worker (replacing Miss Tarrow, who is going on a course) has seen Paul twice at the community home and finds him quite a likeable boy, despite his surly exterior. Paul is bitter about remaining at the community home and, like his parents, feels that he has 'done his time'. The social worker feels that Paul's being in a community home is not helping him to develop: rather it is reinforcing his resentment of authority.

In one month's time the establishment will be holding case conferences on all the young people. At this meeting you would like to recommend that Paul is discharged and returned home, for the following reasons:

a) You feel that Paul has been let down by his previous social worker and that his current behaviour is a reflection of his disappointment.
b) You feel that Paul will not gain significantly from remaining in the community home.

c) You want to work purposefully and practically with Paul over the next few years – you want to give him an opportunity of accepting responsibility and receiving trust and to be able to show maturity.

You discuss this proposal with Miss Tarrow, who is not very hopeful of this being a successful move. Although she had at one stage considered Paul's return home, she felt that it would be too much of a risk and so changed her mind. She feels that the whole family are not really to be trusted in what they say.

In order to gauge the possibilities, you discuss the situation with Paul, without promising anything definite. Paul sincerely promises that, if he were allowed to return home, he would stay out of trouble. Further, he would agree to attend school regularly until he is allowed to leave, even though he is sure he will not like school. He would welcome the opportunity to show that he can be trusted.

At the secondary school Paul previously attended, provisional arrangements are made with the head of year, who agrees to grant Paul a school place. He is willing to give Paul another chance, but – knowing Paul from the past – realistically indicates that he is doubtful about Paul's ability to comply with the arrangement.

You discuss the case with your principal officer and outline your intentions. He is prepared to back you in your decision to request Paul's discharge. (Note: Legally the local authority can withdraw any child from any home at any time – but to do so without involving the community home would be to act in bad faith and jeopardise future relations.)

2. Head of the home (and chair person of the meeting)

You are the head of the community home, which you run on rather strict disciplinarian grounds. Reports from staff suggest that, although Paul made good progress in the first 12 months, his attitude and behaviour have deteriorated recently. You would like Paul to remain in the school at least until his sixteenth birthday, in six months' time, by which time he may have learned to be more responsible and co-operative. You are not anticipating a request for Paul's return home but would object to such a request because of the effect it would have on the other children at the home, if granted.

3. Motor mechanic teacher

You have a good relationship with Paul, who works well and enthusiastically in your group. Paul confides in you occasionally and often talks about his mother, whom he would like to go back to live with. He gets on well with his father and stepfather and agrees that it is a 'funny situation' with them being so close. Paul responds to individual attention and informal instruction.

4. History teacher

You feel Paul that needs to be 'taken down a peg or two'. He is not interested in your lesson and does not respond willingly to instruction. Rather he encourages others to be disruptive. You feel that he needs to understand that he cannot get away with antisocial behaviour.

5. Houseparent

You like Paul but have noticed his recent unco-operative attitude. Paul normally willingly does his share of work in the unit. He was recently involved in a fight with another boy in the unit and had been spoiling for a fight for some days. You feel he should remain in the school and learn to accept disappointments and things which do not go his way.

Task

Take time to identify with your particular role and act out the case conference (about 30 minutes).

The case will begin with the social worker presenting the case for Paul's return home. All members of the group will then make contributions to the discussion. Towards the end of the meeting, Paul's parents will be invited in to the conference to be given a chance to have their say and to learn of the main arguments so far put forward.

Following the role play

Spend some time reflecting on the experience. Consider how the parents waiting outside the room must have been feeling, how Paul was feeling, and whether these parties should have been included from the outset of the case conference.

Exercise 4 – elders residential care allocation

Each of the following people has been recommended by a social worker to the admissions panel of the elderly persons' home. Unfortunately there are only two places available. Which two people do you feel need to be admitted? Consider what community care service may be alternatively provided for those whom you decide not to offer a residential place.

a) *Mrs Musgrove*, aged 83, lives alone in a first-floor council flat. Two years ago she suffered black-outs and is now quite confused, although physically fit. She fell and broke an arm during a recent black-out and has been cared for by her elderly brother and sister, who are both in bad health. Her short term memory is poor and she feels that her neighbours are stealing things from her. She hides objects, forgets where she has put them and then blames neighbours. (In fact she has no contact with neighbours.) Recently she has wandered into the neighbourhood and has been unable to find her way home.

She is visited by a home care aid, has day care for seven days a week, a home help and meal on wheels three days a week. The elderly relatives do not feel capable of providing any more support and would like Mrs Musgrove's request for a fulltime place to be granted.

b) *Mrs James*, aged 85, lives in a ground-floor flat. She suffers severe arthritis and is visually impaired. Since breaking a leg in a fall, she has lost confidence to do anything for herself.

Mrs James is frightened and her anxiety increases when local teenagers congregate outside her flat. It has been broken into once.

Last year her only grandson (20) volunteered to sleep on the settee in her home each night and to make her a cup of tea and her breakfast in the morning. His mother would visit during the day and do the shopping.

Recently Mrs James' grandson obtained a job and he now feels that he needs a proper night's sleep in preparation for the next day and no longer stays with his grandmother. Mrs James' daughter visits less often, as she is experiencing martial difficulties and has been to see the doctor about her anxiety. As a consequence, Mrs James is reverting to previous behaviour – staying in bed all day, unable to do anything for herself and becoming depressed.

Mrs James does not receive any domiciliary services, but her daughter would like her to be admitted to a care home fulltime.

c) *Miss Grant*, aged 64, retired from a responsible job four years ago and lives on her own in rented property where she has been all her life. When she left work she weighed 9 stone. She now weighs over 20 stone.

The loss of her main role in life on retirement reinforced Miss Grant's loneliness and isolation and she became depressed. She began to eat excessively, to the point where she became ill and went into a coma. She went to hospital and her weight reduced a little. On being discharged she became known to the social services. Soon she began overeating again, no longer used her upstairs bedroom and lived in one downstairs room. She had managed to become totally housebound and in need of help. She was on the telephone and often phoned neighbours to request help at any hour of the day.

Domiciliary support services have been brought into the home, but it is now felt that her physical size renders Miss Grant beyond domiciliary care. She is impossible to move by one person.

The social worker recommends that Miss Grant be given a fulltime place in a residential care home where her weight can be slowly reduced and eventually she can be rehabilitated to her own home.

d) *Mr Manning*, aged 91, lives in a ground-floor warden-controlled flat. An ex-alcoholic, he has three children whom he left when the youngest was four and the oldest was ten. They remember him as a violent man. He continued his job but left the family in poverty. Until her death, the children's mother was nursed by the second daughter, who is now 60.

Mr Manning is slightly brain-damaged from alcohol abuse and is lonely and confused. His eyesight is deteriorating. He wants to be looked after. One daughter still visits him occasionally out of a sense of duty. She blames him for her mother's early death and refuses to provide him with the emotional support he craves.

e) *Mr and Mrs Millerman* are aged 79 and 81 respectively. Mr Millerman has always presented a tough image and beaten his wife and daughter. Since he lost the sight of his right eye last year, he has become depressed, neglecting himself and expecting his wife to do everything for him.

Mr Millerman has exhibited characteristics of mental illness, insisting that the lights be turned off because he is frightened of switches. He also insists that his wife stay in the house all day.

The daughter visits, but is contemptuous of her father and speaks only to her mother. Mrs Millerman has recently had a stroke which has led to her being confused.

The social worker has noticed a gradual deterioration of Mrs Millerman's condition and observed her with black eyes and bumps on her head. She claims that these are the results of falling, but the daughter contests this.

The social worker is concerned for Mrs Millerman's physical safety and feels that she would like to get away from her husband.

f) *Mr Latham* is aged 79. His wife is fit, active and very proud of their recently modernised home. Mr Latham was formally a strong man and a 'bit of a womaniser'. Both their children have drifted off and have not been heard of for many years.

Mr Latham has suffered two strokes and lost the use of his left side. He is unsteady on his feet and needs constant care and attention. His wife feels resentful of his behaviour. He uses the commode in front of visitors and urinates when he feels like it. She thinks he is deliberately attention-seeking. Further, his sexual urge seems to have increased and he is making excessive demands on her. He masturbates publicly.

The social worker would like Mr Latham to be considered for a fulltime place, as this is the wish of both Mr Latham and his wife, who is finding the strain increasingly difficult.

Questions for discussion

1. Receptionists in social services departments are normally the first people seen by people seeking help. What kind of skills do you think a receptionist needs in order to deal with clients who might be angry or distressed?
2. You are a nursery officer (nursery nurse), working in a day nursery, attending a staff meeting. The officer in charge would like to encourage more parental involvement in the day nursery. What suggestions would you make?
3. Many older people are supported in the community by relatives and neighbours. Some neighbours offer no help. What kind of assistance could reasonably be expected from the neighbours of a frail 75 year old man receiving day care on six days a week? He is unable to cook for himself but can manage to wash, dress and get himself to bed. His only daughter lives 150 miles away and visits once a month.

4. Social services authorities have been accused of failing to meet the needs of black and Asian communities. What is the evidence of this? What strategies can be developed in order that social services departments (and social work departments in Scotland) do not discriminate against communities and are equally accessible to all?
5. The new role of the SSDs and SWDs as 'enabling authorities' will lead to improvements in the quality of service and encourage a wider diversity of provision. Comment on this statement.
6. 'Child care commentators are agreed that the future depends on how social services interpret "in need". The proponents of centralised services with highly professional but regulatory social workers want the definition restricted to children believed to be immediately liable to abuse. The advocates of supportive child care which maximise local involvement, favour a wider interpretation to allow community support to a range of social disadvantages' (Bob Holman, 'Pulling Together', *Guardian*, 20.1.93). Outline an argument for or against the expansion of community social work.

Further reading

1. *Practice with Care*, Ashri Ahmed (Race Equality Unit, Personal Social Services, 1990). A code of practice which aims to give guidance for managers and practitioners working with black communities within the social services context and give examples of good practice.
2. *The Community Care Handbook – The New System Explained*, Barbara Meredith (Age Concern, 1993). A very readable account of the changes brought about by the community care reforms.
3. *All Equal Under the Act – A Practical Guide to the Children Act 1989 for Social Workers*, Sheilla McDonald (REU, 1991). The main focus of the publication is on race and disability although connections are made and examples given of discriminatory practice which happens on a wider range of issues such as gender, class, sexual identity and poverty.
4. *Assessment and Case Management-Implications for the Implementation of 'Caring for people'*, Virginia Beardshaw and David Towell (Kings Fund Institute, 1990). A clear and comprehensive outline of the functions of assessment and care management.
5. *The Future of Social Work*, Terry Bamford (Macmillan, 1990). This book identifies key themes relating to the future of social work and postulates the positive role for professional social workers.
6. *Homes are for Living In*, Department of Health/Social Services Inspectorate (HMSO, 1989). A detailed model to use for evaluating quality of life in residential establishments.

3

The Probation Service

Introduction

The Probation Service is one of our society's responses to crime, along with the courts, the police and prison services and various smaller agencies. It provides a social work service to the courts in the UK – except in Scotland, where the Probation Service does not exist as an independent agency; its functions are performed by the social work departments (the Scottish equivalent of the social services departments). The work of the Probation Service applies to both the criminal and the family courts of England, Wales and Northern Ireland.

Most of its work relates to the criminal courts and the supervision of offenders in the community. In working towards the rehabilitation of offenders, it also acts to protect the public from the harm that offending causes. In the financial year 1990–91, the Home Office calculated that the average weekly cost of keeping someone in prison was £386, whereas the average weekly cost of someone on probation was £21. Apart from being much cheaper, it is also thought to be more constructive to keep a convicted person in the community rather than in custody.

The Probation Service is a locally, as opposed to nationally, organised service and there are 55 area services in all. In 1992, there were approximately 6600 probation officers, with about 9700 probation services' officers (PSOs) and support staff, most of whom were professionally unqualified. The total cost of the service in the financial year 1991–92 was just under £300 million. Financing of the Probation Service is shared – 20 percent of the total cost is, at present, met by local authorities and the remaining 80 percent by the Home Office from central Government funding.

Although each probation area is locally organised, the service receives official guidelines as to its policy from the Home Office, a part of central Government.

The work of the Probation Service is rather complicated, both professionally and in its financing. Probation officers are social workers and those who become probation officers now must possess the Certificate of Qualification in Social Work (CQSW) or the Diploma in Social Work (Dip. SW), its recently introduced equivalent; both are awarded by the Central Council for Education and Training in Social Work (CCETSW). As well as being social workers, however, they are also 'officers of the court' and they provide much assistance to the courts. This means that not only the Home Office, but also benches of local magistrates (or justices of the peace) and judges have a certain amount of authority over them and the work they perform.

This chapter will provide a brief history of the Probation Service, including recent developments; an account of the organisation and structure of the service; and details of the work performed by probation officers, both for the criminal courts and for the family courts as well as other, more specialised activities. A conclusion will look at what the future might hold.

History

The history of the Probation Service can conveniently be divided into four sections:

1. nineteenth century origins;
2. the period of establishment, 1907–70;
3. from 1970 to 1992;
4. a closer look at some recent developments that will shape the service in the 1990s.

Nineteenth century origins

As with social work generally in the UK, the origins of the Probation Service are to be found in the work of the charitable philanthropists and voluntary pioneers of the late nineteenth century.

During the second half of that century, drunkenness and alcohol abuse were social problems that caused particular concern, especially in the cities and large towns. The abuse of alcohol was often brought about, or worsened, by social deprivations such as unemployment, poverty and appalling housing conditions. People were frequently brought before the criminal courts for drunkenness and other related offences and a large proportion of these people would be sent to prison.

In 1876 a Hertfordshire printer called Frederick Rainer wrote to the Church of England Temperance Society (which still exists today, incorporated into the Church of England Council for Social Aid) expressing his concern about such people. He felt that once a person had been convicted and imprisoned by the court, there was little hope for them – on release from prison it was likely that further offences would be committed which would soon result in a further term of imprisonment. Rainer could see no end to this sad process – which is called 'recidivism' – unless something was done for the offender. He even sent five shillings to help the society start some kind of practical work with offenders.

Rainer was only one of many concerned people and in August 1876 the Temperance Society appointed the first unpaid police court missionary in London. Many more appointments followed and by 1900 what had become known as the police court mission employed 143 missionaries. It is interesting to note that only 19 of these were women.

What did the missionaries actually do? They made enquiries into the background of people who appeared before the courts and, if the courts agreed, they accepted responsibility for the offender's care and supervision. Sometimes they even helped financially, by providing money as a security so that a person could be bailed and not kept in custody. Much of the work performed by missionaries with offenders involved matrimonial conciliation and assisting with difficult children.

The police court missionaries rapidly earned respect and credibility from the courts for their work. And while they were doing so, other interesting developments that came to have a bearing on the history of the Probation Service occurred abroad.

Developments abroad

In Boston, Massachusetts, in 1878, a Probation Act had introduced the appointment of what were called 'probation officers'. Members of the newly formed Howard Association (a penal reform group in Britain) went to the USA to learn about the new ideas in Boston and they returned enthusiastic about what they had seen. Along with others, some of whom actually worked in the British criminal courts, they acted as a powerful pressure group in trying to bring about changes in Britain similar to those in Boston.

In 1887 they met with partial success and the Probation of First Offenders Act of that year introduced a system of releasing a first offender from a possible sentence of imprisonment, provided that they committed no further crimes. It was similar to what we now call a 'conditional discharge' – a person receives no punishment from the court as long as they stay free from further criminal activity.

Although this Act did not authorise supervision of the offender, it was a first move in this direction. The credibility that was gradually being built up by the police court missionaries led, in 1907, to the Probation of Offenders Act being passed, which permitted local authorities, from January 1908, to appoint probation officers whose job it would be to supervise offenders.

The period of establishment, 1907–70

Between 1907 and 1970 the Probation Service became officially established as the agency providing a social work service to the courts.

The Probation of Offenders Act of 1907 contained the basic principles of probation as we know it today. A local authority could appoint probation officers to 'advise, assist and befriend' those people convicted by the courts. Unfortunately, however, it was only 'permissive' legislation – it did not force local authorities to appoint probation officers. Such 'mandatory' legislation was not introduced until the Criminal Justice Act 1925; this meant that local authorities had to appoint probation officers (but many areas were still slow in actually doing so). Nevertheless, these two Acts of Parliament did mean the establishment of the Probation Service as a statutory (that is, an official State-provided and State-funded) service.

From 1925 onwards, the Probation Service expanded and became an increasingly professional service. In fact, the Probation Service pioneered training for social workers. In 1936, the Home Office introduced maintenance grants for students intending to become probation officers. To administer and control this scheme, the Home Office established the Probation Advisory and Training Board. At the same time, it began to inspect the services provided.

Probation officers formed a professional association as early as 1912, the National Association of Probation Officers (NAPO). One of the first debates to take place in the Association is still very much alive today – that of the court officer (or controlling agent) role versus the social worker (as caring agent) role. For many, this debate was (and is) irresolvable, because they believed that caring contained within it elements of controlling, in order to protect people from harming themselves and others.

After the Second World War, the Criminal Justice Act 1948 repealed the original Probation of Offenders Act 1907. The 1948 Act established the organisation of the

Probation Service as we know it today (to be discussed later in this chapter). One of the changes the 1948 Act made was that the insertion of the actual supervising probation officer's name into the probation order made by the court was no longer required.

In 1962, the Government set up the Morrison Committee to examine the work of the Probation Service. As a result of the committee's report, the role of the Probation Service became very much expanded. From being a social work service to the courts, it became a social work service to the whole penal system. Most importantly, it became responsible for the after-care of adult offenders being released from prison. This expansion of role brought about a change of name; in 1965 the Probation Service became the Probation and After-Care Service.

The Morrison Committee's report contained a definition of the Service: 'the submission of an offender, while at liberty, to a specified period of supervision by a social caseworker who is an officer of the court'. 'Social caseworker' is not now an accurate description of the probation officer because the Probation Service increasingly involves others in the care of offenders and utilises other agencies' resources.

As a result of the Criminal Justice Act 1967, the law no longer required that only a female probation officer should supervise girls and women. Two years later the Children and Young Persons Act 1969 introduced a number of changes, one of which was that a probation order for juveniles (in law, those under 17 years old) was to be called a 'supervision order'. It is interesting that the 1969 Act used the same words 'advise, assist and befriend' as had originally appeared in the Probation of Offenders Act 1907 in reference to the supervisor's role.

Since the 1969 Act, either probation officers or local authority social workers supervise young offenders under the terms of a supervision order. Arrangements differ from area to area as to which agency undertakes supervision. Local agreements will determine the age cut-off point at which each agency assumes responsibility. The 1969 Act also introduced 'intermediate treatment' (IT) for juveniles.

The Seebohm Committee's report of 1968 recommended one unified department for social services. In England and Wales the Probation and After-Care Service was to continue and to remain independent, but from November 1969 it ceased to exist in Scotland and became part of the social work department.

1970–92, continued growth

After 1970, the number of probation officers continued to rise until, in 1992 it stood at approximately 6 600. The number of ancillary (now probation services' officers) and support staff also grew dramatically.

Alongside this expansion in numbers, the responsibilities of the Probation Service grew in that, for instance, it increasingly focused on the supervision of people convicted of more serious offences. This development was partly prompted by the Government's desire to decrease the prison population and save money thereby.

The Powers of Criminal Courts Act 1973 gave the service an important step forward in this regard. The Act introduced *community service* for offenders age 17 or over. This required them to perform unpaid work of usefulness to the community, as a sentence of the court. It was, therefore, a form of *reparation*. Often regarded as an alternative to imprisonment, it meant that the Probation Service was now supervising a larger number of people who had committed more serious offences that might have warranted custody.

The number of reports on offenders' backgrounds and criminal activity (known at this time, and until quite recently, as 'social inquiry reports') required of the Service steadily rose during this period. Reports for custodial institutions and reports for the family courts also increased. The preparation of reports is time-consuming; it involves consultation with individuals, which may take place in the probation officer's office or at the person's home. Sometimes the probation officer will be involved in making the often lengthy journey to a custodial institution in which the subject is held. In addition other agencies may need to be contacted and police or probation records checked, for example, in relation to the circumstances of the offence.

The Criminal Justice Act 1982 brought a change in title. It returned the name of the service to what it had been before 1965, namely the Probation Service, and from 24th May 1983, the words 'and After-Care' were deleted. But this did not significantly change the responsibilities of the service; in fact the proportion of prisoners subject to statutory supervision on release has risen.

More centralised direction and control

In April 1984, an event of more significance took place. In that month, the Home Office published a *Statement of National Objectives and Priorities* (SNOP) for the Probation Service. This was the first time such a document had been issued by central Government and there was widespread fear in the Service that it might herald the start of more centralised control and a loosening of local control, of which the service was proudly defensive. The Statement was brief, setting out how the Home Office saw the work parameters of the service at that time and how it looked towards possible future development. At the time, concern was expressed by many (including the National Association of Probation Officers, to which the majority of probation officers belonged) that the Statement gave a low priority to after-care work with offenders released from custody and also to the civil work of the service. In the wake of SNOP, the 56 local services of that time were asked to produce their local version of the Statement, setting out their own objectives and priorities as reflected in their local areas.

The years immediately following 1984 were a time of some uncertainty for the Probation Service. As with other areas of public service, the work and organisation of probation came under scrutiny. However, fears of radical restructuring of the service, widespread privatisation and a move to 100 percent Home Office funding were not borne out. One area was amalgamated; the small City of London service became part of the Inner London Service.

'Cash limiting' came into force for the first time in April 1992, from the start of the financial year. Local authorities still provide 20 percent of total funding, but the Home Office now has more control as a result of a tighter hold over budgets. The devolving of budgets down to senior probation officer ('middle manager') level was also introduced. Area services are expected to set their own objectives, consistent with those of the service as a whole, and in setting targets they have to bear budgetary constraints in mind.

As far as working practice is concerned, two other events have led to more centralised direction and control. Firstly, from April 1989, 'National Standards' began to appear. These were a general attempt to standardise good practice. (They are dealt with in detail in the next section of this chapter.) Secondly, in November, 1992, a *Three Year Plan for the Probation Service* was published. Produced by the Home Office, it covers the financial years 1993 to 1996 and is expected to be the first of many such plans. It stresses the achieving of a cost-effective service that provides 'value for money' characterised by 'efficiency and effectiveness' (p2).

This 'three year plan' supersedes the 1984 *Statement of National Objectives and Priorities*. It is prefaced by a 'statement of purpose' (effectively a 'mission statement') which begins: 'The Probation Service serves the courts and the public by supervising offenders in the community' (pii). The purpose of the plan is set out as being 'the broad direction in which it is expected that area services will move'. Further, 'it will act as a *benchmark* against which the Government will judge progress in the achievement of its (i.e. the Probation Service's) priorities' (pl, Home Office emphasis).

The plan sets out eleven 'goals' for the service, seven of which are called 'operational goals' and four are called 'organisational goals'. The operational goals are:

1. crime reduction;
2. diversion (from prosecution and custody);
3. completing presentence reports;
4. supervising community orders;
5. working with prisoners;
6. providing accommodation;
7. working for 'child welfare' (in family proceedings).

The organisational goals are:

1. achieving equal opportunities;
2. the management of staff and other resources;
3. working in partnership with other agencies or volunteers;
4. 'providing high quality services, which make the most of public money' (pv).

Probation in the 1990s

National Standards

On 1 April 1989 the initial *National Standard for the Supervision of Offenders in the Community* came into force. This related to community service orders (CSOs) and was the first of a series. It contained requirements and guidance concerning the operation of community service throughout England and Wales. It was directed at the Probation Service as the supervising agency of community service. In contrast to the generality of SNOP, the National Standard on CSOs was specific and represented a more stringent form of centralised control.

Between April 1989 and August 1992 several drafts of National Standards on other topics affecting the Probation Service were circulated and were commented on by the service, both by individual officers and by the national bodies representing workers of different grades in the service. There were also workshops held to examine the Standards. This consultation process led to the publication, in August 1992, of the final versions of seven National Standards. The areas of work they cover are:

1. presentence reports;
2. probation orders;
3. supervision orders;
4. community service orders;
5. combination orders;
6. management of hostels;
7. supervision before and after release from custody.

In the official introduction to the Standards (issued jointly by the Home Office, Department of Health and the Welsh Office) it is said they seek to encourage good practice. However their official status is unclear – 'In many respects, the Standards lay down expected norms rather than outright requirements' (p2).

Criminal Justice Act 1991

The full seven standards became operative at the same time (from 1st October 1992) as most of the Criminal Justice Act 1991 came into force. The Home Office claims that the Act offers a 'new sentencing framework' in which sentences should reflect the seriousness of the offence or offences committed and custody should only be resorted to for those who have committed the most serious offences. These will most often be of a violent or sexual nature and in singling out these two the courts are expected to draw a sharper distinction between property offences (burglary, theft, damage) and offences against the person.

The introduction to the *Quick Reference Guide for the Probation Service* (Home Office, 2nd edition, 1992) to the Act reminds probation officers that they are 'officers of the court' (p 2) who 'as never before, statutorily have the central role throughout the whole of (the court) process' (Ibid). Probation officers have this role mainly because they will be responsible for a larger number of reports to the criminal courts on offenders than in the past. These pre-sentence reports (PSRs) are expected to include a proposal to the court as to how the person before the court might be dealt with by way of a 'community sentence'. (*Note*: An example of a PSR can be found in the exercises at the end of this chapter.)

One new development of great importance enshrined in the Act is that for the first time in statute (or written) law, it becomes the duty of all those working within the criminal justice system to avoid discrimination. This duty is contained in section 95 of the Act which specifically mentions 'race or sex or any other improper ground' in regard to anti-discriminatory practice. From time to time the Home Secretary publishes information intended to help people to work in an anti oppressive way. In the Autumn of 1992 short booklets were published on gender and race issues as related to the work of the criminal justice system.

New ways of working

For a number of years there had been a general pessimism around, both within the Probation Service itself and in the wider criminal justice system, a feeling that 'nothing works' in terms of effectively diverting offenders from committing further crime. Much of this pessimism stemmed from the results of the IMPACT research study (Intensive Matched Probation and After-Care Treatment) conducted by the Home Office in the early 1970s. It was based in four probation areas, two of which set up specialised units for the purpose of the research. Briefly, probation officers with drastically reduced caseloads worked more closely with a group of offenders; they met them frequently and involved themselves more in the offenders' home, work and leisure activities. One year after contact ceased, reconviction rates were studied and were found not to be significantly different from those of any other offenders on probation. The report concluded that the research had produced 'no evidence to support a general application of more intensive treatment' (p 22). The IMPACT study has been legitimately criticised for comparing reconviction rates after one year and not repeating the comparison after a longer period had elapsed, when results might have been more encouraging.

No major similar research has since been undertaken in this country. However, the findings over several years of Robert Ross (based at Ottawa University in Canada, along with his colleague Elizabeth Fabiano), working with persistent offenders and using social work interventions such as intensive groupwork, painted a more hopeful picture. Later, in the late 1980s a number of practically minded academics, based in the UK, began to publish findings of a similarly optimistic nature. Peter Raynor, working with the Mid-Glamorgan Probation Service, Colin Roberts with the Hereford and Worcester Probation Service and Gill McIvor at the University of Stirling all produced encouraging material.

Gill McIvor, in an article on such research, refers to the Mid-Glamorgan STOP programme (Straight Thinking on Probation). She summarises the findings thus:

> An intensive group work project employing psychodrama, sociodrama, offence-focused work and problem-solving techniques had lower levels of reconviction after six and 24 months in comparison with a similar group of young offenders who were released from custodial sentences.
>
> (*Probation Journal*, March 1992, p 2)

These techniques are currently being used in probation centres, but in some a shift of emphasis has led to their being conceived as a form of training, rather than traditional social work intervention. In reporting on their work in an Avon Probation Centre, Christine Weaver and John Bensted write:

> It is the opportunity to participate in discussions, moral dilemma exercises and to be intellectually stretched that the participants appear to relish.
>
> (*Probation Journal*, December 1992, p200)

A move to offence-based work

In the past few years, the work of probation officers has become more focused on the offence(s) committed by those they supervise and the wider behaviour which is related to that offending. This behaviour might present a risk or threat to the public or be harmful to the individual offender. Probation officers have also been encouraged to take on more serious offenders who have committed crimes involving, for example, physical or sexual violence.

In response to this change of focus the Probation Service has used more therapeutic programmes based upon lifeskills or social skills training; interventions which involve confronting offenders with the possible outcome of their criminal behaviour; and a greater utilisation of groupwork techniques.

Widespread use has been made of a wide range of cognitive training methods, or problem solving exercises, most prominently gathered together in this country by Philip Priestley, James McGuire and others. Priestley and McGuire's first volume appeared in 1978 and they have published others since. In 1985, they produced *Offending Behaviour: Skills and Strategies for Going Straight*; unlike their earlier, more generalised volumes, this book focused very specifically on crime and what happens when people offend. As with their earlier work, it contained a large number of exercises that some probation officers found extremely useful and relevant.

The use of such offence-based, problem solving material (more traditionally referred to under the titles 'lifeskills teaching' or 'social skills teaching') has increasingly spread through the Probation Service, so much so that some probation areas have devised and published their own material. For example, the Nottinghamshire Probation Service has produced the *Staying Out* pack. It is group-based work founded on Priestley and McGuire's material and it deals with such areas as self-esteem, self-control training and coping with the system (the criminal justice system and wider society). This was followed in 1991 by a pack entitled *Targets for Change* which complements *Staying Out* but is intended to facilitate one-to-one work with clients. It deals with some very practical issues such as accommodation, income maintenance, alcohol and drug problems, as well as self-esteem and personal relationships.

The move to offence-related work is also reflected in probation officers' reports for the criminal courts. The traditional 'social inquiry report' was more of a general personal and social history of an individual offender, often not devoting much space to the offence(s) committed or relevant offending behaviour. The new presentence report has as its main focus the offence(s), relevant information about the offender in regard to the offence(s) and their criminal history, as well as their attitude to the offence(s) committed. Much specifically focused offence-related work is done in probation centres which are dealt with in detail later.

The growth in specialisms

The Probation Service survived the Seebohm Report's recommendations and the creation of the large social services departments in England and Wales at the beginning of the 1970s (it ceased to exist in Scotland). The preferred mode of working for social workers from this time, until recently, was generic, i.e. staff should not specialise, but carry a caseload covering a range of needs and problems. With a few exceptions (e.g. working in hostels) probation officers did the same. A generic caseload would cover criminal work with all types and ages of offender, family work (court welfare work and adoptions), prison visits and visits to custodial institutions for young people, office and court duties (making a Probation Service presence available in the office base and in criminal and family courts).

In the past few years, there has been a move to more specialised work, both in social work and in the Probation Service. In probation, there has been more pressure on officers to demonstrate the skills they have; these are often more easily demonstrated in the form of specialisms. They may specialise as an individual worker within a wider team, e.g. as an employment/education officer to help offenders find suitable work or a

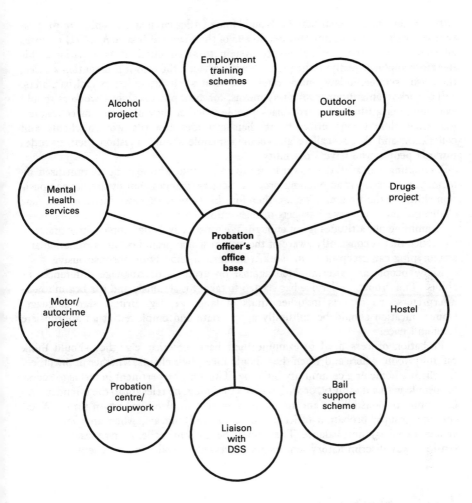

Fig 3.1 Some of the resources in the community that probation officers can draw on. *Note:* Not *all* the above may be available in *all* areas, their availability will depend on local staff and/or management initiatives. Some resources may be partly supported by Probation, e.g. a motor project, others will be completely independent, e.g. mental health services.

relevant college course. It is more likely, however, that they will work in a specialist team, e.g. community service teams, crown court teams, family court welfare teams and through-care teams, working with people while they are in, or released from, custody.

Anti-oppressive and anti-discriminatory practice

Anti-oppressive (also known as anti-discriminatory) practice is integral to the work of probation officers and their supervising of offenders. This is also true for the Home

Office, regarding National Standards and Home Office circulars, and now for the first time it is written into statute law. Section 95 of the Criminal Justice Act 1991 requires all who work in the criminal justice system to avoid unfair discrimination. This therefore applies equally to the police, social services, the crown prosecution service, the prison service, judges, magistrates, magistrates' clerks, solicitors and barristers.

To work in an antioppressive way means, for example, that white workers should examine their attitudes towards black people whether they be clients or colleagues; that men should look critically at their attitudes towards women clients and colleagues; and that so-called 'able-bodied' people should question their attitudes towards people who have a disability.

Examining our attitudes towards groups of people who may be marginalised by mainstream society is an ongoing process. Society changes continually; its composition shifts all the time and we are therefore likely to meet new situations and new challenges that may reveal aspects of discrimination in us.

Examining our attitudes is not enough. We must actively develop positive practice, a practice that is constantly aware of the way in which prejudice, discrimination and stereotyping can creep into our work, whether consciously or unconsciously.

Many people are discriminated against on grounds of language differences or ability. The Probation Service has started to take this seriously and has begun to use interpreters and experts in other kinds of language, e.g. British sign language. Communication should be culturally appropriate and employed at an appropriate level and pace.

Probation officers need to examine their basic practice, e.g. they should think carefully about where and when they should meet their clients, whether in the office, the client's home or a community building. This may be pertinent in terms of access for people with a disability, or with regards to timing, be relevant to the offender who has family responsibilities and needs to be in certain places at certain times. When running groups, probation officers should carefully decide, when appropriate, on gender, racial or ethnic balance. They should be ready to challenge in a meaningful and sensitive way discriminatory sentiments expressed by colleagues or clients.

Equal opportunities

It is extremely important, if the Probation Service is to avoid discriminatory practices, that its staffing composition reflects that of wider society. In other parts of the criminal justice system, women, for example, are grossly under-represented. Home Office figures (published in September 1992) show that less than 20 percent of solicitors in private practice in England and Wales are women; only 19 percent of barristers in private practice are women; only 5 percent of QCs (Queen's Counsel, the elite among barristers) are women. Further, women represent fewer than 10 percent of magistrates' clerks, only 13 percent of stipendiary magistrates (legally qualified, fulltime, salaried magistrates), 5 percent of recorders and 5 percent of circuit judges.

Within the Probation Service the situation is more positive, but far from satisfactory. Fifty three percent of maingrade probation officers are women, but the proportion of women decreases the more senior the grade; 32 percent of senior probation officers are women, 23 percent of deputy and assistant chief probation officers and just 15 percent of chief probation officers (NACRO figures).

Black people currently represent 4.3 percent of the UK population yet only 3 percent of maingrade probation officers are black. As with women, black people are very much underrepresented in higher grades. In July 1992, there were only five black assistant chief probation officers, there were no black deputy chief or chief probation officers.

However, the situation is improving. A NACRO report, *Black People Working in the Criminal Justice System* published in 1992, states: 'All the organisations involved in the Probation Service have been actively addressing the recruitment of black staff' (p15). Of approximately 400 students sponsored by the Home Office to do professional social work courses each year in England and Wales, 14 percent were from 'ethnic minorities' in 1990. In recent years the Association of Black Probation Officers (ABPO) was founded and representatives of this organisation, along with members of the National Association of Probation Officers (NAPO) and the Association of Chief Officers of Probation (ACOP), have recently come together with the purpose of producing joint guidance on antidiscriminatory practice in probation.

Although no figures exist, it is certain that other minority groups, e.g. people with disabilities and people from a working class background, are underrepresented in the service.

The organisation and structure of the Probation Service

The powers and duties of the Probation Service are set down in the laws of this country. They are to be found, in particular, in the Powers of Criminal Courts Act 1973 (as amended by the Criminal Law Act 1977), the Criminal Justice Act 1982 and the Criminal Justice Act 1991. In addition to this legislation, the 'Probation Rules' (which are statutory instruments) also contain official directives for the work of the Probation Service.

The Probation Service is organised both nationally and locally.

National organisation

As far as central Government is concerned, the Home Secretary is the Government minister responsible to Parliament for the Probation Service. Under the Home Secretary's authority is the Probation Service Division, a part of the criminal justice and constitutional department, which is headed by an assistant under-secretary of state. The Probation Service Division is part of the Civil Service. It has a certain degree of control over the Probation Service and it exercises this control, or guidance, by way of circulars and letters of direction sent to the local probation areas.

Also based at the Home Office is the Probation Inspectorate, which has power to inspect local probation areas and make recommendations. It also has a certain amount of responsibility for the recruitment and training of probation officers.

Local organisation

The Probation Service is largely a locally organised service. There are 55 different probation areas. Some areas coincide with county boundaries, while others are simply a part of a large city.

Each probation area is responsible to a probation board, which has to ensure that the work of the service is carried out effectively, and within the budget. Boards have a core membership of 16, made up of the chief probation officer for the area, seven magistrates, one judge, two people appointed by the local authority and five members from the local community who are not judges or magistrates. The latter are appointed by the board itself. Boards can appoint three further members who can be magistrates or judges, to bring the number on the board up to 19.

Members of the board (apart from the chief probation officer) are appointed for a period of three years and can serve a maximum of three terms (i.e. nine years in all). Boards meet regularly and are involved in appointing new staff and disciplinary matters. Each Probation Service has to present an annual report to the Secretary of State which is produced in line with the financial year (April to April).

Probation areas are further divided into smaller areas which are known as petty sessional areas (PSAs). A PSA is an area covered by one local magistrate's court. A group of magistrates in these areas forms a local probation liaison committee. This meets at least three times a year and is an important channel of communication on issues of sentencing, policy and probation practice. Local probation officers are present at these meetings and take part in them. A wide range of matters may be discussed, ranging from the case of a particular individual on probation to more general topics and current issues of interest or concern to either the magistrates or the probation officers.

Structure of a local probation area

The chief probation officer (CPO)

The chief probation officer is responsible for the work of the probation area they are appointed to. The CPO has to liaise with the Home Office and the area probation board and – through assistant chief probation officers and, in larger areas, deputy chief probation officers – has to oversee and organise the work of the Probation Service in the area. Performance-related pay has recently been introduced by the Government for CPOs, DCPOs and ACPOs. This means that a proportion of their salary is dependent upon achieving certain set targets, ag. increasing the number of community orders completed without further offending.

The deputy chief probation officer (DCPO)

Larger, more populous areas and some county areas have one or more DCPOs. They largely carry out the executive functions of the CPO, with a concentration on administration.

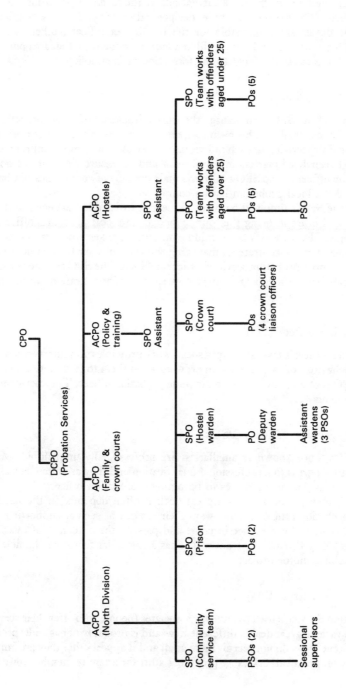

Fig 3.2   A simplified structure of a local probation area (a section of a larger area service).

The assistant chief probation officer (ACPO)

Each probation area will have a number of ACPOs. They will usually be more closely involved than the CPO in the work carried out by the teams of probation officers in the local offices. Their duties can be either general or specific – for example, some with specific duties are responsible for the training of officers; others for hostel provision. Those with general duties will link local teams, ensure that area policies are implemented and assist the CPO in the formation of area policy.

The senior probation officer (SPO)

The main task of the SPO is to manage the work of the team of probation officers for which they are responsible. This means a general overview of the team's work as well as the personal supervision of each individual officer. Another important role is to act as a link between headquarters and the team and to ensure that correct policy is carried out by officers. The SPO is also the main channel of communication between the team and the local probation liaison committee.

Much of the SPO's time will be spent in meetings with other agencies in the local community and often in being the 'public face' of the local probation officers.

Increasingly, SPOs are viewed as 'middle managers'; fewer now carry a caseload of clients because they concentrate on managing the work of their team. The team may include one or more probation services' officers (PSOs). The SPO may be responsible for secretarial staff, although some areas now employ administration officers for this purpose.

The probation officer (PO)

The probation officer's task is to apply social work principles and interventions to the offending behaviour of their clients, in order to assist them to lead more constructive lives. The PO is often known as the maingrade probation officer. They perform direct work with clients.

Probation services' officers (PSOs)

Usually PSOs, once known as ancillaries, are professionally unqualified. Many of them hope to progress to a professional qualification and they are often successful in doing so. This is one of the routes to becoming a probation officer.

The work they perform varies a great deal; it often depends on the needs of a particular probation office. In some ways their job can be seen as supporting that of POs – they represent a presence in court and pass on the outcomes of cases to the service. They may be part of a team which has a particular focus, e.g. homelessness, drug misuse or a motor project.

Voluntary associates (VAs)

The Probation Service's use of voluntary associates (people who offer their services as volunteers) varies a great deal in different areas and is probably not as widespread as it once was. Some areas do not recruit them at all and it appears that they are employed increasingly on practical tasks, e.g. providing a lift for a family member for a prison visit. Having said this, some befriending of offenders does take place and in this regard VAs often bring with them a good deal of life experience and vocational experience which complements the work of the PO.

What the Probation Service does

What the Probation Service does can be subdivided as follows:

a) crime prevention and diversion from prosecution;
b) work in the criminal courts;
c) supervising community orders;
d) supervision of offenders in and after release from custody;
e) work in the family courts.

Each area will now be dealt with in detail.

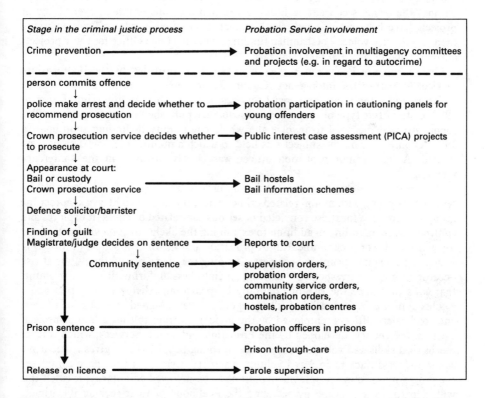

Fig 3.3   The Probation Service in the criminal justice system. Each part depends on the others to do a good job. (With thanks to Robin Parker.)

Crime prevention and diversion from prosecution

Crime prevention

Obviously, in working to divert offenders from further offending, the Probation Service is involved in preventing crime. This might be said to be achieved by the rehabilitation' of offenders, helping them to lead law-abiding lives.

However, the service is increasingly involved in a number of specific crime prevention initiatives. Arrangements vary around the country, so it is not easy to be definitive about the overall picture. The usual situation is that of a multiagency approach, with key agencies such as the police, probation and social services, as well as a number of voluntary organisations, coming together to pool resources and share knowledge and ideas.

Frequently, agencies are grouped into multiagency crime prevention panels, usually with the police taking the leading role. Probation will contribute its substantial knowledge and experience of working with offenders. Sometimes such work will focus on a particular area, say, a housing estate, with the acknowledgement that a more effective approach to preventing crime is likely to be achieved when a number of public agencies come together and work in a co-operative way.

Sometimes the work is targetted at preventing particular kinds of crime. Recent Home Office estimates suggest that nationally, over 1000 motor vehicles are taken without the owner's consent each day. In response to this problem, over 80 motor projects have been set up, with the National Association of Motor Projects giving them a collective voice. Total annual funding from the Home Office for these projects currently stands at £400 000 (*Observer*, 21.3.93).

One example of Probation Service involvement is provided by the Bedfordshire service. As part of the interagency 'County Management Team for Youth Justice', which includes the police and social services, it established an autocrime forum in 1992 to study this type of crime and subsequently published a report about it. This report stressed the need to involve the whole community in finding solutions. In 1993, a conference on the subject was held to which a number of organisations were invited. A local senior probation officer was closely involved in the conference planning.

A number of 'packages' within probation orders are offered by the Bedfordshire service for dealing with motor-related crime. These include an eight-week 'autocrime group' programme for those convicted of serious car-related offences (it explores and confronts such offending in addition to examining the likely effect on victims); a joint 'responsible driver programme' run by probation and the British School of Motoring which targets young people whose past offending may have placed the public at risk because of inept or irresponsible driving; an eight-session 'drink driver programme' that aims to reduce the risk of offending by providing reliable information about alcohol and its effects on driving. The programme was designed by probation officers and road safety officers (employed by the police). Further to this, a 'motor project' exists in the county, developed by the Probation and Youth Services, which teaches mechanical skills and vehicle maintenance to young people. It also gives participants access to 'grass track racing' as a voluntary activity. Even after they have completed the programme, young people may continue to be involved voluntarily; it is felt this will help to prevent crime by reducing the likelihood of their seeking illegitimate outlets on public roads.

Diversion from prosecution

The Probation Service is involved in two important activities concerning diversion from prosecution; these are the established practice of considering cautioning as an option for young offenders, and the newer experiment of 'public interest case assessment' (PICA).

Cautioning panels
Probation is represented on cautioning panels for young offenders, along with the police and social services department. These panels consider whether or not they can recommend a caution for young people who have committed an offence or offences rather than a prosecution; the latter requires a court appearance which invariably brings distress and may involve publicity. Cautioning panels have to take into account the seriousness of an offence, what effect prosecution might have on the young person and how best the public interest might be served. Panels are not involved in the actual cautioning, which is carried out by members of the police force.

Public interest case assessment (PICA)
Under the Prosecution of Offences Act 1985, the crown prosecution service (CPS) has to decide not only whether there is sufficient evidence in a case to justify a prosecution, but also whether it is in the public interest to prosecute. This is covered by the code for crown prosecutors which includes eight listed criteria which, if present in a case, may indicate that a prosecution is not in the public interest. Some relate to the circumstances around an alleged offence, but others involve the age and life situation of the defendant. It may be considered that it would do more harm than good to the defendant if they are prosecuted and; of course, the cost to the public has to be considered.

In 1988 an experiment began in Horseferry Road Magistrates' Court (in the Inner London Probation Service area) in which the Probation Service provided the CPS with relevant information to help them to decide whether or not a prosecution should proceed. A more formal project has since been established as a result of encouraging findings. In October 1991, three other projects started in Coventry, Oldham and Newcastle. The four were the subject of research, for the first year of their existence, by the Home Office Research and Planning Unit.

The Inner London project is staffed by a senior probation officer and two maingrade officers, plus support staff. It is targetted at adults charged with offences that are not particularly serious; for example, disorderly conduct, criminal damage and theft. It covers three magistrates' courts. Defendants are assumed to be innocent until proved guilty and so the alleged offence is never discussed. They have to give their informed consent to take part in the project.

Wherever possible, defendants are invited to be interviewed before their first court appearance, but this occasionally takes place prior to a second appearance. If a defendant wants to take part, an interview is quickly arranged at the project's office. The defendant is advised to bring to the interview any documentation that will verify their personal circumstances, e.g. a doctor's letter or payslip. Later, the Probation Service will make their own independent check on the defendant's personal circumstances and may make other enquiries to augment existing details they have about a defendant.

The circumstances considered by the PICA project are based on the following four criteria: where the offence is not serious and is therefore likely to receive a nominal sentence, e.g. an absolute or conditional discharge or a low fine; where a young adult under 21 would face irreparable harm as a result of the stigma of a criminal conviction; where a defendant is elderly and/or infirm and a criminal conviction would cause them distress (unless the offence is serious or is likely to be repeated); where a defendant is suffering from some form of mental illness which a court appearance might exacerbate.

Early results of the Inner London project were that proceeding with a prosecution was discontinued in one third of cases as a result of the information supplied by the Probation Service. The actual number of cases discontinued, up to March 1992, was 158. It seems likely that PICA projects will continue to grow and be extended to other areas because it appears to be a useful way of diverting certain offenders from prosecution.

Work in the criminal courts

The next section of this chapter will look at the supervision of community sentences made by the criminal courts. This section, meanwhile, examines two other important roles the Probation Service has in relation to these courts: the central one of providing information and assessment of offenders and their offending by way of pre-sentence reports; and the providing of information on defendants at the pretrial stage in order to assess their suitability for being granted bail by the Court rather than being remanded in custody. Schemes that provide this information are known as 'bail information schemes'.

The provision of pre-sentence reports

This area of the service's work has grown dramatically over the past 20 years. Each year the service prepares around 200 000 presentence reports (PSRs) reports for the criminal courts (formerly known as 'social inquiry reports').

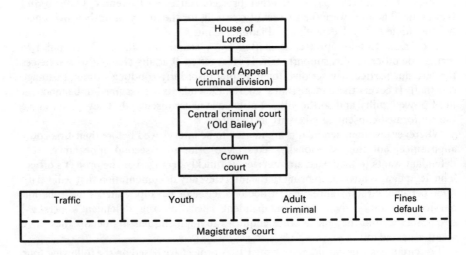

Fig 3.4 Basic structure of criminal courts in England and Wales.

Social inquiry report

I interviewed him twice: once at his home,
once from the back seat of his shooting-brake
with his mangy dog on the soft-top roof,
its tail curling in through the quarter-light.

He'd bought the cars from a friend in Bolton
then sold them. He'd never done a wrong thing
in his life so imagine his surprise
when the law turned up and arrested him.

We sat and watched as the metal crusher
cubed a written-off Morris Traveller
and listened to the panel-beaters send
their muffled echoes into Manchester.

I lent weight to his side of the story
but they sent him down. In the holding-cell
he shook like a leaf but feigned a handshake
to palm me two things: a key to his house

to turn off the water, and a fiver
for dog food and a gallon of petrol.

From *Zoom* by Simon Armitage (Bloodaxe, 1989)

As stated earlier, these are going to increase in number as a result of the enlarged areas of responsibility provided for under the Criminal Justice Act 1991. PSRs are time-consuming to prepare. Each one takes an estimated three to five hours in preparation; it has been calculated that report writing constitutes approximately a third of the total working time of a probation officer.

A presentence report is a written report by a probation officer to a criminal court. In the case of a young person this is sometimes completed by a social worker employed by the social services department. The report provides information about an offender so that the court can make the most appropriate sentencing decision. PSRs should be submitted only after a defendant has admitted an offence or offences or has been found guilty, thus upholding the principle in British law that people are innocent until proved guilty.

Under the Criminal Justice Act 1991, a PSR must be considered before an individual is sentenced to custody (except in serious cases in the crown court where the court regards it as unnecessary, or where the sentence is fixed by law, e.g. life for murder). The presentation of a report is also required in relation to more demanding community sentences, i.e. community service orders, combination orders, or probation or supervision orders that have additional requirements attached to them, e.g. that the offender should reside away from home in a hostel. A PSR is not required where a supervision or probation order has no additional requirements and this concerns many people, because a probation officer will not have met a person in this situation or assessed their needs and difficulties.

The report should focus on the offence, assessing its seriousness with reference to aggravating and mitigating factors. It should provide a summary of the facts, including details received from the crown prosecution service, and convey the offender's attitude to their offending behaviour, and any victim.

The report's central task is to explain to the court what led this particular person to offend, and, if appropriate, what led the person to offend in the past and what kind of intervention might assist the offender to avoid further repetition.

Where the offence is serious enough for a community sentence, the report makes a proposal to the court indicating the sentence considered most suitable for reducing the likelihood of further offending. The more serious the offence, the more the sentence should properly restrict the liberty of the offender. The most serious offences are said to be so serious that only custody can be considered. In other words, the offender's liberty should be very much restricted and the report should comment on what effect this is likely to have. In cases of violent and sexual offences, the report should also comment on the degree of risk to the public that this particular offender appears to pose.

The offender has the right to have access to the report at the court hearing and may well have read it earlier. The author of the report may be asked questions about it by the sentencers or by the defendant or their lawyer.

National Standards require probation officers to 'ensure that proposals for community sentences are realistic and appropriate in relation to seriousness, that PSRs do not stereotype the offender' and that they are 'clear, concise, free of jargon and exclude unnecessary detail' (pp 22 and 18 respectively). Reports should be no more than two pages long. To ensure that reports meet these criteria there is a quality control process known as 'gatekeeping'; this involves the checking of reports by other officers before they are presented to court. Gatekeeping should discover whether reports contain any obvious or unconscious discriminatory remarks. This can help to raise consciousness and be a constructive influence on team building. However, it is not easy and most of us do not find it comfortable to have our work put under the scrutiny of our peers.

As well as National Standards, the Criminal Justice Act 1991 also stresses the requirement that PSRs and the proposals they contain should be free of discrimination on grounds of gender, race, age, disability, sexual orientation, religion or any other improper ground.

Bail Information Schemes

A large number of people are held in custody while they wait to appear in court, either for a trial or for sentence. Of particular concern is the disproportionate number of black offenders held. Those awaiting sentence have, of course, been found guilty of committing an offence or offences. Of those held before trial, however, a certain proportion will eventually be deemed innocent when their case is heard. On any day in 1991, an average of 8246 (7954 males and 292 females) awaited trial in custody. This constituted around 20 percent of the total average prison population (*NACRO Briefing 32*, August 1992).

All people held in custody on remand can suffer a range of problems. They may lose their jobs and, as a 'knock-on effect', their accommodation; and they may be disadvantaged because they cannot contact their solicitors as regularly as they would do if they were free. Furthermore, conditions for remand prisoners are often very poor; they may well be locked in their cells for most of the day. It is also very expensive to the state to hold someone in custody.

One of the fears about people being held on bail in the community rather than in custody, is that they will commit further offences. However, figures from research show the number of people who reoffend in this way to be low. A recent NACRO report states: 'Studies from different areas consistently show that between 10 and 12 percent of persons granted bail by courts are found guilty of offences committed on bail' (*Legislation on Bail*, September 1992, p3).

The Prosecution of Offences Act 1985 created the crown prosecution service (CPS), a body independent of the police, which began operating in October 1986. Its job is to review police recommendations made to it as to whether or not to prosecute. Instead of there being a police prosecutor in court, there is now a representative of the CPS.

Despite the introduction, through the Bail Act 1976, of stronger rights to bail, the number of people granted bail, was felt by the Probation Service to be depressingly low. Totals fluctuated considerably, both over time and also geographically, which seemed particularly unjust.

The Probation Service therefore took the opportunity of the creation of the CPS to set up four pilot projects on bail information. By November 1987, there were eight such pilot projects and since then the growth of bail information schemes has been rapid. All probation areas now have a scheme and some have been set up within prison establishments.

These schemes provide information for the CPS so that it can make a more informed decision on whether or not to recommend bail to the court for an offender. Prior to these schemes the CPS only received information from the police.

Defendants must consent to take part in the scheme which only happens at the pretrial stage. The Probation Service will carry out a structured interview in order to seek positive information relevant to a bail decision. This could deal with community ties, family relationships, employment, special treatment being received for a medical problem or alcohol or drug reliance. Given the disproportionately high number of black offenders received in custody, antidiscriminatory practice is a central feature. Although it is early days, results from bail information schemes are encouraging in their aim of diverting offenders from a remand in custody.

Supervising community orders

The Probation Service is closely involved in four specific disposals of the court included within the category of community sentences and known as community orders. These are supervision orders, probation orders, community service orders, and combination orders. These orders are made by courts in response to offences within a particular range of seriousness. The seriousness of an offence or offences will determine to what extent the court considers there should be a restriction on liberty of the offender.

Less serious offences might warrant community sentences, such as a discharge or a fine, that do not restrict liberty. The most serious offences, many of which will be of a

The range of sentences open to the criminal courts in England and Wales

Note: Ten is the age at which people become criminally responsible.

Absolute discharge

No punishment is involved, but a criminal conviction is recorded.

Conditional discharge

No punishment is involved as long as the person does not commit any further crime for a period of up to three years.

Fine

Can be imposed for any offence, apart from murder and treason. In the crown court, there is no statutory maximum limit, but in magistrates' courts there are various limits which are amended over time. If people fail to pay fines, they can later be sent to prison.

Money payment supervision order

(MPSO) can be made to provide monitoring of, and assistance with, the payment of a fine, for people who have particular difficulties in this regard. Supervised by the Probation Service, this work is increasingly the responsibility of a probation services' officer.

Supervision order

For 10–17 year olds. No minimum length, maximum length three years.

Probation order

For 16 year olds and over. Minimum length six months, maximum three years.

Community service order

For offenders aged 16 and over. A minimum of 40 hours, a maximum of 240 hours to be completed over one year. Requires people to perform unpaid work in the community, as a form of reparation. The National Standard on community service orders states that probation officers should 'make particular efforts to find suitable work for people with disabilities, for women offenders and single parents, and for offenders from minority ethnic, racial or other groups' (p72, para 17). Such 'other groups' include older people and people with limited language and literacy skills. The Probation Service can help with expenses in order to prevent discrimination; for example, childminding fees for single parents.

Combination order

Introduced under section 11 of the Criminal Justice Act 1991, it combines a probation order with community service. The community service can last from 40 to 100 hours and the probation order can last from one to three years and have attached to it additional requirements. This makes for a very demanding community sentence.

Curfew order

Introduced under section 12 of the Criminal Justice Act 1991, this sentence has not, at the time of writing, been implemented. It would require an offender to remain in a specified place or places for a specified period or periods. The period would be not less than two hours and not more than 12 hours in one day, over a maximum of six months. It would apply to offenders of 16 years and over, who would have to consent to it being made. There is also provision in the 1991 Act for the electronic monitoring (known as 'tagging') of the subjects of curfew orders.

Attendance centre order

For ten to 20 year olds. For ten to 15 year olds the minimum number of hours is 12 and the maximum 24. For 16 to 20 year olds, the corresponding figures are 12 and 36. Offenders attend the centre on Saturdays (usually at fortnightly intervals) and take part in sporting activities or education, which may well take a lifeskills/social skills focus, helping the young people to cope better with the demands of life in the community.

Detention in a young offender institution (YOI)

For 10 to 20 year olds, both female and male. The minimum sentence for 15 to 17 year olds is two months, the maximum 12 months; the minimum for 18 to 20 year olds is 21 days, the maximum is the maximum term for the offence concerned (other than life).

Detention under section 53 of the Children and Young Persons Act 1933

Subsection 1 of section 53 was originally introduced as an alternative to the death penalty for young offenders committing murder and allowed for them to be detained for life at 'Her Majesty's pleasure'. Such an individual would only be released from custody when it was considered safe to do so.

Subsection 2 provided for detention for a specified period, for what were referred to as 'grave crimes', such as attempted murder, manslaughter and wounding with intent to do grievous bodily harm. This came to mean offences which, if committed by an adult, could carry a sentence of 14 years imprisonment or more.

Section 53 applies to young offenders aged 10 to 17 years. It can only apply to ten to 13 year olds if they are convicted of murder or manslaughter. For 16 and 17 year old males, it can apply additionally if they are convicted of indecent assault on a woman, although for an adult, this only carries a maximum penalty of ten years imprisonment. The Probation Service will be involved in very careful planning for the release of an offender sentenced under section 53.

Prison

Applies to all those aged 21 and over. There is no minimum or maximum length of sentence. Currently life imprisonment means on average that offenders spend 14 years in prison. However, judges at the point of sentence can make recommendations about the minimum length of time actually spent in prison.

Suspended sentence

As this is a suspended term of imprisonment, it again applies to all those aged 21 and over. It was introduced in 1967. If the offender commits no further offence during a period of up to a maximum of two years, they do not go to prison.

Suspended sentence supervision order (SSSO)

Introduced by the Powers of Criminal Courts Act 1973, they can only be made in the crown court (the maximum term of imprisonment a magistrates' court can impose is six months, whereas an SSSO can only apply to sentences of more than six months). Applies to offenders over 21 years of age. A presentence report is mandatory if such an order is made. Largely, supervision under an SSSO follows the pattern of a probation order and they are supervised by a probation officer.

Hospital order, under section 37 of the Mental Health Act 1983

Can be made by both magistrates' and crown courts for serious offences which are punishable by imprisonment. A criminal court can make a hospital order on the evidence of two doctors, that the offender is suffering from one of the four categories of mental disorder specified by the Mental Health Act (i.e. mental illness, mental impairment, severe mental impairment and psychopathic disorder). The order lasts for six months and can then be renewed for a further six months, after which it can then be extended for one year at a time.

Restriction order under section 41 of the Mental Health Act 1983

This can be made by a crown court that has previously made a hospital order on an offender, if it is deemed that their restriction is required to protect the public from serious harm. At least one of the doctors involved in the hospital order must give oral evidence in court to support restriction. The orders lasts for whatever period the court specifies.

Transfer to hospital from prison under section 47 of the Mental Health Act 1983

The Home Secretary can order such a transfer if satisfied by the evidence of two doctors that such treatment is likely to alleviate or prevent a deterioration of the condition of an offender. The order for transfer lasts for six months, can then be renewed for a further six months, after which it can then be extended for one year at a time.

Deferred sentence

Introduced by the Powers of Criminal Courts Act 1973, it is available in both magistrates' and crown courts. Sentence is deferred, or put off, for up to six months. The defendant must consent to deferment and a date fixed by the court for the next hearing. The purpose of a deferred sentence is to put some onus on the offender to make progress on their own in terms of their life, lifestyle or situation, e.g. finding or staying in employment, accommodation or obtaining treatment.

violent or sexual nature and which will often represent a threat or risk to the safety of the public, will warrant a custodial sentence which profoundly restricts liberty. The four community orders that are dealt with in this section represent an intermediate position between these two extremes. They will restrict liberty to a certain extent.

Offenders who are the subjects of community orders will have to give up time to meet their supervising probation officer. In the case of community service, the court requires that a certain number of hours be spent in doing demanding, unpaid work. These orders, therefore, represent a restriction on liberty.

An offence of less seriousness might attract a probation order of the minimum six month period, whereas an offence of greater seriousness could attract a three year probation order with an additional requirement of residence in a hostel for part of the three year period. The second example represents a far greater restriction on liberty than the first.

Of the four community orders dealt with below, the combination order, introduced by the Criminal Justice Act 1991, entails the most severe restriction on liberty. Not only is the order a combination of community service with a probation order, but the latter can also have additional requirements inserted into it, e.g. attendance at a probation centre or taking part in 'required activities' such as a groupwork programme. It is used for the most serious offenders permitted to remain in the community.

Community orders also vary in the amount and intensity of social work intervention provided. Community service does not offer any, but rather requires offenders to give reparation to the community as part of their rehabilitation. Supervision and probation orders involve the establishing of a professional relationship in which the probation officer will 'advise, assist and befriend' the offender. The aim is to help the offender to examine their offending behaviour, accept responsibility for it and find new, positive ways of behaving in the future without resort to crime.

Supervision and probation orders have a rather different focus from each other. The former, involving as it does younger people, aims in part at assisting development into adulthood. Unlike a probation order on an adult, the probation officer will not only work with the subject of the order, but be more involved with their parents, family and wider social network.

We now look at each of the four community orders in more detail.

Community service order

Anyone over 16 years of age can be sentenced to community service (CS). Community service organisers locate opportunities for offenders on CS to perform suitable unpaid work in the community. The type of work varies but is usually of a practical nature, involving physical activity, e.g. gardening, decorating, clearing footpaths. The offender may work for individuals in their own homes or in some kind of local authority premises, or in public space or public property. It is a form of generalised reparation to the community for the harm or damage caused by offending. The number of hours ordered by the court reflects the seriousness of the offence. The minimum is 40 hours, the maximum 240 hours and they must be completed over a one year period.

Work should begin within 10 days of the making of an order, with a work-rate minimum of five hours per week, a maximum of 21. Offenders should receive written information about community service, in a language they can understand. Records have to be kept of hours worked by each individual and a brief weekly report should be provided for each of them informing them of the number of hours they have

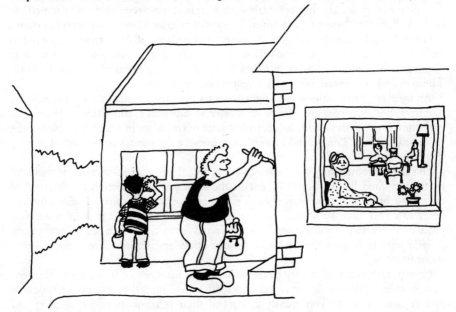

Community Service allows offenders to be more positively involved in their local community.

worked, set against the total required, and giving them a brief comment on their performance.

Breach proceedings may be taken against anyone who fails to comply with a CSO. Failure might include lateness, failure to attend, unacceptable behaviour, or poor quality of work. The Home Office requires an explanation to be sought of any failure within two working days and this must be recorded. Warnings can be given on the first or second incidence of failure, but on the third, breach action is normally expected. If returned to court on breach, the court has several options: it can take no action; punish the offender for the breach; revoke the order and sentence again for the original offence.

Combination order

This order combines community service with probation. The former can last from 40 to 100 hours, the latter from one to three years. The order is only available to the courts for offences which are punishable by imprisonment. Additional requirements can be inserted in the probation order, e.g. residence in a hostel, attendance at a drink or drug therapy clinic. An offender must consent to the making of such an order and a court must have available to it a presentence report before imposing it.

A combination order is a single order of the court and must be supervised by a single probation service, ideally by a single officer. The community service and probation elements of the order will be operated and supervised in the same way as if they were separate orders. The same rules and expectations apply.

Supervision order

A supervision order can be made in regard to young offenders aged ten to 17 years inclusive. The Criminal Justice Act 1991 extended its application to 17 year olds. The situation now is that both supervision orders and probation orders can be ordered by the criminal courts for offenders aged 16 and 17 years. The onus is on the court to assess the young offender's 'maturity'. Broadly speaking, mature 16 or 17 years olds would be more likely to receive a probation order and be supervised by a probation officer, less mature 16 and 17 year olds are likely to receive a supervision order and be supervised by a social worker from the social services department.

Home Office advice on the question of 'muturity', as contained in the National Standard on supervision orders, refers to the clearest difference between the two orders as being thus: 'the supervision order is also intended to help a young person to develop into an adult, whereas a probation order is more appropriate for someone who is already emotionally, intellectually, socially and physically an adult' (p 51). It does go on to say, however, that a supervision order 'may often in practice be the more suitable', because many 16 and 17 year olds 'are still very much in the stage of transition into adulthood' (ibid).

The Criminal Justice Act 1991 has abolished the Juvenile court and introduced the youth court for children and young people. In legal terms, 'children' are under 14 years of age, 'young people' or 'young offenders' are 14 to 17. ('Juveniles', who were dealt with by the old juvenile court, were 14 to 16 years old.)

The fact that 16 and 17 year olds can be dealt with by either the Probation Service or social services departments means that there must be much closer liaison than previously in regard to this age group. Some areas (e.g. Leeds) have set up multi agency teams made up of the Probation Service and the local authority social services department to service the youth court. Practice with regard to interagency co-operation differs widely across the country.

Table 3.1 Persons supervised by the probation service, by type of supervision (Totals as at 31 December and % changes from the previous year)

TYPE OF SUPERVISION	1986	1987	1988	1989	1990	1991
Probation order	52 490 (–4%)	52 160 (–1%)	52 420 (+1%)	52 740 (+1%)	54 558 (+3%)	51 827 (–5%)
Community service order	21 930 (–4%)	23 920 (+9%)	23 930 (–)	24 390 (+2%)	26 985 (+11%)	30 409 (+13%)
Supervision order (C&Y P Act 1969)	8450 (–23%)	6690 (–21%)	5250 (–22%)	4040 (–23%)	3429 (–15%)	2610 (–24%)
Money payment supervision order	7340 (–5%)	7760 (+6%)	7270 (–7%)	8060 (+11%)	8194 (+2%)	8422 (+3%)
Total statutory after-care	23 880 (–4%)	24 510 (+3%)	24 640 (+1%)	23 140 (–6%)	21 916 (–5%)	22 459 (+2%)
Voluntary after-care	27 480 (+3%)	30 020 (+9%)	31 820 (+6%)	31 670 (–)	29 694 (–6%)	30 651 (+3%)

Source: Probation Statistics, England and Wales, 1991. Such statistics are published annually by the Home Office.

Table 3.2 Availability of a range of criminal sentences and ages at which they are applicable

Age	10–13	14	15	16	17	18	19	20	21 or over
Absolute discharge	*	*	*	*	*	*	*	*	*
Conditional discharge – up to 3 years	*	*	*	*	*	*	*	*	*
Fine – Limited fines in magistrates' court, unlimited in crown court	*	*	*	*	*	*	*	*	*
Supervision order – no minimum length to maximum of 3 years	*	*	*	*	*				
Probation order – from 6 months minimum to 3 years maximum					*	*	*	*	*	*
Community service order (CSO) – from 40 hours to 240 hours					*	*	*	*	*	*
Combination order – CS from 40 to 100 hours – probation from 1 to 3 years					*	*	*	*	*	*
Attendance centre order – under 16, 12 to 24 hours, 16 to 20, 12 to 36 hours.	*		*	*	*	*	*	*	*
Detention under CYPA. 1933 S.53	* [2]		*	*	*	*			
Detention in a young offender institution (YOI) – 15 to 17, minimum 2 months, maximum 12 months: 18 to 20, minimum 21 days, maximum is the maximum for the offence concerned (other than life)			*	*	*	*	*	*	
Imprisonment (including a suspended term and life)									*

Notes:
1. All apply equally to females and males
2. Murder and manslaughter only

A supervision order can be made for a maximum of three years. There is no specified minimum period. The court does not require the consent of the offender for a supervision order to be made, unless it has certain additional requirements specified. These might be being ordered to refrain from certain activities (e.g. attending football matches) or required intermediate treatment (IT). IT was introduced by the Children and Young Persons Act 1969 and the Criminal Justice Act 1982 made it a duty for local authorities to provide IT schemes. It was 'intermediate' in that it was a provision which bridged the gap between supervision in the community and a custodial sentence.

Intermediate treatment involves a wide range of activities, often undertaken in groups. 'Outdoor pursuits' have figured a good deal, motorcycle groups have been run and some sporting activities have taken place. In recent years, the Probation Service's involvement in IT has decreased and, in many areas, social services have taken complete responsibility for it. This is partly due to the decreased number of young offenders being supervised by the Probation Service.

Home Office guidelines recommend that the first meeting between a probation officer or social worker and the young offender should take place within five working days of the making of a supervision order. If possible, this meeting should be arranged after the court appearance, before the offender leaves court. A supervision plan should be drawn up within two weeks of sentence. This will contain what the probation officer or social worker hopes to achieve with the offender and it will be developed in co-operation with them. Both will sign the order and the offender will be provided with a copy. A review of the order should take place every three months, with a final review on completion. An order can be terminated early if good progress is made. Probation officers are advised to consider early termination after two thirds of the term of the order.

Arrangements for young offenders in Scotland

The criminal justice system in Scotland is very different from that in England and Wales. The Probation Service in Scotland ceased to exist from November 1969 and its work was taken on by the social work departments. Offenders in Scotland, therefore, are supervised by social workers. These new arrangements were introduced by the Social Work (Scotland) Act 1968.

Children under 16 years old in Scotland will be considered for prosecution in court if they fall into one or more of a number of categories:

a) If they have committed serious offences, such as murder or assault, that endanger life;
b) If they are jointly accused with adults;
c) If they are involved in offences where disqualification from driving is possible.

However, it is by no means certain that children involved in such offences will be prosecuted in court. Instead, they may, if the public interest allows, be referred by the procurator fiscal to the reporter for a decision on whether or not they can be dealt with by a children's hearing. The reporter is a local authority official and they will then decide which of three courses of action to pursue:

1. To take no formal action;
2. To refer the child voluntarily to the social work department for advice or assistance;
3. To refer the child to a children's hearing because the child is, in their view, in need of compulsory care.

Children who commit less serious offences than those mentioned above, along with children who are beyond parental control, who are not attending school, who are engaging in solvent abuse or who are not receiving adequate care from their parents, can also be dealt with before a children's hearing. These hearings were one of the radical changes made in Scotland by the 1968 Act. In April 1971, the hearings took over from the courts most of the responsibilities for dealing with children under 16 on both care and criminal matters.

The people who make a decision on a child at a hearing are drawn from children's panels (the nearest equivalent in England and Wales are magistrates). There is a balance between women and men at a hearing and a wide range of ages represented. In Scotland there are about 1650 panel members.

Procedures at children's hearings are far more informal than in a court setting. Each hearing has a chairperson and all the participants usually sit round a large table. The child must attend, except when domestic matters that might cause distress are being discussed. Both parents' attendance is compulsory by law. The press can attend, but must not disclose the identity of the child in any later report. Approximately 63 per cent of all referrals to reporters each year involve alleged criminal offences.

The hearing has to decide on what measures to take in the best interest of the child. In order to assist it, a report from a social worker on the child will be available and this will often include a school report. Psychological or psychiatric reports might also be present. Most of the time at the hearing is taken up by discussion between all present. If it is decided that compulsory care is necessary, the child can be placed under supervision and this can run until the individual is 18 years old. The child might remain at home or be sent to local authority accommodation or accommodation belonging to a voluntary organisation. A hearing does not have the power to fine either the child or the parents; this can only be done by a court.

When a supervision requirement has been made by a hearing, it lapses after a year, unless it is renewed by a review hearing. At a review hearing, the supervision can be discharged, renewed or altered. A child or their parents can appeal against the decision of a children's hearing. This system is considered by many to be more child/family orientated and more appropriate for young people than the courts that operate in England and Wales, although the recently established youth court is expected to create a degree of informality.

Probation order

A demand for justice must go beyond retribution for the offence and reparation for the victim. It has to include a demand for *understanding* the offender.
(*Recession, Crime and Punishment*, S. BOX, p29; author's emphasis)

A probation order can be made on any offender aged 16 years or over. Originally introduced as an alternative to a sentence of the criminal courts, it has been made a sentence in its own right by the Criminal Justice Act 1991. This change has been made so that the probation order can now be combined with a fine or another community sentence, e.g. community service. The length of a probation order varies from a minimum of six months to a maximum of three years. It legally requires the person on probation to keep in touch with the probation officer, as requested by the officer, and to notify them of any change of address. Anyone placed on probation must consent to such an order in court. In Scotland, social workers of the social work department supervise people on probation.

The National Standard on probation orders sets out the three official purposes of such orders. They are:

1. to secure the rehabilitation of the offender;
2. to protect the public from harm from the offender;
3. to prevent the offender from committing further offences. (p 31)

In order to facilitate this, the probation officer aims to establish a relationship with the offender which is based upon the officer setting out to 'advise, assist and befriend'.

Guidance contained in the National Standard states that a first meeting should take place between the probation officer and offender within five working days (Mondays to Fridays) of the making of the order and if possible, this meeting should be arranged before the offender leaves court. At this first meeting, the offender should be given written information about the requirements of being on probation, including the possibility of breach which requires the offender to return to court for punishment if they fail to comply.

Probation officers are advised by the National Standard to formulate a supervision plan (the equivalent of a social worker's individual care plan) within two weeks of sentence (four weeks at the latest). This should be done in co-operation with the offender. It is in part an assessment that sets out the needs and problems of the individual; it also identifies the resources that are to be used in meeting the objectives set. Frequency of contact and time limits on the achievement of objectives should also be set. Both the offender and supervising probation officer should sign it and each should retain a copy. The supervision plan should be reviewed every three months and there should be a final review on completion of the order. Written records should be kept of all reviews.

Probation orders can be terminated early if good progress is made, but not normally before the half-way point. Probation officers are, however, encouraged to consider termination at a point two thirds through the total length of the order. Up-to-date records of all contact must be kept and it is considered good practice to share these with the offender. If the guidance contained in the National Standard on probation orders is not adhered to, the Home Office now requires a written record stating the reasons for the non-adherence. This is a clear example of an increase in central control.

Having said this, a probation officer still has a large amount of autonomy as to how they work with an offender; and freedom to act as one thinks best invariably increases job satisfaction. The said freedom applies particularly to the officer's right to select the kind of social work intervention they think most appropriate (see Chapter 8 'Strategies for Helping').

We now turn to look at some of the specialisms that probation officers might be involved in as part of the additional requirements that can be inserted in probation orders. These may include a particular kind of social work intervention, e.g. groupwork, or a particular kind of offence, e.g. autocrime, or a specific setting, e.g. probation centres or hostels.

Groupwork

Few probation officers will specialise in groupwork in the sense of doing it all the time to the exclusion of other kinds of work, e.g. one-to-one work, but it is a skilled activity nevertheless and can be very specialised. It is practised in a variety of settings. It can be, and has been, a traditional aspect of a 'straight' probation order (one with no additional requirements), but it is also now increasingly used as part of the programme of a probation centre (see below) involving intensive probation supervision. Groupwork can range from a discussion group, which might be open, informal and leaderless, to a very focused, intensive experience dealing with specific issues such as male violence towards women, sexual offences, alcohol or drug misuse. Groupwork is therefore a neutral helping technique that can have a host of applications, regimes, power structures and programmes.

It is possible to identify three kinds of groupwork which are most common in the Probation Service:

a) Groupwork involving problem-solving, social skills or lifeskills work which focuses on offending behaviour. Sometimes the umbrella term 'cognitive training' is used for such groups; it signifies that they are about helping offenders to learn new ways of reacting and new ways of behaving when facing difficulties or challenges. If the process is successful, group members who break their offending pattern will then be directed towards new interests and activities. Philip Priestley (himself an ex-probation officer) and James McGuire (whose background is in psychology) particularly have promulgated this type of groupwork and the exercises within it, in the Probation Service.

Groupwork based on this material will usually be carefully structured and time-limited (it will run for a fixed term) with a programme planned and set down in advance. Issues it may explore are self-esteem, self-control and anger management, including an examination of the roots of anger and violence. Since the majority of offenders are male groupwork based on this model can usefully question how masculinity relates to offending and to what extent issues of power and the male ego are relevant.

b) Groupwork that takes place in drop-in or reporting centres. Such groups, run on a weekly, time-limited programme, will be attended by offenders who are released from custody and are subject to licence or are on probation orders. Licences require that offenders attend such centres, but once there, they may well have a degree of choice as to which groups they opt for. Group activities might well centre round money advice, health education (including taking precautions against HIV infection) or a job club for people attempting to find work. Literacy and numeracy help might also be offered. The atmosphere within such centres is likely to be a relaxed one, with facilities such as darts, pool and refreshments available.

c) Groupwork for offenders who have committed particular categories of offence (e.g. alcohol or drug-related, sexual offences, persistent violent offenders). This kind of groupwork is often open-ended, i.e. it is not time limited. There will be much open discussion in such groups, involving disclosure of personal histories and behaviour which may often result in confrontation. This approach is used to good effect by probation officers who work in custodial institutions.

It is of key importance that such groups are led skilfully and sensitively, therefore there is a great deal of reliance on the officer's intuition. This is so for two reasons: firstly, they do not have a structured programme to rely on; secondly, much of the material revealed by the group will be of a very personal and intimate nature. Being open-ended has its usefulness because group leaders and members can decide for themselves when issues have been resolved or when to extend the life of a group. More details of groupwork techniques can be found in Chapter 8.

Autocrime work

Crime involving motor vehicles is, at present, the fastest rising type of crime. This may involve theft, the competitive and reckless driving of stolen vehicles (called joy-riding by some, death-riding by others), and drinking and driving. Many probation areas have now set up specific projects to deal with offenders committing such crimes. They go under a number of different names, e.g. 'responsible drivers courses', 'drink-impaired drivers courses'.

Several techniques are used in these projects. They include groupwork in which offenders share experiences and are helped to explore their reasons and motivation for offending. They also include lifeskills work intended to inform, educate and encourage more responsible, mature attitudes, say, towards drinking and driving. Much of the work involves confronting male offenders with the link between masculinity and crime: of joy-riding, Bill Downie, a probation officer, says: 'It is a power thing. For the first time in their young lives they have control over something when they drive a car. It brings them into adulthood . . . They want to grow up as quickly as possible.' (*Hendon and Finchley Times*, 10.10.91).

Probation centres and intensive probation programmes

Additional requirements can be added to a probation order to cater for particular needs and/or to 'toughen them up'. There is now a more general awareness that keeping a person in a custodial institution may be destructive and often counterproductive as regards an individual's progress (certain people have to be imprisoned order to protect the public from danger). Custody is also very expensive. There has been a drive, therefore, both by central Government and by the courts and Probation Service to keep more people in the community. The Probation Service has, as a result, taken on the supervision of offenders who have committed more serious offences ('high tariff' offenders). Such supervision can be made more demanding, in one of two ways:

a)   General additional requirements can be added to a probation order (PCCA 1973 section 3(1) inserted by Criminal Justice Act 1991, section 9(1)). This kind of requirement would mean an offender taking part in activities as a condition of the order. These activities may take place in a range of locations. Examples are someone dependent on alcohol or drugs attending a specialised substance abuse project; drink/ drivers or autocrime offenders attending a motor project.

b)   As an alternative to custody for the 'highest tariff' offenders who remain in the community, they can be required to attend a probation centre for up to a maximum of 60 days, as a condition of a probation order (PCCA 1973, schedule 1A, para 3). The only exception to this is for someone convicted of a sexual offence who can be required to attend a group at any time during the full length of their probation order. Prospective attenders at a centre are carefully assessed prior to an order being made; they will meet with probation staff either at the centre or in custody if they are being temporarily held there on remand.

The length of programmes in probation centres varies around the country. Thirty to forty days is common, with an attendance pattern of three or four days a week. Home Office National Standards suggest that a full day's attendance should last at least six hours. Some centres will run a daytime regime for unemployed people and an evening programme for those who have work.

Centres will have clearly laid down rules relating to attendance and time-keeping and will stipulate no alcohol or drugs on the premises and no threatening or violent behaviour. Offenders can be breached for non-compliance, in the same way as any person on probation.

Hostels

The Probation Service began running hostels for young offenders in the 1920s. Some fifty years later, in the early 1970s, it introduced hostels for adults. They cater for both females and males, many of whom may have committed quite serious offences. Broadly, there are two types of hostel: approved probation hostels and bail hostels.

a) An offender might move to live in an approved probation hostel as a condition of a probation order or under the terms of a licence on release from custody. There are about 120 in England and Wales. They are 100 percent funded by central Government, through the Home Office. The person in charge, the warden, will be a senior probation officer and their Deputy will be of maingrade probation officer status. All such hostels will accept offenders on bail if they are being considered for residence as a requirement of a probation order, or simply as a condition of bail. The former arrangement would constitute a trial period, in order to see if a longer period in a hostel would be appropriate; a move to a hostel could be a traumatic change in a person's life, particularly if it is the person's first experience of life away from home and their local area.

The pattern of provision of approved hostels has changed in that there has been an expansion in recent years in the number of places available; there has been an increased in what are known as 'core and cluster hostels'. The Probation Service has purchased ordinary houses in the community to form a 'cluster' around the 'core' of an original hostel. This is a constructive way of normalising offenders' experience of living; it is less stigmatising and helps them to cope better with conventional daily life.

Hostels are administered by a management committee consisting of area probation staff and lay members of the local community. The committee is required by the Home Office to have an equal opportunities policy in place which must ensure that there is no unfair discrimination against any staff or residents and ensure equal access to all the facilities provided. Regimes within hostels vary a great deal; much depends on the staff's attitudes towards care and control.

b) There has been an increase in the numbers of bail hostels and places available for offenders on bail and the government currently plans further expansion. Bail hostels are a much cheaper resource than keeping someone in a custodial institution. Courts set the conditions for bail and hostels must closely adhere to them in order that the bail system does not become discredited in the eyes of sentencers. All bailees are subject to a curfew; usually residence in the hostel is required from 11 p.m. until 6 a.m. the following morning. Hostel staff are required to notify the police, on the same day, if a resident fails to arrive at the hostel or is known to have committed a further offence.

The Probation Service also uses a range of other accommodation, including hostels run by voluntary organisations, specialist projects dealing, for example, with alcohol or drug misuse, and private households.

Supervision of offenders in and after release from custody

Probation officers do not only supervise community orders and work with offenders in the community, they also work with offenders who are sentenced to custody: before they go 'inside'; during their imprisonment; and after their release back into the community. This is also referred to as THROUGH-CARE. In addition, probation officers provide custodial institutions with information about offenders.

Reports for custodial institutions

As well as presentence reports, the Probation Service also prepares reports for custodial institutions. For offenders subject to automatic conditional release, a probation officer prepares a brief predischarge report based on a proforma which is sent to the institution in question. It will set out the circumstances the offender will return to on discharge. It will also cover any conditions the home probation officer considers should be inserted into the licence the individual will be subject to on release.

For those offenders subject to discretionary conditional release, the home officer will send a longer, more detailed report to the institution concerned. This is known as a parole assessment report; it will help to inform the parole board's decision on release and the timing of it. Something of particular importance here is the issue of child protection from abuse, whether physical or sexual. If a particular offender has committed offences of this nature, it is important that the home probation officer checks out release plans to ascertain, for example, whether the prisoner is returning to a home containing children. Other details a report may contain are the attitude of the offender's family or community to their release; the former's response to previous supervision; whether any special help is required by the offender with, say, accommodation or managing alcohol or drug misuse; and whether or not there is a likely risk of reoffending.

Probation work in custodial institutions

There are two main kinds of custodial institution in England and Wales: young offender institutions (YOIs) and prisons. In addition there are secure establishments where offenders are held on remand, awaiting either trial or sentence, e.g. Risley Remand Centre, Cheshire, for young offenders and Brixton prison in London for adults. Earlier types of institutions for young offenders were Borstal institutions (which were supposed to give training in a trade), abolished in May 1983, and detention centres (some of which provided a so-called 'short, sharp, shock' regime); the latter ceased to exist from 1 October 1988 when the new sentence of 'detention in a young offender institution' came into force.

Young offender institutions (YOIs)

Both female and male offenders aged 15 to 20 years can be sentenced to detention in a YOI. For 15 to 17 year olds, who will be dealt with in the youth court (changed in name from the juvenile court by the Criminal Justice Act 1991, on 1st October 1992) or the crown court, the minimum term is two months, the maximum 12 months. For 18 to 20 year olds, the minimum term is 21 days, the maximum is the maximum term for the offence concerned (other than life); they are sentenced in the magistrates' court. All young offenders under 22 are subject to at least three months supervision by a probation officer on release from a YOI, except that it will never go beyond an individual's 22nd birthday. Those sentenced to 12 months or more (or more than 12 months if under 18 years) are subject to statutory supervision by the Probation Service on release, under rules which apply to all those aged over 18 who are released from custody.

Regimes, programmes and activities in YOIs vary a good deal, depending on age and on the length of custody. Shorter term inmates will usually face a busy and brisk programme with a full, structured daily timetable. There will be an emphasis on education, including physical education. Longer term offenders will take part in similar activities, but will have a programme geared to their individual needs.

The probation officer from the home area remains responsible for those serving a sentence in a YOI; they will visit them while they are 'inside' and will supervise them on release. In recent years, the Probation Service has tended to draw back in terms of its involvement within young offender institutions. This is to allow prison service officers to get more involved with their charges and, hopefully, to more fully 'humanise' such regimes. The Probation Service's presence inside YOIs is now mostly limited to one probation officer of senior grade. Much of their work will involve liaising with the Probation Service outside the institution.

Inside the YOI, prison officers act as a 'personal officer' to each offender; in the early days of the sentence, a sentence plan will be drawn up in co-operation with the inmate. In their role of personal officer, the prison officer will attempt to make the offender's time in custody as constructive as possible and they will help with any problems the offender may have and plan for a smooth release.

Prisons

The United Kingdom currently has a higher prison population than any of the other twenty countries of the Council of Europe. On 1st February 1990, it stood at 53 182 which represented 93.3 prisoners per 100 000 population. The country with the second largest prison population in Western Europe is West Germany (51 972 on the same date) and the third largest, France (46 798 on the same date). The Home Office expects, and is planning for, an increase in the number of prisoners in this country. By the year 2000, it expects a prison population of 57 500, a depressing and expensive prospect.

Even so the Government has attempted to reduce the number of people held in prison, both those on remand (by encouraging bail information schemes and by increasing the number of bail hostel places available) and those serving sentences (by certain measures in the Criminal Justice Act 1991). Under the Criminal Justice Act 1991, courts are encouraged to consider imprisonment only as a last resort and keep offenders as much as possible in the community. Prison should be used mainly for offenders who represent a threat or risk to the public, particularly if they have committed a violent or sexual offence.

Any offender over the age of 21 can be sent to prison. There is no minimum or maximum length of sentence (people can receive a number of 'life' sentences). A magistrates' court is restricted to six months imprisonment on any one offence.

The age and state of the fabric of prisons varies greatly, from old Victorian prisons based on the 'wing system' (a number of 'wings' radiate from a central core) without decent sanitation (therefore requiring 'slopping out') to relatively, more comfortable, modern buildings equipped with electronic surveillance and security devices. Some of the more modern prisons offer industrial work regimes, e.g. metalwork, contract laundries.

The first privately run prisons have now opened. There are different categories of prison ranging from open prisons (for those regarded as no security risk or those preparing for release) to top-security institutions which often have a 'prison within a prison' for detaining the most serious offenders, e.g. those who have committed murder or acts of terrorism.

Some prisons will have specialist units within them, say a psychiatric wing or a wing for sex offenders, for segregating such offenders from other prisoners. One prison – Grendon Underwood, in Buckinghamshire – is known as a psychiatric prison; it offers various therapeutic programmes with a high utilisation of groupwork, often of a confrontational kind.

Probation officers in the home area of a prisoner retain responsibility for maintaining contact with the prisoner both in prison and on release. Letters or visiting will be the means of communication and the officer will aim to facilitate contact with families at home as well. Being in prison will almost always cause great strain and difficulties in relationships, especially as visits are normally only permitted once a month and are of a short duration.

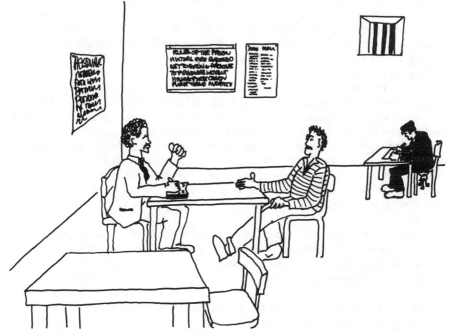

Probation officers provide a necessary link between the prisoner and the outside world.

In addition to home probation officers, others work fulltime in prisons as prison probation officers in probation departments. They help offenders to keep in touch with the outside world and are involved in a range of social work interventions within the establishment. As with probation work in the community, there is a greater stress on offence based work and an increased use of groupwork techniques. There may be groups run on specific topics such as anger management or controlling violent behaviour, or they may be targetted at particular categories of offender, e.g. sex offenders. An increasing amount of this work is shared working, with the prison service or with outsiders who come into the prison such as teachers or psychologists. As in YOIs, the Probation Service is encouraging prison officers to get more involved in closer working with offenders and thereby extend their role from mere 'turn-keys'.

There are three major concerns relating to imprisonment. Firstly, there is a greater awareness that a disproportionate number of black people are being remanded in, or sentenced to, custody. Secondly, there is a disturbing number of 'mentally disordered' offenders who are inappropriately spending time in prison. And finally, there is the long-standing concern that the physical environment in many prisons needs to be drastically improved.

Supervising prisoners released on licence

The Criminal Justice Act 1991 has introduced a new concept with regard to custodial sentences. Such a sentence is now seen as being served partly in custody and partly (after release from custody) in the community. The offender is now liable to recall to custody, right up to the end of the sentence. The Act has abolished remission (time taken off the period in custody, as long as the offender behaved co-operatively) and made important changes to the parole system (a discretionary early release arrangement, if certain criteria are met). The parole system had fallen into particular disfavour because judges became concerned about the variations of time spent in prison; it was noted that some prisoners served markedly different terms from other prisoners who had committed similar offences. It thus affected morale in prisons and proved to be a control problem.

All adult prisoners serving 12 months or more and all young offenders (i.e. under 21) are subject to compulsory supervision on release under the terms of what is called a 'licence'. Young offenders released from a YOI receive a minimum of three months supervision by either a social services department social worker or by a probation officer (depending on which agency had been in contact with the family earlier). The period of postrelease supervision is intended to help offenders resettle in the community and avoid reoffending. In this way the public will be protected.

There are three categories of prisoner (both adults and young offenders) who are eligible for early release:

1. **Short term** prisoners. They are further divided into two categories: those serving under 12 months and those serving from 12 months to under four years.
2. **Long term** prisoners. This is classed as four years or more.
3. Those serving a **life** sentence.

Taking each in turn, the diagrams below illustrate what proportion of time will be spent in custody and in the community:

1. **Short term prisoners serving less than 12 months**. These are covered by what is called an automatic unconditional release (AUR) scheme:

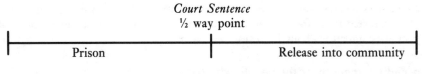

Court Sentence
½ way point

| Prison | Release into community |

If convicted of a further imprisonable offence during this period, a court may order the outstanding term to be served in custody, in addition to the sentence for the new offence.

Short term prisoners serving from 12 months to under four years. These are covered by what is called an automatic conditional release (ACR) scheme:

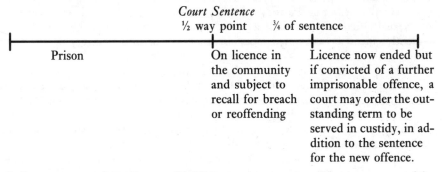

Court Sentence
½ way point   ¾ of sentence

| Prison | On licence in the community and subject to recall for breach or reoffending | Licence now ended but if convicted of a further imprisonable offence, a court may order the outstanding term to be served in custidy, in addition to the sentence for the new offence. |

2. **Long term prisoners, serving four years or more**. These are covered by what is called a discretionary conditional release (DCR) scheme, which involves the parole board making a decision as to when release is suitable:

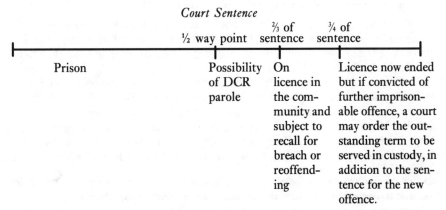

Court Sentence
               ⅔ of   ¾ of
½ way point   sentence   sentence

| Prison | Possibility of DCR parole | On licence in the community and subject to recall for breach or reoffending | Licence now ended but if convicted of further imprisonable offence, a court may order the outstanding term to be served in custody, in addition to the sentence for the new offence. |

Note: Those prisoners in this category who are *not* released before the two thirds point will automatically be released at the two thirds point. They will be under licence until the three quarter point, as with other prisoners.

3. Those serving a life sentence. There is no specific time set to be served in prison, but a court (it will always be a judge sitting in the Crown Court) can specify the period that must be served in custody. All those sentenced to life are subject to supervision on release by a probation officer, under the terms of a life licence. At the present time, the average period spent in prison by those sentenced to life imprisonment is about 14 years.

Special arrangements for people who have committed sexual offences

The Criminal Justice Act 1991 allows for some offenders who have committed sexual offences to be supervised on licence until the end of their sentence. It is at the discretion of the sentencing judge to stipulate this. Some offenders who have committed particular kinds of sexual offences are referred to as schedule one offenders and special arrangements apply to them. The term refers to the first schedule of the Children and Young Persons Act 1933. This set out a number of offences against children or young persons; murder or manslaughter, infanticide, assault, abandoning, neglecting or cruelty. Special arrangements exist also for offenders released from custody who have been convicted of crimes covered by the Sexual Offences Act 1956 (e.g. intercourse or attempted intercourse with a girl under 16, incest or attempted incest by a woman or man, buggery or attempted buggery, abduction or causing or encouraging prostitution).

Under the Children Act 1989, which came into force in October 1991, if a schedule one offender were to be released into a household with a child, it would be possible to allege that the child 'is suffering or likely to suffer significant harm' (section 31). Such a situation, therefore, requires close liaison between the Probation Service and local authority social services departments, who have widespread responsibilities for children. Prison-based probation officers write to directors of social services notifying them that a schedule one offender is to be released to a certain address in their area. The local home-based probation officer confirms to the SSD that the address is correct and continues to liaise closely with social services over release plans.

Official requirements regarding release from custody

Some offenders will have a short period of home or prerelease leave prior to their final release from custody. This is intended to facilitate their resettling in the community. Supervising home probation officers will want to use this time to meet the offender and further the plans for release.

For those offenders in the automatic conditional release category, a brief predischarge report will be completed by the home probation officer, using a proforma. It must be sent to the custodial institution one month before release. It will include details of any needs the offender might have for specialist provision after release, e.g. help with illegal drug use and any special conditions that may have been added to the licence. There are six possible core conditions set out by the Home Office. They are:

1. to receive treatment from a medical practitioner, psychologist or psychiatrist;
2. not to engage in any work or activities (say, a youth club) which involve a person under a certain age (the age will be specifically mentioned in the licence);
3. to reside at a certain address (it might be a hostel) which the offender must not leave without the prior permission of their probation officer;
4. not to reside in the same household as a child under a specified age;

5. not make contact or communicate with particular people (e.g. wife, former wife, children). Anybody can be specifically named for this purpose. If the offender wishes to make contact they must seek prior approval from their probation officer and any social services department that may be involved. This would particularly apply to contacting children.
6. to co-operate with any arrangements a probation officer might make to help the offender with a particular problem, e.g. alcohol, drug or solvent abuse, gambling, debt, anger or violent behaviour or a sexual problem. The licence must specify the location where activities are to take place. This might be a probation centre or a probation office, or anywhere a group may be run.

A predischarge report will also contain reporting instructions stating the time, date and place where the offender will meet their supervising probation officer.

For offenders in the discretionary release category, a parole assessment report is prepared by the home probation officer and sent to the parole board, and a copy is sent to the custodial institution. The contents of this report will be known by the prisoner, the probation officer having involved them in discussions during its preparation. Such a report may contain a great deal of detail and may recommend any of the special licence conditions set out in the list above. The details covered will include the offender's family's attitude to the offender and their home coming; prospects for finding work on release; the offender's response to any previous periods of supervision; the risk of reoffending; whether there is any risk to children and if so, whether there has been liaison with social services. The compiler of the report will also recommend whether or not, in their view, release should be granted.

When the offender has been discharged, they should have face-to-face contact with the supervising officer on the day of release. When, in exceptional circumstances, this is not possible, they must meet on the next working day after release. The objectives of licence supervision, as set out in the Home Office National Standards, are: 'i) protection of the public; ii) prevention of reoffending; iii) successful reintegration into the community' (p109). On release, the aims of supervision should be worked through with the offender and they should be reminded that breach of the licence conditions can be punished by a fine or recall to prison, or both.

The probation officer should visit the offender at home, within five working days of their first meeting after release. Probation officers are vulnerable when home visiting; there has been a growing awareness of the potential danger to staff, particularly when the probation officer visits alone. There have been a number of examples in recent years of violent attacks on both probation officers and social workers, therefore employers are taking increased precautions. These might be arranging for the visit to take place at a certain time during daylight hours or having the member of staff accompanied by a colleague.

A second meeting should take place within ten working days of release, to discuss the plans for supervision. This programme should include the objectives to be met and their time targets; frequency of contact should also be decided upon and any restrictions on movement made clear to the offender. For the first four weeks of release, travel abroad is not allowed and after this period staying abroad can last no longer than three consecutive weeks. People on licence will not normally be permitted to permanently leave the country to live abroad.

After the second interview, the supervising officer should confirm to the chief probation officer that release has taken place and state the address at which the offender is living, as well as the length of the licence period (with dates). The CPO must then pass this information on to the chief constable of the area, within five working days of receiving it.

Work in the family courts – the Court Welfare Service (CWS)

Family court work has increasingly become a specialism within the Probation Service. Whereas 10 years ago civil work was commonly a part of a probation officer's generic

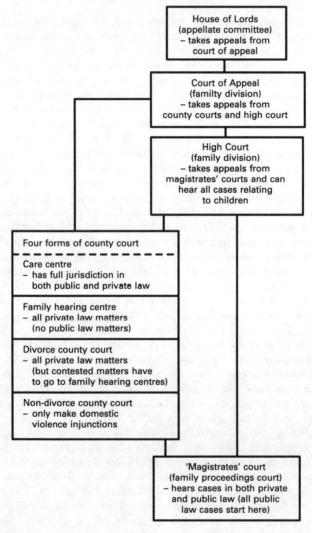

Fig 3.5   Structure of the family courts in England and Wales.
   Note: Both private and public law matters *can* start in Magistrates' Courts, County Courts or the High Court.

workload, it is now almost certain to be the responsibility of a team of officers referred to as a family court welfare unit. Such a team will be headed by a senior probation officer, called a senior court welfare officer, and will comprise a number of probation officers known as court welfare officers. A substantial number of them work on a part-time basis.

Not only has family work become more and more a specialist activity, it is acknowledged as being particularly stressful and time-consuming because of its nature. The work constitutes just under 10 percent of the Probation Service's total workload. In 1990, the service provided 27 940 reports on children in families broken by separation or divorce. This represented some 6 percent of all separation/divorce applications. In the same year it began work on 11 370 conciliation cases. This was an increase of 9 percent over the previous year and the highest figure ever recorded.

Family work is centrally concerned with issues affecting the children of divorcing and separating parents. The Children Act 1989, which came into force in October 1991, is an important piece of legislation of relevance to the work of probation officers as court welfare officers (as well as social workers). The Children Act makes a distinction between private law and public law. It is private law which most concerns the Probation Service, as its work deals with the private world of families and the arrangements made within them (sometimes with outside support) for the care of children, following the separation or divorce of parents.

Social services departments are mostly concerned with public (or care sector) law, which focuses on the protection of children who are at risk of neglect, harm or abuse. The term 'public law' acknowledges that as a society we have some responsibility to use public money and resources (e.g. community homes and foster homes) to care for children whose parents, either temporarily or permanently, are unable to care for them. We have a duty to protect those who are too young to care for, or who are incapable of caring for, themselves. The Probation Service would only rarely be involved in the public law aspects of the Children Act, e.g. if a supervision order is made under the Act and the Probation Service was already involved in the formal supervision of another family member.

Under the Children Act 1989, the welfare of the child or children involved in any family matter is to be considered paramount. It must be put before any other consideration. This is known as the 'welfare principle'. Antidiscriminatory practice should be central to court welfare work and the Children Act specifically deals with avoiding discrimination. Section 1(3) and section 22(5) stress that decisions concerning children should always take into account a child's racial origin and cultural and linguistic background and their religious persuasion. When they have reached a certain age, or maturity, young people's wishes must be listened to and taken seriously.

Court welfare officers can be involved in family work in three different courts: the family proceedings court, a local court in which magistrates who deal with family matters sit; and the county court and high court in which judges sit (see Figure 3.5). If the court is concerned in any way about the arrangements for the child(ren) officers can be requested to make enquiries about the situation: about the parents' plans and shared responsibility for their child(ren); the child(ren)'s own feelings and wishes; and to advise about the future residence and caring arrangements for the child(ren). A key task for the welfare officer is to assist the parents to reach agreement between themselves about these arrangements and to advise the court if these are thought to be appropriate to the child(ren)'s needs.

The court welfare service process (CWS)

Applicant goes to a solicitor and completes an application.
Respondent files an answer.
Court arranges a directions appointment hearing.

This can lead to:

1. seeking agreement between the two parties;
2. referring to a conciliation service;
3. asking for a welfare report.

If (3) happens, then the CWS is further involved. Outcomes could be:

a) the parties are helped to negotiate their own agreement;
b) the parties cannot agree;
c) further work is needed, but there is no more time under the timetable.

So the court arranges a second directions appointment hearing (lasts 10–15 minutes). There are two possible outcomes:

1. agreements are endorsed;
2. the length of time for a full hearing is decided upon.

At the **full hearing**:

a) an agreement is negotiated, with the help of solicitors/barristers and/or court welfare officer(s);
b) the issue is decided by the bench/judge;
c) a family assistance order (FAO) could be made, giving either the CWS or social services department a remit to do further work with the parties.

In 1992, the average time taken to prepare a report was over ten weeks and this is of concern to all involved. The Children Act stresses that delay in court proceedings is harmful to the welfare of a child and all efforts should be made to avoid it. In response the court welfare service is calling for more resources.

In making enquiries, meeting with and interviewing the people involved, whether in an office setting or at the home, the court welfare officer must apply what is termed the 'welfare checklist'. This acts as an aide memoire to the court and the CWS and is contained in section 1(3) of the Children Act. Particular attention must be paid to seven factors, which are:

1. the ascertainable wishes and feelings of the child concerned, taking into account their age and understanding;
2. the child's physical, emotional and educational needs;
3. the likely effect on the child of any change in circumstances;

4. the child's age, sex, background and any characteristics that the court considers relevant; this might be racial or ethnic background, culture or whether the child has a physical or learning disability;
5. any harm the child has suffered or is at risk of suffering;
6. how capable each of the child's parents is of meeting the child's needs. This could apply also to other people who have care of a child;
7. the range of powers available to the court under the Children Act 1989, that might be applied to the current proceedings.

Other important concepts the court welfare officer must bear in mind is the new one created by the Act of 'parental responsibility'. This is the 'rights, duties, powers, responsibilities and authority' embodied in being a parent (Section 3(1)). It applies to both parents, if married (and it can be acquired by an unmarried father, if applied for), whether or not they are living with the child. The concept relates more to the welfare of the child than it does to the rights of the parents.

No order should be made by a family court unless it is absolutely necessary. It will only be necessary if it positively contributes to the child's welfare. Intrinsic to the Children Act is the belief that children are generally best looked after within the family, both parents playing as full a part as possible in their care and welfare. Court proceedings should therefore be a last resort. It is preferable for arrangements to be made by the consent of all involved, whether they be parents or other relatives.

The orders the court can make which most involve court welfare officers are contained in section 8 of the Children Act. They are as follows:

1. *Residence order*. This fixes arrangements for the person or persons with whom the child is to live. A shared order can be made if a child is to spend lengthy periods of time with each parent or is to be with one parent for weekdays and the other at weekends. When one parent is granted a residence order, it does not take parental responsibility away from the other.
2. *Contact order*. This requires the parent (or person) with whom the child lives to allow the person named in the order (usually a parent, but it might be another relative) to have contact with the child or to have the child to visit or stay in their home. 'Contact' may be by telephone, letter or by sending gifts. Although loosely based on the old access order, it is a stronger order and it is also positive, i.e. it cannot be used to *deny* contact.
3. *Prohibited steps order*. This means that a particular action (or 'specified step') which could be taken by a parent in carrying out their parental responsibility shall not be taken without the court's permission. It could be applied, for example, to prevent a child being taken out of the country without permission. It relates to a single issue and can be made against anyone.
4. *Specific issue order*. This gives the court the power to resolve a specific question or problem which arises in relation to the parental responsibility for a child. It can be made in relation to a residence or contact order or stand on its own. It might involve issues such as a child's education or medical treatment; and if it chooses to, a court can give very detailed directions for the resolving of the issue.

All the above four orders can be applied for by parents (or other persons) or be made by a court of its own volition. A further order, which can only be made at the instigation of the court and then only in exceptional circumstances, is a *family assistance order* (section 16(1)). This can last for up to six months. It enables a court welfare officer (or a social worker) to 'advise, assist and befriend' (the traditional phrase applied to the criminal work of the Probation Service) any person named in the order. This should not be recommended lightly by the CWS because voluntary contact might prove just as useful and be less obtrusive. The order is a new one created by the Children Act 1989, to be supervised for the most part by court welfare officers. One example of its usefulness might be to sort out 'teething troubles' with contact arrangements.

Directions hearings

These take place prior to the full hearing of a family court case and are becoming increasingly common. They are useful for a number of reasons and it is felt that the court welfare service can be constructively involved in these directions hearings in that it can actively support the principles of the Children Act 1989 (e.g. support the court's reluctance to make orders).

By being in court, the CWS can help with the timetabling of family cases, which is becoming increasingly important as courts try to cut down on delay; offer advice to the court or to parents and in so doing facilitate the making of an agreement; be involved in the decision as to whether or not a welfare report is necessary; refer parents and families to advice and conciliation schemes.

Conciliation

Prior to the Children Act 1989, the CWS had begun to establish conciliation schemes which offered assistance to parents considering separation or divorce. It was an attempt to break with the adversarial approach in the family courts, in which divorce proceedings became a fight or contest between the two parties to see who could get the better deal. The aim was to encourage parents to make as many arrangements as possible by mutual consent, thereby involving the courts as little as possible. In this area of work, the court welfare officer acts very much as a mediator.

The Children Act 1989 gives a great impetus to this work, often called 'in-court' conciliation, because the CWS becomes involved at the request of the court, following a directions hearing.

Whereas in-court conciliation focuses on the welfare of a child in a family broken by separation or divorce, a number of voluntary groups provide 'out of court' advice and conciliation (e.g. Relate, once known as local marriage guidance councils) and these groups may well deal with the partners' relationship as well as the child's welfare. The CWS many refer families to such helpful advice services for out of court assistance.

Some concluding thoughts on family work

Family work is not easy and is rarely straightforward. Eve Northey, a senior divorce court welfare officer in Somerset, sums up some of the pressures involved: 'The welfare officer has to be at one and the same time probing, sympathetic, objective and, above all, a listener, demonstrating a capacity to help people through a period of crisis' (Community Care 9.1.86).

There have been problems with the service the CWS provides, particularly regarding time delays. The number of welfare reports requested by courts has risen, but finances and staffing differ very little from pre-Children Act 1989 levels. Although the work of the CWS is overseen by the Lord Chancellor's department (responsible for the appointment and work of judges), it is funded, like the rest of the Probation Service, by the Home Office. There is a feeling within the CWS that the Home Office is more interested in the criminal work of the Probation Service and as a result the CWS has been, and is, somewhat marginalised. There have been fears in recent years that there might be a 'hiving off' of the CWS out of Probation Service control. In relation to these fears the Association of Chief Officers of Probation (ACOP) and the National Association of Probation Officers (NAPO) have jointly pushed for increased funding for the CWS and for local probation committees to 'cost family work as a discrete area of work to be accounted for separately within the overall probation budget' (ACOP/NAPO Paper, February 1991). The work of the CWS is greatly valued both inside and outside the Probation Service. It is felt, however, that its unique experience and expertise should receive more official support, in terms of both morale and practical resources.

Adoption

The Probation Service has a very small involvement in court proceedings relating to the adoption of children. The Guardian Ad Litem and Reporting Officers (Panels) Regulations 1983 set up local authority administered panels who appoint reporting officers and guardians ad litem in adoption proceedings. If a probation officer is a local panel member, they can be appointed to act in either of these capacities. The person appointed must be independent of any agency that has the child in its voluntary or compulsory care.

Basically, the reporting officer represents the natural parents and, in completing a report to the court, must ensure that any agreement by the parents to allow their child to be adopted is given 'freely and unconditionally'. If a parent refuses to give their consent, then a guardian ad litem will be appointed by the court to safeguard the welfare of the child. The guardian ad litem must interview all relevant family members and all professionals involved and present a report to the court. Of crucial importance in the report will be the wishes and feelings of the child. The guardian ad litem is expected to provide their assessment of the case in their report and go to the court hearing to present it.

Conclusion

The most recent period of the Probation Service's history has been hallmarked by change and uncertainty. The service has been under scrutiny from central Government, while that the same time the Criminal Justice Act 1991 and the introduction of National Standards have made new demands upon it. The pace of change has been unsettling and fears about more central direction at the expense of local autonomy have adversely affected morale, particularly that of maingrade officers.

The 1991 Criminal Justice Act has meant the Probation Service is being asked to provide more reports for the criminal courts. It has also meant the service is supervising a growing number of offenders, either on community orders or on licence after release from custody, who have committed more serious offences. There

TIME	MONDAY	TUESDAY	WEDNESDAY	THURSDAY	FRIDAY
9	Magistrates' court	Administration	Present report in local youth court	Office duty: report and record writing (+ 2 clients seen who called in on off-chance)	Attend fines default court with 2 clients
10	duty	full staff meeting			
11					3 clients seen in office
12			3 clients seen in office		
1					
	LUNCH				
2	5 clients seen in office + phone calls	Visit to local YOI to see 2 clients	Attend case conference (with SSD) to discuss a mutual client	Talk to tertiary college class on work of probation	'Gatekeeping' meeting with 5 colleagues
3					
4					Home visits to 2 clients
5				2 clients seen in office	
	TEA				
6	Late reporting evening (6 clients seen – 2 for PSRs)				
7					
8					
9					
10					

Fig 3.6   An example of a week in the working life of a fieldwork team probation officer.
Note: A probation officer's hours may fluctuate a good deal, although the official working week is 37½ hours. When crisis occur concerning clients, the week's plan will be disrupted as the officer responds to the immediate situation.

is concern, at all levels of the service, that inadequate new finance and resources have been invested.

Despite these reservations, there are reasons for optimism about recent changes and the future of the Probation Service. The Criminal Justice Act 1991 encourages courts to make less use of custody which, for the majority of offenders, is a thoroughly negative experience.

Both the Act and the National Standards make antioppressive practice a requirement and there is a heightened awareness amongst probation officers of the destructive effects of unfair discrimination and stereotyping. The service can continue to learn from the monitoring and gatekeeping procedures it has established.

In addition to containing much good practice, the National Standards also encourage probation officers to be more accountable to their clients. Offenders have strengthened rights to be involved in devising their supervision plans; this can have the effect of empowering clients. Meanwhile, the move to offence-based work means that offenders are given greater opportunity to express their motivations for offending in their own words and to seek new, more constructive ways of behaving that they can 'own' and understand.

The Probation Service is being encouraged to work in closer partnership with the voluntary sector. Increased involvement and co-operation will have the positive effect of drawing more deeply on the considerable skills, knowledge and experience of a range of voluntary organisations. In the financial year 1993–4, each area Probation Service is to allocate 5 percent of its revenue budget to 'partnership schemes' and from 1994, grants to outside bodies can be made in return for a range of services.

Finally, the growing amount of research evidence that indicates that social work intervention, particularly if offence-focused, can have positive results in diverting offenders from crime is very encouraging. Thoughtful, well-planned use of group-work techniques and the development of 'intensive probation programmes' have regenerated faith in the social work base of probation work. This provides an important counter to pressures for a more punitive, correctional approach. It also keeps the Probation Service true to the police court missionaries' aim of advising, assisting and befriending offenders.

Appendix 1 — office duty in a fieldwork probation team — a morning's work

9.30   Two homeless men who had earlier been waiting for the office to open, enquiring about cash help and possible accommodation. Phoned the local night shelter and made arrangements for them to go there.

10.20   Mother in with 15 year old son. Worried about his court appearance in ten days' time. Explained youth court procedure and generally tried to calm and reassure her. Told her a duty probation officer or youth court team social worker would meet her and speak with her at the court, on the day.

11.00   Another probation officer's client arrives, very distraught because the expected girocheque from the DSS had not arrived this morning. Telephoned the DSS and managed to arrange a special interview for this afternoon, with the possibility of an emergency payment being made.

11.35   Young woman from London (50 miles away) arrived. She is on probation there and has moved to live here without notifying her officer. She was concerned about this. Telephoned her officer in her presence and they spoke together. She will come to see me on a weekly basis and if she looks like settling we shall arrange for the order to be transferred to this office.

11.50   Telephone call from social services department, enquiring as to whether we have had any contact with Mr and Mrs Johnson, as Mrs Johnson has applied to be a childminder. Checked our records and phoned back to say we did not know them.

12.30   Local crown court (probation) team phoned to check whereabouts of presentence reports on individuals appearing at crown court over the next few days and whether or not probation officers would be attending with their reports. Clarified what details we had and promised to phone back later with the remainder.

Appendix 2 – The Rehabilitation of Offenders Act 1974

This Act applies to England, Wales and Scotland. It relieves the burden of past criminal conviction on offenders, most relevantly when they are applying for work. If an offender remains free of further convictions for a specified period of time (the Act calls this the 'rehabilitation period'), she or he becomes, in the terms of the Act, a 'rehabilitated person' and the conviction becomes 'spent' or forgotten.

For example, if placed on supervision or probation, the rehabilitation period is one year or until the order expires, whichever is longer. If sentenced to imprisonment of more than two and a half years, this never becomes 'spent'.

As regards applying for work, the Act means that an employer cannot refuse to employ someone (nor dismiss someone) because of a 'spent' conviction. However, several jobs and professions are excluded from the Act, including working in the caring services. Any job which gives substantial access to people under 18 is excluded, so this means that teachers, social workers, youth and community workers and probation officers all have to declare even 'spent' convictions. The health service, police force and prison service all work under the same arrangements. If convictions are not disclosed to the prospective employer, the employee could be dismissed at any time if these are later discovered.

Exercise 1 – a pre-sentence report

Fordshire Probation Service

Presentence Report to Old Town Magistrates' Court

Date of hearing – 1st August 1993

Date of report – 26th July 1993

Concerning – Keith Ramone Hendry

Address – 13 BASILS ROAD, OLD TOWN, FORDSHIRE TW1 1GG

Date of birth – 4.4.71 *Age* – 22

Offences – Burglary × 2 (3.2.93, 18.3.93)

Basis of report – This report is prepared on the basis of two interviews with Mr Hendry, both at my office. I have had sight of witness statements and case summary, as well as records of previous convictions. I have also had a telephone conversation with staff at a local drug rehabilitation unit.

Report by – Robin Downie, Probation officer, Oldtown Probation Office.

Current offences

1. Mr Hendry appears before the court convicted of two burglaries of commercial premises. His account of what happened is consistent with police statements.
2. Both burglaries he planned and committed alone in the early hours of the

respective mornings. He broke into both warehouses via ground floor windows. In the second burglary, he was apprehended by police whilst still on the premises, their having been called by a security guard in an adjacent warehouse. In the first he got away with electrical goods worth £550, but the police later recovered these at his home address.

3. He accepts full responsibility for his actions and acknowledges that the offences are serious ones. He regrets his involvement in such criminal behaviour. He has indicated that his key motivation for committing the offence was his need for money, largely to buy drugs (cocaine), his use of which has grown, so he informs me, during recent months.

Relevant information about the offender

4. The offences before the court occurred whilst Mr Hendry was subject to automatic unconditional release, following his discharge on 28 January 1993 from HMP Clinktown, having received a six month custodial sentence in October 1992. This sentence was for burglary × 3, all of domestic properties.

5. Mr Hendry has been unemployed for 18 months and is currently receiving £67 per fortnight Income Support. After paying £5 per week on a catalogue (for clothes), he has the remainder of his money for normal living expenses. He lives in lodgings, paid for by Housing Benefit.

6. He tells me that his use of cocaine began some two years ago when a number of his friends started to use the drug for recreation. His use of it has increased of late, he believes, because he has become increasingly bored by having no job and more pessimistic about his future. My own impression would confirm the truth of this. It is encouraging to be able to report that he has made contact, of his own volition, with a local voluntary group who support drug users.

Conclusion and proposal

7. Mr Hendry appears to be an amicable and sensitive young man who has grown increasingly pessimistic about his lack of opportunity of paid employment. He has become more isolated and reliant upon his use of drugs as a result, withdrawing from what was a reasonably large number of friends. These offences are serious enough to warrant a community sentence, although Mr Hendry realises that he is at risk of receiving a further custodial sentence today. He expresses a resolve to remain free of further criminal activity, but this may be a vain hope without some kind of support, given his apparent vulnerability.

8. The court will be aware that the defendant has a reasonably long history of minor property offences. As far as disposals are concerned, he has thus far only spent one period in custody.

9. In determining sentence, having regard to the defendant's breach of automatic unconditional release, the court may well be considering the imposition of a further period of custody. Such a sentence would punish Mr Hendry, it would do

little, if anything, to support him. He might well be increasingly vulnerable on his future release into the community.

10. If the court were to consider the imposition of a community sentence, I do not consider that a period of community service would provide Mr Hendry with sufficient support nor fully address his offending behaviour. I believe that a two year probation order would prove the most appropriate community penalty and would have the following aims:

a) to provide support to Mr Hendry, most importantly, in his efforts to become drug free. In regard to this, the court might feel that an additional requirement might be inserted into the order, requiring Mr Hendry to attend a group running in a local drug centre, which is administered by a voluntary organisation which specialises in drug-related therapy. I can confirm that a suitable place would currently be available; b) weekly appointments with Mr Hendry for at least the first three months of the order would allow time to analyse and challenge his offending behaviour. This would examine the effects of his behaviour, both for himself and others with the aim of establishing an offence-free lifestyle and thus reducing the risk to the public; c) to assist and support him in finding work or a suitable college course, which might lead to future employment. This could include referring him to the Probation Service's employment/education officer.

The conditions and expectations of such an order have been explained to him and he is aware of the commitment it will require from him and of the serious situation he would face if he was to breach such an order.

This report is a presentence report under the Criminal Justice Act 1991 and has been prepared in accordance with the requirements of National Standards issued by the Home Office in August 1992.

Robin Downie
Probation Officer
26th July 1993

Questions

1. If you were the magistrates reading this report, how would you sentence Mr Hendry? (You can use the guide to sentencing on to help you. Read the section through completely before trying to decide.)
2. Give reasons for your sentencing decision.
3. If you were a magistrate, to what extent do you think you would be influenced by previous convictions?
4. Do you feel Mr Hendry needs control or care or a mixture of both? Imagine you are Mr Hendry. How do you think you would feel about your present situation and your future?

Exercise 2 – public interest case assessment and bail information scheme

Read the following case notes. In part (a) of the exercise you are to decide whether to recommend the discontinuance of prosecution, taking into account the public interest and the individual's situation. In part (b) you are to decide whether or not to object to the granting of bail.

a) The defendant is a single man aged 55, with no previous convictions. He is charged with theft of goods (shoplifting) valued at £25. He is alleged to have stolen food from a supermarket. In interview with the police, he admitted the offence and said that he had committed similar offences on approximately six occasions.

   The defendant was made redundant some four years ago from his poorly paid job as a school caretaker. The school closed. He has been seeing his GP for medication to relieve depression. He told the police that he could not afford to live on Income Support and had thus been forced to steal.

Questions

1. Would you consider this case suitable for Public Interest discontinuance? If so, give your reasons.
2. Do you require further information in order to decide? If so, what and why?

b) The defendant is male, aged 26. He is charged with deception to the value of £300. He used a stolen credit card. He has three past convictions for theft and one for deception committed over the past two years. The latter offence was committed whilst on bail.

   The police are recommending a remand in custody because:
   i) the amount involved is a relatively large sum;
   ii) he has committed a past offence whilst on bail.

   The case papers tell you that the defendant lives with his partner and child (aged two and a half years) in council accommodation. He is unemployed, after being made redundant some 18 months ago. When you interviewed him he seemed depressed and feared being separated from his family.

Questions

1. On the above information, would you object to bail or not? Give reasons for your response.
2. Do you feel you need further information before you can decide? If so, what and why?

Exercise 3 – a parole assessment report for a custodial institution

The subject of the report is eligible for release on parole in three months' time.

To – The Governor, HM Prison Springtown

Re – Tony Barton 55013 (C Wing)

Home address – 21 Bute Crescent, Newtown

Age – 24

1. Mr Barton received a four year prison sentence for causing grievous bodily harm to a youth aged 18. In December 1991 he was transferred to Springtown, having served four months of his sentence elsewhere. I understand that staff at the prison feel that he has settled in and made good progress and he is given various responsible jobs on the wing.

2. He had married only six months before he was sentenced and a baby girl (Ruth Bernadette) was born just two weeks before he entered custody. He has received regular letters and visits from his wife, whom I have visited at the matrimonial home, and I believe their relationship is a sound one. He has also had regular visits from members of his own family.

3. Successful at school, he gained two A-levels and had found work in London as a computer programmer. He commuted from Newtown to London each day, a journey of two hours each way. I feel that it is because he was one of six young men involved in a fight at a local disco that the crown court decided on a fairly severe penalty.

4. I also know that the youth whom Mr Barton struck in the fight has moved with his parents to live in the west country, so there is no possibility of problems involving reprisals on his release.

5. I do not believe that his remaining in prison any longer will serve any useful purpose. He very much regrets what he has done and being deprived of the company of his wife and daughter, as well as the loss of his well-paid job, has been a punishment in itself.

6. Mr Barton has a stable home life and family to return to. He has experience as a computer programmer, so his chances of finding work may be reasonably optimistic, despite his prison sentence. I shall consider referring him to a job club if he has problems finding employment and here he will get professional advice. I shall see him at least once a week for the initial two months after release. I have no hesitation in recommending that he be granted release on parole.

Charles Paulson
Probation Officer

Questions

1. If you were a member of the local parole review committee, would you have any hesitation in recommending to the parole board Mr Barton's release? Give reasons for your decision.
2. As a professional carer or social worker, would you agree with the probation officer's conclusion? Why/why not?
3. Should society punish people for crime as well as think about their welfare? Why/why not?
4. Do you feel that violence towards other people is more serious than other crimes (theft, burglary and fraud, for example)? Give reasons for your opinion.

Exercise 4 – priorities

You are a probation officer and have just returned to work on a Monday morning after three weeks' summer holiday. You are greeted by your secretary, who informs you that there have been several crises involving your caseload while you have been away and that, as a result, there are urgent things you need to do! The specific problems you are faced with are as follows:

1. Ten days ago an 18 year old who has abused drugs for over two years telephoned the office to say he intended to take an overdose in order to 'do himself in'. Although a colleague has visited his home three times since, he could see into the flat and there appeared to be nobody there. Repeated knocking at the door met with no response.
2. Mr and Mrs Cawthorne came to the office four days ago in a very agitated state. Their daughter Melanie (aged 17) had, by her unruly behaviour and staying out late at night, driven them to despair. They were also angry with her and were threatening to exclude her from home if her probation officer did not intervene quickly on his return. Mr Cawthorne is disabled and he and his wife are at home all day.
3. Just ten minutes before you arrived at your office this morning, the police telephoned to say they had picked up Jill O'Sullivan (on probation for shoplifting) on the hard shoulder of the motorway, during the early hours. They had soon discovered that she had been physically beaten and sexually assaulted and was near collapse. She had been rushed to the local hospital and a doctor there had asked that her probation officer be consulted and should come immediately.
4. In the waiting room on your arrival at the office is Fred Skerman. On seeing you enter, Fred hurries to tell you that he requires £4 immediately for the train fare to a place three stations down the line. As usual Fred is penniless and if he does not catch the train in 12 minutes, he will miss the opportunity of travelling to Brighton for some labouring work – his first chance of paid employment in two and a half years.

Questions

1. Which of these four problems would you deal with first? Why?
2. Order the remaining problems and describe how you would deal with them, giving reasons for your decisions.
3. If you were a probation officer, what would you regard as a real emergency? Why?

Exercise 5 – role play – a probation office staff meeting

Setting

A local fieldwork team – the weekly staff meeting which usually lasts about three hours every Tuesday morning. All who should be are present.

Roles

1.	Stuart	senior probation officer
2.	Sue	
3.	David	
4.	Sally	
5.	Talib	Probation officers
6.	Karen	
7.	Novelette	
8.	Charlie	
9.	Carol	
10.	Geoff	Probation services' officer (PSO)

The Meeting

Most of the 'business' of the meeting has been dealt with – for example, allocating new work and discussing the agenda for the probation liaison committee meeting later in the week. The team is now turning to a thorny problem which it has to resolve.

Discussion background

Bob (aged 45) and Andy (aged 52) are two homeless men who both have a drink problem. Both have appeared in court on several occasions and they are well known to all the local probation officers. They spend nearly all their time together. At night they sleep wherever they can – in a derelict building or any makeshift shelter. During the day (when they have money) they drink together, usually sherry or cider. They sit around the town centre, trying to attract the attention of passers-by, even begging for money from them on occasion. Only rarely do people become upset by their behaviour when approached by them – they are usually inoffensive.

It is February and the weather is very cold. As a result, Bob and Andy are spending more and more time during the day sitting in the probation office waiting room. Sometimes they chat together; at other times they may take a nap, having lost sleep during a rough night outside. However, recently they have upset one or two people who were waiting to see probation officers – their language has been very bad, they have occasionally demanded money or cigarettes and some people have found their lack of personal hygiene offensive.

The team's attitudes

Karen and *Charlie* feel very strongly that, as team policy, Bob and Andy should be excluded from the office, except when they have a specific need to see a probation officer.

David and *Novelette*, who have responsibility for seeing Bob and Andy respectively when they come into the office, adamantly disagree.

Geoff also disagrees. As the team PSO he has special responsibility for a local single homeless project.

Stuart, as the office senior, is mindful of the public accountability of the office and tends to feel that Bob and Andy should be excluded if they are upsetting other people.

Sally and *Carol* are keen that the office should be a 'community resource' and feel that the team should therefore pursue an 'open-door' policy.

Talib and *Sue* do not feel very strongly about the issue either way, but they are both good at raising useful points which move the debate along.

Task

Allocate the ten roles and set the discussion in progress. You have 30 minutes and must resolve the problem today.

Following the role play

As a group, you might like to consider how you reached a decision. If you were unable to decide, you could examine why. You might also like to think about how you felt in your role and how you dealt with these feelings. Sharing in the group in this way will probably mean that you are looking at issues about teamwork and at general questions about how teams or groups come to make decisions. Study the process of reaching a decision.

Questions for discussion

1. A shift of emphasis in recent years has seen probation officers moving away from direct one-to-one work with clients towards being more of a case manager or resource finder for clients. In the light of this, can probation officers in the 1990s still regard themselves as social work professionals?
2. The idea of antidiscriminatory practice with offenders is a nonsense – in committing crime, they put themselves out of the sphere of society and should be discriminated against as part of society's punishment of them.
3. In late 1992, John Major, the prime minister, said that society should 'understand a little less and condemn a little more' those who commit crime. Discuss.
4. Most offending is committed by males. Many crimes, e.g. 'joyriding' and crimes of violence, appear to be of a 'macho' nature, fitting with public perceptions of 'toughness'. To what extent is crime an expression of masculinity?
5. For many black people, the probation service represents an establishment agency of repression. Given this, how would you set about attracting more black people into becoming probation officers?
6. The concept of the probation service delivering 'punishment in the community' is a false one. What offenders really need in order to divert them from crime is sensitive help of some sort.

Further reading

1. *The Penal System – An Introduction*, Michael Cavadino and James Dignan (Sage, 1992). A useful introductory guide to the wider criminal justice system, including the Probation Service.
2. *Racism and Anti-racism in Probation*, David Denney (Routledge, 1992). Analyses the differential treatment received by black people from the Probation Service.
3. *Living Dangerously – Young Offenders in Their Own Words*, Roger Graef (Harper Collins, 1992). A group of young offenders attending an intensive probation programme speak about their lives and experiences.
4. *The Probation Handbook*, Alison Jones *et al.* (Longman, 1992). A general guide for those wanting to join the Probation Service.
5. *Offending Behaviour – Skills and Stratagems for Going Straight*, James McGuire and Philip Priestley (Batsford Academic, 1985). A practical handbook of exercises which focuses on offence-based work.
6. *Jarvis – Probation Service Manual*, edited by Alan Sanders and Paul Senior (Pavic Publications, 5th edition, 1993). Now in three volumes, this is the standard reference work, comprehensive in its coverage.

Note: In addition, NACRO produces a lot of useful material in accessible form – factsheets, handouts, etc. on all aspects of the criminal justice system, including probation. Many of their short publications are free. For more information write to: NACRO, Information Department, 169 Clapham Road, London SW9 OPU.

4

Other Statutory Services

Introduction

In addition to the social services authorities and the Probation Service, there are other agencies that provide services within the caring network. Some of these services are run by voluntary, community and private organisations and others are provided by statutory agencies. This chapter will focus on the services provided by the statutory agencies and will include the work of those in the health service, local authority education departments and the local authority housing departments.

The work carried out by State-funded community projects and the role of community workers will also be outlined and there will be a brief look at community police work.

Just as the work of the SSD's, and to a lesser extent the Probation Service, has been greatly affected by recent legislation so the remainder of the statutory sector has needed to respond to the diminishing providing role of the local authority and the extension of the mixed economy of care provision.

Statutory organisations are those bodies which have been set up following specific legislation and are obliged by law to provide and maintain services to the community. More simply, the word 'statutory' refers to services which are run by the state via local authorities or by regional offices of central Government.

The National Health Service (NHS)

The health service is concerned with the nation's physical well-being and, in the case of psychiatric disorders, its mental health. Care is provided in various medical institutions: the general practitioner's surgery, health centres, clinics, hospitals, hospices and nursing homes and increasingly, in a person's own home in the community.

The NHS came into being in July 1948 and was intended to provide a comprehensive range of care for all those who required it. The service was to be free at the point of consumption and was to be funded largely through general taxation. But since its inception there has been much concern about the cost of providing an equitable National Health Service that is accessible to all citizens regardless of geographical location or financial or personal circumstances. In 1948 expenditure on the NHS represented 3.9 percent of Britain's gross natural product (GNP) and in 1984 this had risen to 6.2 percent of GNP. Attempts aimed at reducing the costs and/or improving efficiency have resulted in the NHS having to be restructed on several occasions: in 1974, 1982, 1985 and finally in 1991.

The White Paper *Working for Patients* (1989) proposed a reorganisation of the NHS with the declared objectives of ensuring that:

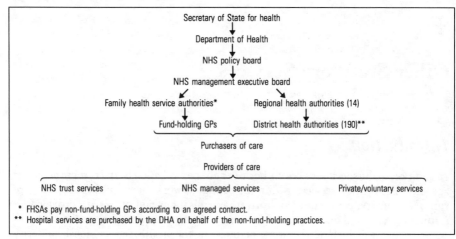

Fig 4.1   Current structure of the health service.

1. patients were given 'better health care' and a 'greater choice';
2. those working in the health service have an opportunity to receive greater satisfaction.

The principal changes introduced in order that objectives could be more easily reached were as follows:

1. district health authorities (DHAs) to be allocated funds by the regional health authority (RHA) according to population size, health, age distribution; and service providers are paid by the DHA in whose area the patient resides;
2. the creation of hospital trusts within the NHS hospitals that may choose to 'opt out' from the NHS. These trusts take responsibility for their own affairs including conditions and rates of pay for staff. They earn revenue by selling their services to other hospitals, health authorities and fund-holding GPs;
3. large general practitioner (GP) practices with over 9000 patients may hold their own budgets to obtain a defined range of services directly from hospitals. GPs to be paid by the RHA in which the patient resides;
4. the creation of an internal market within the NHS and a separation of those who purchase and those who provide care; the providing agents being directly managed hospitals, community services, NHS trust hospitals and the private sector hospitals and the purchasing agents being the district health authorities and GPs who opt out and become fund-holders, and private purchasers such as employers or insurance companies.

The 'inverse care' law

The health service can be conveniently divided between those services which are provided in the community, known as *primary health care,* and those services provided by hospitals, both acute and long stay, known as *secondary health care.*

In terms of expenditure the acute services, i.e. hospital inpatient care, still dominate the health budget, despite attempts made by successive governments to shift the balance towards community provision. 'Furthermore, client groups are differentially treated with regard to resourcing, with hospital and maternity services accounting for the majority of funds whilst 'Cinderella specialisms' such as mental health and learning difficulties are less well resourced' (*Health and Health Care in Later Life* Christina R Victor, Open University Press, 1991). Older people are disproportionately the main users of the health service: 'Those aged 85+ represent 1 percent of the total population and account for 8 percent of NHS expenditure' (ibid.) and 'Those aged 65+ account for 48 percent of all NHS expenditure' (ibid.). It is well known that there are geographical variations in health provision and studies have shown that middle class people tend to derive more benefit from the NHS than their working class contemporaries. This is related to the tendency for the more affluent areas to be better endowed with health care provision, their greater awareness of services and middle class people's ability to articulate need.

Ann Oakley, in her recent study of the health care experiences of 'high risk' mothers, showed that middle class mothers experienced shorter waiting times for both hospital and GP prenatal care and saw fewer other health care professionals and therefore had a greater continuity of care treatment. She concludes her study by saying that her findings, like those of many others, demonstrated the 'continued operation of the inverse care law within a nationalised care system, i.e. that those with the greatest need have least contact with appropriate medical care' (*Health Service Research*, 26 (no 5), 651–69).

Similarly it can be seen that black people, who are disproportionately over-represented in areas of social deprivation, underuse the health service. Access to health care is made unnecessarily complex where language barriers exist and when discriminatory practices operate within the NHS. This is well documented: 'There is a growing body of evidence that black people receive a qualitatively and quantitatively worse service' . . . 'The response of the health service has in all but a few cases been either to neglect or marginalise the needs of black populations' (Safder Mohammed, *Share, Health and Race*, issue No. 1, November 1991).

Primary and secondary health care

'Primary health care' refers to the work that is carried out in the community by medical personnel. It includes, for example, work provided by GP surgeries, child development clinics, family planning clinics, community psychiatric and midwifery services. It is now more common for health service workers to be based in health centres and increasingly they are working together in teams.

A primary health care team involves co-operation between GPs, health visitors, district nurses and practice nurses. Meetings are arranged with the purpose of co-ordinating their schedules and observations for the benefit of the people whom they mutually serve. (In cases where a social worker is attached to a GP's practice, they will also be included in the team.) Observations made by, say, the district nurse may be useful to the GP, health visitor and social worker alike. Each person's role is clearly prescribed, but each person will benefit from an appreciation of the involvement of other professional carers.

'Secondary health care' refers to work carried out in hospital settings and sometimes the term 'tertiary' is used to describe the health care provided in long stay institutions.

The general practitioner (GP) or family doctor

GPs have always been independent of the NHS and have been remunerated through contracts based on the number of patients registered with them. Contracts are met by the family health service authority (FHSA) and were formerly paid by the, now defunct, family practitioners' committee. The FHSA does not restrict the number of patients on a GP's list to reflect the health needs of the community. As a result the NHS has never had power to match the supply of doctors to areas of demand. Consequently, the provision of GP services throughout the country remains patchy and varied.

The GP's traditional 'knowledgeable' role within our culture and the prevailing belief that there are 'pills for all ills' encourages many people to initially seek help from their local GP. Since most people are already registered as patients, they will find their local doctor easily accessible and some may have developed a trusting relationship through previous contact.

On the other hand, some patients may be reluctant to reveal an inability to cope to a doctor whom they have known for some time – they may choose to go elsewhere, or even not look for help with something they interpret as personal failure. Yet it is important that people suffering psychological stress are helped at an early stage, before an escalation of the problem occurs. Other people may feel that they need to present a legitimate symptom (a cold or headache, for example) before concerning the doctor with an underlying anxiety.

The inter-relationship between psychological and physical illness is now more widely recognised. Some physical illnesses are known to bring on associated psychological disorders and similarly there is evidence that stress and anxiety can induce secondary physical illness. The word 'psychosomatic' is frequently used but often abused in describing this relationship. It refers to an illness which has definite physiological symptoms, but psychological factors also can be associated with the development, maintenance and treatment of the illness. For example, a person suffering from an ulcer may not have experienced any psychological stress – the illness will be independent of the person's life style. For other ulcer sufferers, stress factors will be seen to contribute to their physical condition and a reduction in their anxiety level will result in improved physical health and a more rapid recovery.

The work of a GP ranges from the diagnosis of serious illness and monitoring of chronic diseases to treating common ailments and the prevention of disease through screening, identifying risk factors and health education. Doctors are restricted by time – it is common for GPs to see their patients at intervals of less than five minutes. Longer sessions with individual patients will mean an increased delay for those in the waiting room. It is therefore often impractical and inappropriate for the GP to undertake a counselling role.

Not all GPs have been trained in psychiatry or have gained counselling skills, but since 1983 all doctors wanting to become GPs must undergo vocational training involving two years in a hospital setting and a further year spent attached to a general practice; thus it is possible for an interested GP to develop skills in this area. Nowadays it is less common for GPs to work singlehanded – most are based in group practices, often in health centres. This arrangement enables doctors to share their areas of expertise.

A patient suffering from the effects of anxiety may be prescribed tranquillisers by the doctor in the hope that the resultant reduction of physical discomfort may enable that person to deal with the causes of the problem. This treatment, plus the knowledge that there is nothing physically wrong, may be sufficient to encourage some people to combat their difficulties themselves. However, not all psychological states respond well to drugs – a course of counselling may be necessary in addition to, or instead of, medication.

An important role of the GP is to refer patients to more relevant agencies – some people suffering from psychological/social problems may be directed to voluntary counselling agencies, the Probation Service, or Relate. Sometimes a GP will refer a patient to the social services department, either to the local office or, where possible, to the social worker attached to the group practice, particularly where practical information or resources (day nursery places, for example) are required. Because of their training, social workers are more likely to be 'non-directive' in their counselling compared to GPs, who may tend towards being authoritarian, given their preoccupation with speedy diagnosis.

GPs can also refer patients to a clinical psychologist when anxiety states and emotional difficulties are seriously affecting someone's everyday life. However, there are certain severe mental disorders that are more than just more serious forms of unpleasant emotional states – they are regarded as mental illness. Where the illness is of a psychiatric nature (such as schizophrenia), the GP will refer the patient to a psychiatrist. All general practitioners are required to work within the 'section' procedure of the Mental Health Act 1983 with those people who are suffering mentally to the extent that they are a danger either to themselves or to other people.

Following the White Paper *Promoting Better Health* (DHSS, 1987) a new contract was imposed on family doctors with the stated intention of improving the standard of general practice and changing the way in which the GP practice is structured and financed. GPs now have to retire when they reach the age of 70. They have to set various health care targets and undertake specific activities, including the obligation to annually screen each patient over the age of 75. This health check is to cover six dimensions: mobility, mental condition, physical condition including continence, sensory functions, social environment and use of medicines.

More recently a Patients' Charter has been drawn up which informs patients of the standards of care they should expect. Increasingly it is felt, however, that these expectations should be matched with an understanding of what is reasonable behaviour on behalf of the users of the service. A doctor's charter might include attending appointments on time, informing the surgery of cancelled appointments and calling the doctor out of hours for urgent problems only.

Finally, a further White Paper *The Health of the Nation* (1992) sets out targets for the promotion of health and the prevention of disease in the population. Those expected to play their part in promoting health include, in addition to the NHS, statutory and other organisations, the health education authority, voluntary bodies, employers and employees and the media.

The practice nurse

Practice nurses are being employed by more and more GPs and their role is expanding. As well as carrying out practical treatments, many will see and diagnose patients with minor ailments, run immunisation, and well-person clinics and in addition, give family planning advice.

The clinical psychologist

Today clinical psychologists can be found in every setting of the health service where they are providers of specialised care. In 1976 the Trethowen Report recommended a ratio of one clinical psychologist to every 25 000 of the population. However, the implementation of this recommendation has varied from district to district. Some health authorities or trusts have little psychology service of their own, whereas others have developed large departments and have demonstrated the need for more than the recommended number of psychologists.

Clinical psychologists are not medical doctors – they do not prescribe drugs or give injections, for example. They are trained in the science of behaviour, cognition and emotion and in the conduct of research in these fields. Their purpose, therefore, is to further this knowledge and apply its principles to the assessment and treatment of people with psychological difficulties throughout the human lifespan.

Some clinical psychologists are involved in the support of people with learning difficulties. The psychologist's expertise as a behavioural scientist is used in order to help the person with learning difficulties to achieve their maximum potential and independence. They often work alongside parents, teachers or special employment training centre workers in creating the most suitable conditions for development.

Other clinical psychologists will specialise in working with children and families. For example, a family may be counselled in order to work out the factors involved in a child's drug use, bedwetting or other forms of 'maladaptive' behaviour. The psychologist can assist the family to discover ways in which it can promote more suitable activities and relationships.

The majority of psychologists, however, work in the area of adult mental health; they may work with a person individually or they may work with people in groups. They treat people suffering from anxiety states and phobias; they provide counselling or psychotherapy for people who find themselves repeating unhappy relationships; and they help severely mentally ill people in the community to cope with everyday tasks. Another application of their work is in helping groups of smokers, drinkers or compulsive eaters to reduce their dependency.

A growing division of psychologists is concerned with health psychology, or psychology applied to physical illness, healing and medicine. It has been found that people recover better from a physical illness, such as a heart attack or even a simple broken leg, when their psychological needs are taken care of. Psychological needs may include being kept informed of progress; being allowed to express anxieties; and being more actively involved in one's own treatment.

Related to health psychology is the work of the neuropsychologists who are concerned with the cognitive, behavioural, emotional and social effects of an injury

Service	Intervention
Learning difficulties	Work with parent(s) on structured learning programme of social skills for child with learning disabilities.
Children and families	Work in family therapy team (including social worker and community psychiatric nurse) with the family of a teenager who is misusing drugs. Advise parent on how to respond to their four year old child's 'tantrums'.

Adult mental health	Teach anxiety management to person with phobia of travelling in lifts.
	    Help patient with schizophrenia to plan and organise day.
	    Offer counselling to recovering person with anorexia.

Health psychology	Present information to surgical nursing staff on psychological needs of patients before and after operation. With physiotherapist, run class for back pain sufferers, learning to apply relaxation and correct posture.
Neuropsychology	Assess mental abilities of motorcyclist who is recovering from head injury. Offer counselling to a man who has had a stroke, and his partner, concerning expectations of recovery and reorganisation of home and/ or work responsibilities.
Older people	Consult with social worker on availability of community social facilities for clients who feel isolated. Counsel couple on redistribution of home responsibilities now that husband has retired.
Research activity	Conduct research project into the psychological burden on family of caring for dependent relative in the community.

Fig 4.2   Examples of a clinical psychologist's work.

to the brain (for example, head injury, stroke or multiple sclerosis). The neuropsychologist's duties include using psychological tests to detect and measure cognitive impairment (for example, memory loss); helping a patient relearn skills in daily living; assisting a person to maximise their recovery; and assisting the person to make important emotional adjustments to a new life which may have quite different challenges and limitations.

Finally, psychologists work with older people who may be having to make adjustments to their lives. For example, some older people, particularly women because they marry younger and live longer than men, may find themselves living alone for the first time in their lives. And some older people who suffer from a chronic ailment may find themselves becoming increasingly reliant on others. There are other elders who are left to care for a dependent relative who is either older than themselves or is younger than themselves but more disabled through illness. Worry and depression can become disproportionate in these circumstances but with skilled support an older person can be helped to regain a fulfilling life.

The psychiatrist

The psychiatrist is a medically qualified doctor who has completed, or is undergoing, further specialist training in psychiatry. They are normally based either in a general hospital with psychiatric facilities or in a psychiatric hospital (a 'mental hospital'). For some of the time they may also work in a general practitioner health centre, a psychiatric day hospital, in prisons or other security units or in special hospitals (such as Broadmoor). The psychiatrist also liaises with group homes and day centres within the community.

Referrals may come from a GP; the patients themselves, either directly or via the casualty department; other medical practitioners in hospital; psychologists; or social workers.

Psychiatrists may work individually or as part of a multidisciplinary team where their work is shared and may overlap with that of other professionals involved.

Problems dealt with by the psychiatrist

The main problems dealt with by the psychiatrist are as follows:

a) *Major psychiatric illness* – including schizophrenia, manic depressive illness and dementia.
b) *Less serious illnesses* – anxiety, phobias, depression, obsessional illness and psychological problems of surgery or physical or mental disability.
c) *Alcohol and drug addiction.*
d) *Self-injury/overdose.*

Functions of the psychiatrist

Initially the psychiatrist is concerned to assess patients referred and make a diagnosis of the mental disorder, if present. They will then go on to make a treatment plan. This may involve the patient being admitted to hospital as an inpatient, a day patient or an outpatient – depending on the severity of the illness. The psychiatrist will consider the possible involvement of other professionals, including the psychologist or social worker, and the use of any appropriate community resources. The use of drugs or other physical treatment will be decided upon and the psychiatrist will make long term plans based on diagnosis, response to treatment and likely prognosis as well as the availability of follow-up support within the community.

Method of assessment

On seeing the patient for the first time, the psychiatrist will take a detailed history of the problem as the patient sees it and will note previous illnesses or psychiatric problems. They will then gather information about the patient's family and personal history before making an assessment of the patient's current mental state. Once the diagnosis is made, a proposed plan of action will be outlined and discussed with the patient and others involved – including members of the family. Some people have no insight into the mental illness they are suffering and may not recognise the seriousness of their condition. Where the psychiatrist feels that such a person is a danger either to himself or others, they are empowered to recommend compulsory admission and detention in hospital under section 2 and 4 of the Mental Health Act 1983, as outlined in Chapter 2.

A typical week in hospital-based practice

A typical week for a psychiatrist working in a hospital might include the following tasks.

a) *Assessing patients referred from casualty departments* – those who have taken overdoses or have tried to injure/kill themselves, and those who seem 'psychiatric' to the casualty doctor, such as an old person who has fallen at home and is suspected of being demented or depressed.

b) *Seeing newly referred patients at clinics* – interviewing and considering appropriate further action, including investigations of alcohol consumption or physical disease which may cause mental problems, such as thyroid disease.

c) *Meeting with patients on the ward or in a day care setting* and discussions with staff about such patients' progress.

d) *Outpatient clinics for regular attenders* – these are mostly people who have been inpatients at some time and have recovered or those who have always been treated as outpatients. With the increased emphasis on community care, more people are being seen as outpatients throughout their illness rather than being admitted to hospital, as removal of someone from their home environment can be counterproductive.

e) *People at home* – visits to a person's home are carried out by psychiatrists. This practice is particularly relevant for older people, who are best assessed in familiar surroundings – this is known as a domiciliary psychiatric assessment.

f) *Teaching and administrative work* – this involves consultation with other staff and attendance at case conferences with staff or with particular patients and other workers.

In all circumstances, the psychiatrist is responsible for the medical aspects of treatment, including physical well-being and the action of drugs and their side effects. They also have some legal responsibility for the care of the patient and for ensuring, for example, the safety of a patient with a mental disorder or that of others who may be in contact with the patient.

Mental disorders and illness with which psychiatrists may be involved

It is not within the scope of this book to explain the details of the different forms of mental illness but, for the purpose of familiarity, the main classifications are outlined below and some explanation is given concerning the meaning of some of the terms used.

a) *Learning difficulties* Learning difficulties may result from brain damage or early deprivation, often from birth, but it is not a mental illness – although people with learning difficulties may also suffer mental illness.

b) *Psychoses* These mainly include schizophrenia and manic depressive illness (mania and depression) – see below for explanation.

c) *Neuroses* These include anxiety states such as hypochondria and phobias, anxiety/depression and depressive neurosis; obsessional disorders; and hysterical neurosis.

People with neuroses have some insight into their problem, which may be an exaggerated form of their normal behaviour.

d) *Personality disorders* This term refers to problems of personality and character development.

e) *Drugs* This category includes alcoholism and drug dependency involving both illicit drugs (such as heroin) and prescribed drugs (such as tranquillisers).

f) *Organic states*, including confusional states such as delerium and dementia.

Psychosis corresponds to the general image of 'madness' or 'insanity', with a breakdown in understanding of the difference between real and imaginary events.

Mania is a state of overexcitement, with unrealistic optimism, grand plans (but poor execution), increased energy, and reduced sleep and food consumption. People with mania often have episodes of depression at some time – hence 'manic depressive' psychosis. Manic depressive illness is a disorder of mood which tends to recur, a number of episodes being separated by periods of well-being.

Schizophrenia is a term for a group of various conditions in which the thinking process may be disorganised, alterations of mood and perception may occur, and unrealistic ideas (such as that all someone's thoughts are being recorded and played back to others) or hallucinations may be experienced as definite realities. There may be changes in the personality and behaviour, even when the other experiences are not present. Some people recover fully from an episode of schizophrenia; others need long term treatment and have some disabilities in between the episodes of obvious illness.

About 1 per cent of the population (of any race, country or sex) can expect to suffer from schizophrenia at some time in their lives and rather fewer from manic depressive illness. There is a tendency for both disorders to have a hereditary element.

Most people with 'depression' do not have manic depressive psychosis but have a depressed mood, often associated with adverse factors in their lives. This may be known as reactive depression.

Psychosis generally requires psychiatric treatment with antipsychotic medication. Occasionally other physical treatments including electroconvulsive therapy (ECT – 'shock treatment') or, rarely, psychosurgery may be used for severe intractable depression. Many other psychological treatments including psychotherapy and other 'talking therapies', and physical treatments may or may not play a part.

The health visitor (HV)

The health visitor is essentially concerned with the promotion of health and the prevention of ill health within the community. They will visit people in their own homes, mainly expectant and nursing mothers and families of children under-five. The health visitor's task is principally educational – they will advise on child care, child needs and child development.

The health visitor has a statutory obligation to visit all newborn babies. They normally take over from the midwife ten days after the birth of a child and continue to visit the home of the child until the child reaches school age (when responsibility for the child is transferred to the schools health service).

Referrals from the midwife form the bulk of a health visitor's caseload, but they are not always exclusively involved in the care of the under-fives. The health visitor may be required to identify the needs of elders or disabled people within the community and to visit them in their own homes to offer medical and dietary advice to those in need and those who care for them.

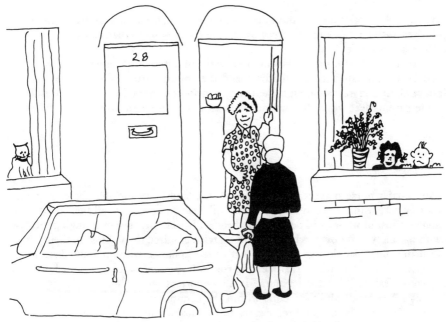

A call by the health visitor is often welcome

The HV may be based geographically, covering a specific area, or they may be attached to a GP's practice, in which case clients will mainly consist of those on the doctor's list. They are, however, an independent professional with the responsibility of deciding whom, and how often, they need to visit and they are free to accept referrals from outside the health service (from social services or voluntary organisations, for example).

The size and nature of the health visitor's caseload will to some extent determine priorities with regard to frequency and duration of visits (similar to field social workers). They will need, for example, to closely monitor suspected child abuse situations. Because of the HV's early involvement with families and their training, they are in a good position to detect early signs of non-accidental injury and may undertake preventive work before the situation becomes more serious.

Not all of the HV's work is done in clients' homes – part of their promotional health role is to hold group sessions at health centres (mothers' groups, anti-smoking groups and anti-stress groups, for example) or to provide health talks to schools, with which they may be in regular liaison. The HV also visits disabled and older people in residential establishments as well as children in local day nurseries and nursery schools. Some health visitors specialise in working with minority ethnic groups within the area.

An essential part of a health visitor's task is to ensure that a child's progress is normal – physically, emotionally and socially – and to offer help and support to the family. They are not required to provide counselling for non-health issues, but must be able to respond sensitively to distress.

Because of their general helpful advisory role, the HV may soon gain the confidence of the parents whom they visit and they may express their concern about any social or emotional difficulties they are experiencing. The health visitor may be able to offer advice, but at the same time they need to be aware of the role of other caring agencies and resources within the community so that they can refer when this is appropriate.

Although a health visitor has no legal right of entry into someone's home, most people welcome their practical advice and the opportunity of having their anxieties about child care resolved. In some cases, a visit from the HV reduces the isolation some parents feel when they are at home all day with no adult company.

The district nurse

The district nurse may head a team of nurses, and is responsible for carrying out nursing care within the community. They will visit sick people of all ages in their own homes, most of whom will be older or chronically sick. Because of changing lifestyles within society, it is now less common for married children to live close to their parents so many older people live alone, or with their spouses, without immediate family support. This often means that a caring role is forced on someone who is limited by personal frailty. The district nurse is an important social contact who is able to monitor a person's ability to cope within the community.

The GP and the hospital refer cases to the district nurse where home nursing is necessary. They visit to apply dressings, give injections, generally attend to medical needs and to encourage the development of independence and rehabilitation. When attending to the terminally ill, they need special skill in helping the patient's relatives come to terms with the prospect of the imminent death of the family member. They will enrol the help of other agencies in some cases – for example, they may request respite care in a social services home where a partner, or the family, is feeling the strain of providing continuous care.

The community psychiatric nurse

Community psychiatric nurses are principally concerned with enabling people who are suffering mental illness to remain in the community and stay out of hospital. They follow up patients discharged from hospital and visit them in their own homes, where they may administer injections or check that prescribed drugs are being taken. They will look for signs of deterioration and will be able to observe behaviour changes and any signs that medication is not being taken regularly.

Psychiatric nurses need to be aware of community resources, local voluntary mental health organisations, group meetings and services offered by other statutory bodies. Liaison will be made with disablement resettlement officers (DROs) with the aim of helping people find work if possible or a place in a sheltered workshop. The debilitating effect of being out of work and the related social isolation can adversely affect someone's chances of recovering from mental illness.

People who have spent periods of time in psychiatric hospitals may lack confidence socially and may also need encouragement to combat the social stigma or prejudice that society sometimes attaches to those who are known to have suffered mentally. Here the community psychiatric nurse may work as an advocate, attending a job interview with a client to ensure that their personal qualities are understood by a prospective employer. With the current employment situation, not everyone can hope to find work, but it is harder for those who are vulnerable in some way.

Community nurses may also receive referrals from GPs who have seen patients in their surgeries and require a fuller psychiatric assessment to be carried out in a person's home. In some areas community nurses are used to support people who would otherwise be on medication, encouraging social involvement and an ability to cope without drugs.

Liaison between the hospital and half-way houses and other hostels for assisting the recovery of people who have been mentally ill will also be done by community psychiatric nurses, who may also visit people in the hospital wards for a period before they are discharged.

Occupational therapists

Occupational Therapists (OTs) function as part of a multi-disciplinary team, serving a wide range of clinical specialities, including cardiology, orthopaedics, neurology and general medicine. They work on both an in-patient and out-patient basis.

Essentially OTs use a 'problem solving' approach to their work. This begins with the assessment process, when OTs, governed by the specific needs of the patient, select from a range of established assessment techniques. For instance, a neurological assessment may be undertaken on a stroke patient. Range and pattern of movements, muscle tone and posture are some of the features that would be looked at.

Using the information gleaned from the assessment of OT will develop an *individual treatment plan*. Long and short term goals are set with the patient. Treatment goals directly relate to the patients assessed needs and are prioritised so that the most important issues are dealt with first i.e. those that will enable the patient to leave hospital and return home. Sometimes it is not possible for patients to go back to their homes, in which case a residential setting, usually via a social worker, may be sought.

OTs play a vital role in assessing a patient's level of independence for discharge. They may conduct a *home assessment* to identify whether the patient can manage safely and independently at home. This also provides the opportunity to arrange necessary home adaptations prior to the patient leaving hospital or following discharge. Home trials may be implemented for patients who are considered to be at extreme risk.

The OT may refer patients to other community services, for example, home care, or district nursing, and may offer to follow up care in the day hospital or outpatient rehabilitation centre. Each OT attends the appropriate ward rounds and team meetings along with other nursing and medical staff; staff nurse, community liason sister, doctors, social worker and physiotherapist. These meetings have goal setting and review functions for patients undergoing rehabilitation.

Medical social workers

Some medical social workers (MSWs) are based full or part-time in hospitals or other health care settings; they may be attached to GP practices, special clinics or work in hospices. They are paid by the local authority and their main area of responsibility surrounds the patient's social needs as opposed to their medical needs. It is not always possible to distinguish between health-related difficulties and social needs because of their essential inter-relatedness. Social needs may be described thus: emotional, psychological, cultural, interpersonal, practical and financial.

Some hospital-based social workers will specialise in working with a particular client group: paediatric, psychiatric or geriatric. Others work generically. Because they work in a secondary setting, medical social workers are accountable to both the health authority and the local authority social services authority. This arrangement may restrict the social worker's personal freedom of working. They need to be mindful of the medically orientated approach of health professionals, the medical priority of the patient's immediate health and the operation of busy treatment schedules. At the same time the MSW needs to be conscious of their own responsibilities concerning the client's social and emotional welfare.

It is common practice nowadays, in hospitals, for professionals to work in a multidisciplinary team; the social worker will be an integral member of this team. The MSW is responsible for regular liaison with other team members and will often undertake joint work, for example with an occupational therapist or a psychologist. The team will meet together at set intervals. At these meetings information is shared, patients are reviewed and action plans are made.

MSWs are often involved in direct counselling of patients and their families, or carers. Much of their work is centred around loss counselling with people who have reduced mobility; undergone radical surgery; had limbs amputated; learned that they have a terminal illness; experienced a miscarriage or still birth, or have given birth to a sick or disabled child. They will also be involved in counselling people who have chronic illnesses, for example, respiratory diseases, and they will counsel women who have to decide whether or not to terminate a pregnancy.

On a more practical level MSWs will work alongside other professionals such as the occupational therapist or local authority environmental health officers, in preparing for a patient's rehabilitation. In some instances the MSW may refer the patient to a medical rehabilitation centre for a period of intensive therapy. The patient may have been involved in a serious road traffic accident or have suffered a stroke and may need training to maximise their mobility and independence. When a patient returns from such a centre, the MSW will assess and plan for their discharge from hospital and arrange appropriate support services. Unless the patient is expected to return to the hospital on a frequent and regular basis the MSW will refer them to the local authority community social work team, should this be necessary.

There is always a good deal of pressure to vacate a hospital bed as soon as the occupant no longer needs immediate medical treatment. This is most apparent with older people who still need care but are often seen as 'blocking beds' for others. The MSW may be engaged with the family in trying to find alternative care arrangements, perhaps in sheltered accommodation a care home or nursing home if it is apparent that the patient requires long term nursing care. MSWs may arrange support services for patients and their carers in order that patients may be discharged directly home.

Radical changes to the structure of the NHS and local authority social services departments, brought about by recent community care legislation, have caused changes in social work in health care settings. For instance, some MSWs are employed directly by hospital trusts, and in some areas local authorities have reduced the number of MSW posts. There is still a crucial role in contributing to the mix of in depth investigation; practical assistance, personal counselling and liaising with statutory and voluntary organisations.

An example of a multi-disciplinary team

Many health care services are planned and delivered by multi-disciplinary teams. This arrangement promotes co-operation, prevents overlap and co-ordinates the service to the patient and the patient's family. The following example of a *paediatric HIV team* based in a specialist hospital demonstrates the value of an interdisciplinary approach.

HIV infection in children can disrupt their lives by causing recurrent illness (or AIDS) and by devastating their family and social life. Daily medications, regular visits to hospital clinics, frequent absenses from school and occasional periods of separation from parents due to admission to hospital all contribute to their unhappiness and distress. Some will even become orphaned within their childhood. The hardship is compounded by society's general lack or sympathy and the stigma surrounding AIDS which forces families to restrict who they tell, often hiding the diagnosis from friends and other family members.

The specialist team will work with the following: babies born to known HIV positive mothers from the antenatal period onwards; children known to be infected with HIV; babies and children who need further investigation and testing for HIV; and they will give general counselling and support for parents and carers. The team may comprise a non-medical co-ordinator, a consultant paediatrician, a paediatrician, a social worker, a ward sister, a health visitor and a clinical psychologist. They have distinct roles but there is overlap in some instances.

Co-ordinator

The role of the co-ordinator is to act as assistant to the consultant who leads the team and to be an office-based contact for the families. Confidentiality is important when providing services for people with HIV and their families and so families should have to deal with as few people as possible. The co-ordinator will also liaise with outside organisations such as HIV voluntary agencies.

Consultant

The role of the consultant is to provide the most appropriate medical treatment in a sensitive and caring way, but the actual clinical management of the patient is only a small aspect of this role. HIV is a complex disease about which very little, as yet, is known. It is also a 'family disease' since it affects all family members who share the stress and uncertainty. Very often there is also an ill parent and this amplifies the effect of the disease on the family as a whole; it is harder for an ill person to care for, or visit, another ill member of the family and the illness itself can be a great strain on a family's financial resources. The consultant will share the treatment plans with other team members.

Paediatrician

The paediatrician will also be responsible for the clinical management of the child and will also provide a sensitive service to the family. They will be responsible for making a diagnosis and will provide appropriate treatment. Further responsibilities include counselling patients about the positive status of their child and helping parents come to terms with this; even the parents' own health status will be part of the paediatrician's role. The following case study illustrates the doctor's involvement.

A baby boy was breastfed and remained in good health for three months, but then frequent visits to the GP were required following episodes of diarrhoea, lack of weight gain and constant colds and coughs. At five months this developed into a severe respiratory disease and the baby's weight was 3.5 kilos. The child was placed in an incubator ventilator and later was diagnosed as having HIV. The parents were then consulted and tested themselves. The mother was shown to be positive and the husband negative. The prognosis for the child was poor but he began taking oral feeds and gained some weight. The child reached his first birthday developmentally delayed and is still receiving treatment.

The above case touches on the despair and uncertainty faced by HIV positive children and their families. Many HIV positive babies have died but there are instances of young children, infected from birth (via their mothers), who are attending secondary school. For some children it is possible to live with HIV but nobody knows for how long.

The ward sister

Is in charge of providing a safe environment for children and their families, developing a knowledge base and encouraging family contact. Confidentiality is ingrained into their code of conduct. In some cases families will receive some of their treatment in local hospitals and clinics and this will be co-ordinated with resident periods in the specialist hospital. The ward sister will encourage parents to visit and to stay over if necessary. It is important that a ward in which babies and young children sometimes die remains a positive place for children to be in and is not devoid of happiness and humour.

The social worker

May also be involved in counselling parents of children with HIV. Many families have financial problems which may have been brought on by the onset of their child's illness; parents may have to give up work; they may be involved in frequent visiting and may be ill themselves. Families may also have housing difficulties. They may need help in coming to terms with their situation or practical support in the form of rspite foster care or babysitting services which may be provided by the local authority or by voluntary organisations. The social worker will be aware of relevant voluntary organisations including specialist black organisations. Black and ethnic minority people may experience more distress in instances where there is a language barrier; when they have temporary resident status; where they have no extended family; and when they are faced waith the hostilities of racism. They may prefer to deal with black professionals. The social worker will need to help people to overcome any fear they may have of welfare organisations and decide when to step back and when to become more involved.

The specialist health visitor

Will be involved in advising, counselling, informing and assessing families. They may undertake pretest counselling and will outline the full implications of being diagnosed as positive. They are responsible for disseminating information concerning hygiene, safety, first aid, safer sex, keeping well and diet. Parents will need to plan for times of illness and the health visitor may assist them in this preparation. They will liaise with one member of the primary health care team, (usually the GP who will be aware of the child's and family member's HIV status) and with other relevant organisations. Above, all the health visitor provides support by regularly contacting the family, either by visiting their home or by telephoning them; this provides an element of consistency, of 'being there' for the family. Their role is to keep children well and out of hospital and enable them as far as possible to live with HIV.

The clinical psychologist

Not every team will have a fulltime child clinical psychologist. Where there is one they may have a dual role of research and clinical practice. Research will be undertaken into the psychological aspects of the HIV illness, such as at what stage parents inform children. Parents may need help in carrying out the process of informing children. Psychologists will work with children, both those infected and those affected, and may use play and art therapy. Children's drawings will be interpreted and analysed and their meaning shared with the children, particularly with brothers and sisters who are not infected and whose needs often go unmet.

Local authority education departments

Local authority education departments (LEAs) have a statutory duty to ensure provision of education for all children between the ages of five and 16. In addition to this, where children are considered to have 'special needs', the range of facilities is extended to accommodate children from the age of two and occasionally earlier. Educational provision for those with special needs is made beyond the school-leaving age, usually up to age 19.

A child's educational needs are related to their learning ability and to social, emotional and physical factors. The education department provides caring services in recognition of this.

Today, the local authority has a diminishing influence on the day-to-day running of schools now that so many schools have been encouraged to 'opt out' of local authority control. Many schools are now responsible for managing their own budgets and implementing decisions under the local management of schools (LMS) arrangement that was introduced following the Education Reform Act 1988. School governors are more directly concerned with the immediate day-to-day educational decisions and practices, whereas local authorities are responsible for regulating and co-ordinating provision.

The under-fives

Education departments are not legally required to provide education services for ordinary children under five, but many do. In 1991, 26 percent of the UK population aged three or four attended nursery schools or classes; the majority of these attended on a part-time basis.

Nursery schools and classes

Nursery schools and classes help prepare children for ordinary school and soften the transition from home to school. Some nursery schools exist in accommodation separate from infant schools and are devoted solely to children between the ages of three and five. More commonly, educational provision is offered in reception and nursery classes that are part of a primary school. They provide the same functions and are staffed by teachers who are responsible for planning the day's activities. The teachers are assisted by qualified nursery officers, who will help to create a stimulating, secure, caring environment aimed at meeting children's emotional, social, cultural and intellectual needs.

For those children whose home situation lacks stimulation and parental encouragement, an educational nursery setting is of particular benefit because it is designed to help them develop skills and so catch up with more fortunate children. However, places in nursery schools and classes are not allocated according to social need – they tend to be determined by availability. For example, in 1990 Brent education authority provided full-time or part-time places for 2371 children under five, whereas another London borough, Bexley, provided only 857. In the same year, Nottinghamshire county council offered a total of 12,671 places, compared with 84 places provided by Somerset county council (DES Statistical Bulletin 7/91, April 1991).

Many nursery schools will encourage the involvement of parents by inviting them to participate in the classroom and or in school social activities. Attention will be paid to the needs of those children from non-English-speaking families – books, stories, pictures, food and the celebration of their festivals will reflect the diversity of the multicultural society in which we live. Children will also be encouraged to take part in a wide range of activities, to engage in fantasy play and to develop practical skills that avoid restrictions of sex role stereotyping. Boys will be encouraged to express their caring nature, for example they will be allowed to nurse dolls, to play in the home corner and to join in cookery sessions. Similarly, girls will be encouraged to develop practical skills and to express their physical nature, for example play with cars, bricks and so on. Even by the age of five, children will have picked up what is expected of them by the adults in their lives and a nursery class gives them an opportunity to challenge their ideas of expected social behaviour. For example, a boy who refuses to wash up during fantasy play because 'my dad never does the washing up' can be encouraged to question this and develop a broader recognition of what other mothers and fathers do in the home.

Nursery centres

Nursery centres are a recent development, run jointly by the social services and the education department; they aim to combine education and social care in the same setting. Some education authorities have taken over responsibility for running the day centres that were previously the responsibility of the social services departments with the purpose of unifying the service provided for young children.

Primary schools

A primary school may provide a young child with their first experience of a large social setting. It may also be the first time they have been outside the familiarity of their home environment. The transition from home to school is best made gradually – it is therefore considered desirable for parents to share their young children's initial primary school attendances. Children who can build on playgroup or previous nursery experience are at an advantage compared to those who are separating from home and family for the first time and who may suffer distress at this.

Although the major role of teachers is an educational one, because they see children for so long and so often they are in an ideal position to observe disturbed behaviour and to recognise deprivation and distress. They may feel the need to refer children to education social workers, educational psychologists or the social services. Owing to their proximity, especially at times when children change for PE lessons, they may also identify signs of non-accidental injury and report this to the agencies concerned.

Most children settle and enjoy their initial school experience and although absenteeism is known to occur, it is not usually a significant problem early in a child's school life.

Secondary schools

Secondary schools are essentially concerned to meet the educational needs of pupils within the school and teachers are responsible for pupils who are in their charge. However, a child's formal education has to be seen within a social and emotional context. A child whose family life is stressful and disturbing may present behaviour difficulties at school which may be seen to affect educational progress. At the same time, it is possible for children to be suffering a disadvantaged home life but for their social problems to go undetected because their behaviour is not outstandingly different from that of other pupils.

The teacher

Most secondary schools make provision for counselling and pastoral care, giving teachers time to be available to children to help with all matters, including academic issues.

Class tutors

These will normally be responsible for between 15 to 30 children and – rather like the form teacher of the past – will be concerned with regulations, reasons for absence, discipline and notes of trips and school events. The teacher may see a child on an individual basis at the beginning or end of the school day as part of a structured personal and social education programme. Children who present serious difficulties or who require disciplinary action can be referred to the year tutor.

Year tutors

As head of year, the year tutor will have a reduced teaching load to allow them to carry out a pastoral care role. They will be involved in the usual straightforward disciplinary action for standard misbehaviour and also in the more serious matters which may involve outside agencies. The year tutor will need to be aware of the functions of other organisations and will liaise regularly with outside personnel including the education social worker, whom they may see weekly.

Occasionally year tutors will make home visits to see parents (when the parents are genuinely unable to visit the school), but their involvement can only be limited. In some cases they will, when appropriate, refer to other organisations (such as social services). It may be that some pupils feel more comfortable disclosing their problems to another member of the teaching staff and where this is the case the information will be relayed to the year tutor, as it is important that they are aware of the difficulties that children in their year may have. Serious disciplinary cases will be referred to the deputy head (pastoral) and may even go beyond, to the head of the school or to the board of governors.

Special needs

Since the Education Act 1944, local authorities have had an obligation to provide education for children who are disabled in some way. Following the Warnock Report in 1978, the Education Act 1981 extended the designation of 'special needs' to a wider range of children and stressed that, where possible, education should be provided within an ordinary school setting.

Classification

In the past, children with 'special needs' were rather narrowly defined and included the more obviously physically disabled – the blind and partially sighted, hearing impaired, epileptic and physically disabled children. Crude labels describing children as 'educationally subnormal' (ESN) or 'maladjusted' are no longer used. Special needs categories are now more wide-ranging and include those children with learning difficulties. Learning difficulties are currently classified as mild, moderate, severe and specific. These may be associated with physical and sensory difficulties, speech and language difficulties or emotional and behaviour difficulties.

As a consequence of the Education Act 1981 (section 5), all children who are considered to have special needs have the right to be made the subject of professional assessment and have a *statement* drawn up outlining their needs. Once this statement is made, it is maintained and reviewed throughout the child's life. The early detection of a child's needs is crucial, so the obvious priority for education departments at the moment is to consider those children under the age of five. However, there are some children who have experienced schooling without their special needs being catered for, so education departments are also concerned with current 13 to 16 year olds.

A statement of special needs can be made at any stage in a child's life at the instigation of parents, the education department or any outside body. A child's own feelings have to be taken into account and parental involvement is considered essential at all stages of the child's education. An appeal procedure is available for parents wishing to challenge educational decisions made on their child.

It is estimated that one in five children will need some form of special education during their school lives.

Within an ordinary secondary school there will probably be a teacher responsible for special education. In most cases they will be the *named* person statutorily concerned with the maintenance of the child's special needs statement and for liaison with the parent and the child and other agencies.

The educational psychologist

An educational psychologist may play a principal role in the assessment of a child's special needs. As a non-teaching member of the education department, the educational psychologist can be seen as neutral, so the child may more freely indicate their needs and express whether or not they are being met by the school. The psychologist is also equipped to scientifically test a child's educational ability and to consider the most appropriate form of provision. There will be other agencies involved in assessing a child's needs – for example, a full medical report is required; however, usually it is the educational psychologist's responsibility to co-ordinate the assessment.

Integration

The Education Act 1981 stressed that, where possible, children's special needs should be provided within *mainstream* education. This recognised the mutual benefit and increased understanding that disabled and ordinary children would gain from interaction within an ordinary school setting. It is not, of course, possible to accommodate all special needs within mainstream education, so alternative provision has to be made available.

Types of provision

The following types of provision are made for children with special needs.

Within the ordinary school

After a child has been 'statemented', attempts will be made to provide for the child's needs within the school. For example, if a child is unable to climb stairs because they suffer from asthma but is required to attend school in a high-rise building, they may have their timetable altered so that they can attend lessons at ground level. Similarly a child with impaired hearing may be able to attend an ordinary school with the aid of a special radio microphone (which transmits only to them) which they pass on to successive teachers. Some schools will act as a resource for a child with particular disabilities and may have a lift installed in order to meet the needs of wheelchair-bound children. It must be stressed that physical disability is not viewed as a drawback to learning ability.

The majority of children with special needs are not, statemented because their needs are not so severe. It is felt that non-statemented children miss out on appropriate support because resources are focused on statemented children.

Peripatetic teachers for behavioural support

The behavioural support teachers may offer support to pupils in mainstream schools whose behaviour is 'interfering with their own academic progress or that of their peers'. A vital part of the team's role is the examination of the cause of behaviour difficulties in the context within which they occur. This involves classroom observations and discussions with all relevant teachers. Following this, a plan of the intervention is agreed. The parents of individual pupils must give their written consent for the team to be involved. In turn the teachers regularly monitor the progress of the intervention programmes through discussions with the class/form teachers, parents and pupils.

Peripatetic teachers for specific learning difficulties

Teachers will provide additional help for children who are identified as having specific learning difficulties that are hindering the progress of their literacy skills. Amongst this group of children are those who are sometimes called 'dyslexic'. The teachers will carry out assessments on the pupil's reading and writing skills and offer individual or small group support. Most of this support is offered within the school or, less commonly, by part-time withdrawal to specialised centres.

Tutorial classes

May be offered to pupils of primary school age and, in exceptional circumstances, to secondary aged pupils whose emotional development is interfering with their progress in mainstream school. The emotional difficulties may manifest themselves in many ways, e.g. under-achievement; disruptive behaviour; inability to communicate; inability to form relationships, or displaying lack of confidence.

Pupils attend classes for a maximum of three sessions per week and must be on the roll of, and attending, a mainstream school. They are offered a programme of individual learning and groupwork which is aimed at their successful full-time reintegration into the mainstream school. Teachers work closely with parents, educational psychologists and other professionals who may be involved.

Individual support teachers

The teachers provide support for pupils in mainstream school who have a statement of special educational needs under section (V) of the Education Act 1981. They work in mainstream infant, junior, primary and secondary schools. By working closely with mainstream colleagues the teachers aim to enable pupils with special educational needs to gain full access to the curriculum and to achieve their full potential.

Support teachers are allocated to individual pupils by the teacher in charge according to the provision required by the statement of needs. The support which they offer in schools covers a wide range and accords with the needs of the pupil, as determined in part 2(ii) of the statement of special educational needs. The nature of the support provision is determined by local discussion between the school, the parent(s)/guardian(s) and the teacher in charge.

Outside school provision

Under the Education Act 1944, local authorities have had the power to provide 'Education otherwise than in school' (s56). This 'education otherwise' provision, as it is known, provides for children who are permanently excluded (expelled); school phobic, provided this is supported by medical evidence; and children who have psychiatric difficulties. This power, however, is no longer optional. The Education Act 1993 has made it mandatory for local education authorities to establish referral units for all children who are not attending school.

Off site centres

This provision may be made for disaffected secondary pupils, usually aged between 14–16, whose behaviour and relationship with the school has deteriorated to such an extent that they are in danger of being permanently excluded. Children with a history of truancy or school refusal and children who are perceived to be in danger of care or custody may well be provided for outside the school. The education programme should offer access to the full National Curriculum with emphasis placed on developing interpersonal skills; it also offers the opportunity for progression to further education and the world of work.

Formal education may become an irrelevance in the lives of some teenagers, particularly if they are not making academic progress and the prospect of finding paid work upon leaving school seems bleak. Alternative, out of school provision, which is smaller and more intimate, aims to meet the needs of a limited number of disaffected young people. An imaginative example of this is the current pilot project devised by Lewisham council and Millwall football club, whereby 12 young people receive their education on a part-time basis on the premises of the football club. So far as is possible the National Curriculum is related to the activities and organisation of the football club. Mathematics, for example, is taught with reference to match takings, receipts and ground capacity. Similarly aspects of science are related to the work of the physiotherapist who personally gives lessons to the pupils. Pupils negotiate and set targets which, if reached, result in a ticket to the next home match. The local authority has been able to attract outside funding to keep this arrangement alive for a limited period of time and the idea has interested other football clubs.

Individual tuition

This is a short term provision for primary and secondary pupils, many of whom have major difficulties and cannot (as opposed to will not) attend mainstream school. Such pupils can be referred for several reasons, e.g. pregnant schoolgirls; schoolgirl mothers, children who are long term sick or permanently excluded. The aim of the tuition is to offer pupils an education which will prepare them for a successful transfer to school, to further education, or to the world or work. Pupils may receive tuition of up to ten hours per week at their home, in hospital or at an educational centre.

The school psychological child guidance service

Before the Social Services Act 1970, this provision was part of the school health service, but following the 1974 reorganisation of the National Health Service, the school psychological and child guidance service became administered by the education department. It is a multidisciplinary service – social workers are employed by the SSD but seconded fulltime to the education department; similarly, child psychiatrists will be paid by the district health authority to work within the educational setting.

A typical team might include a senior social worker, three or four social workers (usually experienced and level 3), five educational psychologists and three specialist teachers (tutors). Child psychiatrists may attend on a sessional basis and be available for consultation by the team. An open referral system is in operation whereby anybody can refer, including the parent or the individual child involved. In practice, most referrals come from the school via educational psychologists, education social workers, head teachers or year tutors and from social services and general practitioners.

Regular meetings ensure collaboration between team members and at allocation meetings the team decides on which worker is to become involved with the child and their family. This decision will be made after investigation into the nature and location of the problem. If the behaviour difficulties are considered to be closely related to a child's home life, it is likely that a social worker will be involved initially.

Social workers may see the whole family and engage them in family therapy sessions; alternatively, they may work individually with the child using simple behaviour modification techniques. For example, a child with an enuresis problem will be encouraged to develop control over their bedwetting by the use of a 'star chart' or something similar. In using this approach, the social worker will draw up a chart with the days of the month outlined. This chart will be displayed in the child's own home and they are then able to record (with a star or tick) each dry night and thus observe progress. The involvement and co-operation of parents is important to the success of this exercise – for example, the child's progress may be positively reinforced if the child is given praise or more tangible rewards. Sometimes a child's bedwetting can be seen as a symptom of family stress and it may be more appropriate for the social worker to work with the whole family and help them deal with their difficulties and so reduce the anxiety felt by the child. In other cases, social workers might work with groups of parents, children and other professionals.

Educational psychologists are also involved in therapeutic measures, but they are primarily concerned in the assessment of a child's learning difficulties. Each educational psychologist is allocated to a certain number of secondary schools and their feeder primary schools. Because of their regular contact with schools, educational psychologists are the main source of referrals. They are themselves involved in special needs assessments and in recommending residential schooling where appropriate. Parents have to give their permission for an educational psychologist to be involved with their children and this consent can be dispensed with only in very exceptional cases where it is felt that without intervention a child would be deprived of their educational needs.

Teachers who are part of the child guidance service team may see children at the child guidance centre or in the school. They may involve children in regular group activities in either setting. In addition to normal educational instruction, they may also be responsible for the continued observation and assessment of behaviour. Children who respond to such close and individual attention may eventually advance sufficiently to be able to continue their education in an ordinary school.

The schools' psychological and child guidance service is a specialised agency primarily concerned with children's problems that are manifested within an education context. Various methods of intervention are used, including goal-setting, task-focusing and contract-based work. Because of the intensive nature of their involvement, child guidance workers have restricted caseloads. Parents are encouraged to be involved and are informed of the agencies' proposals concerning their work with the child. In many areas of the country there are waiting lists for children who need to be helped in this way.

The careers service

Youth advisory services existed in many forms before 1973, but in that year the Employment and Training Act placed a mandatory duty upon all local education authorities to provide a careers service, defined as 'an employment service for persons attending or leaving educational institutions other than universities although university students may use the service'. The service was also to be open to those people who had ceased fulltime education.

Careers officers are involved in a two-way process of trying to assess and match the needs of both young people and employers. Their work involves seeing pupils in schools, beginning when they are making significant subject changes at the end of the third year and also concentrating on helping those about to leave school. Pupils may be seen on an individual basis, so that the careers officer can take note of and assess their ambitions and inclinations and comment on the practicality of their choices. Alternatively, interested pupils may be seen on a group basis. At the same time, in order to keep up-to-date, careers officers will visit industry, the professions and other services and will advise about the employment of young people and also canvas for vacancies in the current job market.

The work of the careers service is a continuous process and is available to young people once they have left school – its liaison with further education establishments and familiarity with Government training measures for unemployed people are of course essential. Careers officers may be involved in starting young people on training schemes and be responsible for monitoring them while they are undergoing selected courses. In addition, the careers service produces literature, holds conventions, gives talks and generally contributes to the dissemination of information relating to employment opportunities.

Most careers workers see a wide range of young people with differing abilities and ambitions. Others feel the need to specialise, in order to be up to date and to be able to provide an expert concentrated service. Some local authorities have teams specialising in helping disabled young people and people who are unemployed.

Team working with disabled young people

Employment opportunities are problematic for many young school leavers, but finding employment is even more of a problem for young people who are disabled in some way. Employers of more than 20 people are legally obliged to make available at least 3 percent of the workforce vacancies to registered disabled people. In many cases a person's disability in no way interferes with job performance and they may go about a job in the normal way. They may, however, need support and intervention to counteract any prejudice that employers may have.

Young people with learning difficulties have a harder task in finding work, but they can be assisted in their search and also be advised about various training opportunities that exist in some further education colleges or adult rehabilitation centres. Although capable of employment at different levels, young people with learning difficulties are dependent, initially, on a sympathetic and understanding employer.

Team working with unemployed young people

Careers officers working with unemployed young people will be concerned with those who have been unable to find permanent work since leaving school or since following a youth training scheme course. Many of these young people will be keen to seek help from careers officers and others will respond after some encouragement from them. However, some older young people may be so disenchanted by their unsuccessful efforts to find work and lack of hopeful prospects that they may resist any help offered and make no attempt to seek official help. In response to this problem, careers officers may make home visits and try to encourage young people to take part in the specialised prevocational programmes that they run. These involve some counselling support, practice interviews, role play exercises and advice and guidance on job applications.

Careers services are provided by each local authority, but the standard of provision varies. More committed authorities will have special provision for disadvantaged young people and some have extended the service to adults. They will encourage young people who want to cross existing traditional boundaries to employment by offering positive support to girls seeking jobs in engineering and to boys wanting positions in caring work. Such authorities will have done much to reduce the bureaucratic and formal image of the careers service by making it more acceptable and more accessible to users.

The education welfare service

The education welfare service stems from the work carried out by the late nineteenth century 'school boardmen' who were appointed to ensure the school attendance of children between the ages of five and 13. Recruited largely from the police force and military sources, these men were generally disciplinarians concerned simply with the enforcement of the law. However, as a result of their investigations they became aware of the poor living conditions and severe poverty in which many families were living and were able to bring this information to the attention of the authorities. The need for child care and welfare, in addition to formal education, began to be recognised.

Today the role of the Education Social Worker, formerly known as Education Welfare Officer, has been greatly extended, but they are still primarily concerned with school attendance. The education welfare service provides social work support to the school or schools to which Education Social Workers are allocated and which they visit on a regular basis. As well as scrutinising registers in order to identify pupils who are developing problems of irregular attendance, the Education Social Worker will talk to teachers or heads of year about children who are causing concern because of the problems they are presenting. They will also help teachers to appreciate the difficulties experienced by particular families at home.

Home visits are made by Education Social Workers in order to establish reasons for absence and records of their involvement will be kept. Consultation and supervision are provided by senior staff who may themselves carry a small caseload.

Most education welfare services are run by local education authorities, but in some cases the service is based within the social services department.

Under the Education Act 1944, it is the duty of every parent to see that his or her children receive fulltime education between the ages of five and 16. (This need not necessarily take place within a school – where the parent is a qualified teacher, for example, it is possible for that person to educate his or her children in their own home. However, education is concerned with more than simply imparting knowledge, and to educate children exclusively at home would be to deny them the social opportunity to mix and make friends with other children of their own age.) The Education Social Worker may summon parents to court under section 39 of the 1944 Act if they feel that they are failing in their duty to ensure that their child receives fulltime education. Following the Children Act 1989, applications for care orders on the ground of non-school attendance can no longer be made..

Legal measures are taken only as a last resort, when all other forms of help have been offered. However, it is to often the case that the actual implementation of the court procedure is itself enough to encourage improved attendance.

Children absent themselves from school for many reasons, which range from difficulties experienced at home to general disaffection with the school. Although not unknown in primary schools, most attendance problems occur within secondary schools. It is part of the education social worker's role to ascertain the root cause of the continued absence and to offer help accordingly. If the cause of the problem is felt to lie within the school itself, then the school may be able to provide alternatives and make changes in the curriculum or organisation.

Like other professional workers involved in schools, Education Social Workers have a responsibility to identify children 'at risk educationally' and may recommend a child to be considered for a special needs statement. In certain cases, a change of school will be beneficial for a child and the will arrange this.

The education welfare service provides financial benefits in the form of grants for essential school clothing, travel allowances and free school meals for children from low income families. Educational Social Workers can advise about these benefits and also offer advice to parents on the availability of preschool provision, special education and the procedure for school transfer. In addition, they can outline for parents the work of the child guidance service, the careers department and other educational support services as well as give information about the type of help offered by other agencies. Sometimes this information is made available at education welfare adult centres situated within the community. In providing benefits, the education welfare service is the only agency outside the Department of Social Security (DSS) to supply direct financial assistance to families (although the social services also have limited resources which they can use to help a family if this diminishes the need for a child to be brought into care – section 17 of the Children Act 1989).

Finally, the Education Social Worker is responsible for checking that school age children are not being employed illegally, either under age or beyond the maximum hours they are legally permitted to work. As well as responding to allegations of illegal employment made by individuals within the community, the Education Social Worker will patrol likely areas – such as markets – outside of normal office hours if necessary.

The Franks Report

The 1973 Franks Report is the only official report on the work done by Education Social Workers. It concluded that the most relevant professional training for an Educational Social Worker is social work training, although their work is clearly different from mainstream social work because of its educational setting. The report led to the education social workers being upgraded from a clerical to a social worker grade.

The youth service

Local education authorities employ youth workers to provide a service aimed at encouraging the personal development of young people in an informal setting. There are separate provisions for children between eight and 13 and for young people between 13 and 25.

Some youth centres are based in schools and may be open to the local community on one or two nights in the week as well as to those who attend during the day. Others, operating from community education centres, may be open day and evening. These

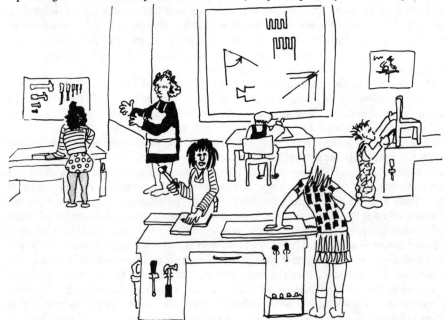

Youth centres may provide girls with an opportunity to be involved in new activities.

centres often incorporate a youth club, play schemes, women's groups and sessions for unemployed people within the same building complex.

Although youth clubs provide essentially recreational activities, they also aim to advance a person's general education. Through involvement in supervised group activities, young people can develop relationships which may encourage them to challenge their existing perceptions of others and of society. Issues such as racism and sexism can be confronted informally in settings unrestricted by timetable requirements. The available advice counselling offered by youth workers is founded on a trust relationship which is built up through association. Young people are encouraged to make decisions and are supported in accepting responsibility. The youth worker will respond to initiatives that stem from the group and will organise activities accordingly.

Outreach work

This is undertaken to gauge the unmet need for youth work in the area. It involves the youth workers going out into the community and talking to particular individuals, to schools and to other agencies in order to establish what should be offered to young people. In some areas, special projects have been set up under such headings as 'girls' work' and 'Asian youth groups' among others, in an attempt to extend resources to hitherto neglected young people. More people are therefore given an opportunity to engage in interests and activities within a supervised setting.

Detached youth workers

These go further towards trying to meet the needs of young people. They may be based in a local centre, but much of their work is done on the streets, in cafés and other meeting places where they attempt to reach more isolated individuals. Some young people may lack sufficient confidence to join a youth club or may simply be unaware of the resources which are offered.

Community education

Community education has developed from the adult and youth and community services. It derives from the 1970 Youth Service Development Report and from the 1973 Russell Report on adult education. It aims to provide wide-ranging educational opportunities to all members of the community, particularly those groups who have traditionally been excluded. However it has been severly cut back in recent years.

Many people's educational experience is restricted to the time they spent at school. For a number of reasons – lack of confidence, ignorance of courses on offer, added responsibilities or lack of time or money – they may have been unable later to fulfil their educational desires or needs.

Community colleges include all the local further education, adult education and community education sites within a specified area. They are now in the process of extending services to more people and involving the community in policy decisions. This move has meant that community colleges have had to develop more flexibility with regard to timetabling and the nature of courses offered, in order to respond to felt needs within the community. The main groups identified as having a special need within the community include women, manual workers, people with difficulties, ethnic minority groups, unemployed people and older adults.

Since April 1993 colleges of FE have become independent from the local authority and are responsible for generating much of their own income; less emphasis is being placed on developing community needs; more is being placed on meeting the needs of industry and obtaining outside funding.

Women

Although more men are becoming involved, society still lays responsibility for child care firmly on the shoulders of women. With the general lack of fulltime day care facilities for children under five, many mothers spend much of their lives attending to the needs of children. For some this is an ideal way of using their time, but others may feel the need to develop their particular interests and may feel trapped in what can often be an isolating activity. It is estimated that twice the number of women would seek work or some form of education if adequate day care facilities were available.

For community colleges adequately to meet the needs of parents – mothers in particular – they need to be able to provide crèche facilities and shorter courses (between 10 a.m. and 3 p.m.) so that children can be taken to and from school. In a stimulating educational setting, women can develop interests, grow in confidence and prepare themselves for the time when their children have grown up.

Manual workers

Most manual workers are unlikely to have participated in any further education and usually they left school with few or no qualifications. Sometimes this is regretted.

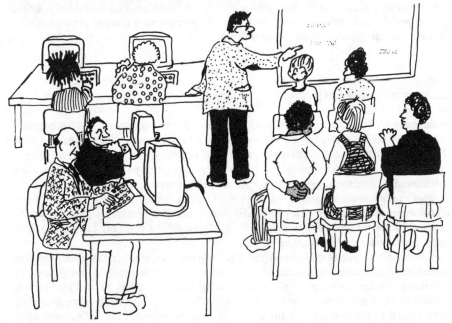

Community education aims to give everyone the chance to develop new interests.

Furthermore, during the course of their adult lives, people often discover that they possess talents or interests and an all too often frustrated desire to develop them. This is where community education can help. Some people may see no relevance for them in the courses already offered and it is part of the role of community education to ascertain people's needs and to get together in designing appropriate courses. It is regrettable that some people carry their negative school experiences with them throughout their lives.

Adults with learning difficulties

The Warnock Report recommended that educational provision for people with learning difficulties should be extended, so young people finishing school are now encouraged to take up additional education. Link courses to adult residential homes are made and courses are offered to adults with learning difficulties living in the community. Courses vary in their range from some form of basic education to basic NVQ courses to more sophisticated work in computer workshops. Many people with learning difficulties find the facilities more stimulating and the atmosphere friendlier in a community college than in an adult training centre, say, and in turn their presence contributes to a greater social integration.

Black and Ethnic minority groups

Members of black and ethnic minorities have a right to preserve their distinctive identities, culture, language, religion and social values. Many community colleges have responded by introducing changes in curriculum, procedure, practices and provision to meet this need.

It is recognised that a high proportion of children from black and ethnic minority backgrounds have underachieved at school. This is seen partly as a result of the difficulty some children have experienced in trying to come to terms with the values of two different cultures – those of their parents and those of the wider society in general. This is particularly evident with regard to language. For example, an English child born of West Indian parents may speak one language at home (patois) and another with their friends (a mixture of patois and English), but academically their linguistic proficiency is measured purely in terms of the dominant wider culture. It is, of course, important for everybody that Standard English is learned, as it is the basis of communication in society, but where children have been given no additional help they will inevitably leave school disadvantaged.

For social work and other caring organisations to reflect the attitudes of the population as a whole, professional representation needs to be made from all the various groups which make up our society. In a deliberate effort to encourage the recruitment of caring practitioners from different backgrounds and cultures, some colleges have developed *access courses*, linked to training courses at universities and other higher education establishments, and have restricted entry to ethnic minority members. These access courses aim to enable students to reach the academic level required for professional training.

Most access courses, however, are open to everyone over the age of 21 but those restricted to ethnic minority members are an example of *positive action*, aimed at counteracting previous less obvious *negative discrimination* which for a long time went unrecognised.

Increasingly, some ethnic groups are involved in providing their own educational courses within the traditional adult educational structure. For example, in some areas the Asian communities run courses in Urdu and other languages as well as wider aspects of their own cultures.

Older adults

Increased opportunities for early retirement and a shorter working week mean that some people have greater leisure time. Education is not simply about obtaining formal qualifications – it is concerned with developing potential within individuals, with the overall aim of enriching and improving their quality of life. Community colleges are involved with meeting intellectual, physical and creative needs as well as with the acquisition of relevant skills. Well planned pre-retirement courses in particular can enable individuals to adjust to changes in lifestyle.

Unemployed people

There are few more debilitating or demoralising experiences in life than being unemployed, particularly over a long period of time, or having been made redundant at a late stage in life with little hope of re-employment. Without the sense of usefulness and social involvement attached to economic activity, people may become despondent and feel unfulfilled. A wide range of courses aimed either at specific retraining or broader personal development are available to help people back into the job market or at least assist them to live their lives in a more constructive and satisfactory manner.

There are, of course, other groups within society who could benefit from extended educational provision – the above list is by no means exhaustive.

In order to ascertain need, committed community colleges are involved in *outreach work*, talking to individuals and community groups to find out what people want. Some colleges offer a *drop-in* service where people may call at any time during the day, either to participate in a particular interest group (for parents and toddlers or unemployed people, for example) or to seek advice about the availability of educational opportunity. Systems of *open learning* have extended educational provision to more people, with the development of individual work packages as part of course modules and the availability of tutor support. Through open learning, people are able to work at their own pace to complete chosen courses of study. This may be done in the college workshop or at the student's home or place of work. In this way it has been possible for a person working in a remote situation, such as an oil rig, to continue their education and to consult a tutor by post or by attendance at the college during shore leave.

The inclusion of ordinary members of the public on neighbourhood education management committees enables individual participation and allows the public to actively affect the kind of educational provision being made.

Local authority housing departments

Although this book is mainly concerned with social work as seen from the perspective of the practitioners, this approach is not possible when dealing with the work of housing departments owing to the uniqueness of each local authority housing department. Each housing department differs in regard to structure, functions, responsibilities and approach to its work.

Historically, housing has been taken for granted and to a certain extent left to the individuals to provide for themselves. In the nineteenth century when the state became involved in housing, it did so initially from a concern with public health. However, few local authorities made any substantial provision until after the First World War (the Addison Act 1919), when the Government committed itself to providing 'homes fit for heroes' and provided subsidies in the form of grants to local authorities to enable them to provide low cost rented accommodation. Since then subsidies have been withdrawn and reintroduced at intervals. The period following the Second World War saw a boom in building local authority accommodation. Some housing, especially in the 1960s and early 1970s, was built with scant regard for customer preferences and concentrated on quantity of household units at the expense of quality.

Since 1979, the Government has demonstrated a commitment to the extension of a 'property owning democracy'. Various measures have been introduced to support private ownership and reduce public provision of housing. In 1980 the Government gave council tenants the right to buy their homes from the council and made it mandatory for local authorities to sell stock to existing tenants at a reduced rate according to length of residence. In 1988 legislation was passed to encourage more property owners into the private rented sector which had been in decline and also encouraged local authorities to sell housing estates under 'tenants' choice'.

The Government envisages the role of the housing department, as with other local authority departments, to be an enabler rather than a provider. It is expected that housing associations and the private sector generally will expand to fulfill the provider role formerly undertaken by the local authority. At present, as a result of a combination of factors including demographic changes, economic hardship and the depletion and deterioration of public housing stock, demand for local authority housing greatly exceeds supply.

The current workload of a housing department is complex and varied. It has a number of statutory obligations to private and council tenants alike. Some areas of work which are pertinent to social work and social care are outlined below.

Access to local authority housing

People who wish to be considered for local authority accommodation must register on a housing waiting list. The local authority will request details of the applicant's personal circumstances and their accommodation needs. In the past local authorities would allocate their resources on a date-order basis, i.e. to those individuals and families who had waited the longest, but this is no longer possible.

Nowadays, most local authorities use a points system in an attempt to prioritise applicants who are, in theory, in most need, so that they may be given accommodation first. A points system may be idiosyncratic and may reflect the circumstances of the local authority, their existing housing policy and the values and beliefs of the people who have designed it.

Some authorities will operate restrictive practices; for instance they may not admit owner occupiers onto their waiting list or they may require an applicant to be resident in the authority's geographical area for a specified length of time before applying. Some authorities may take this 'waiting time' into account. Nevertheless the points scheme in all its variations remains the fairest method available for allocating resources which are becoming increasingly scarce. A comprehensive points scheme will reflect the whole picture of the applicant's circumstances. Areas which may be considered are:

The points system

Attempts to quantify the urgency with which people need to be rehoused may involve an assessment of the following conditions:

a) *Overcrowding* Points for overcrowding are awarded on a sliding scale calculated on the relationship between family size and the number of rooms in the house at the time when the housing department is first notified of the condition.

b) *Medical* Applicants whose household includes one person who is suffering unacceptable hardship due to the structure of the building (a severely disabled person having to negotiate stairs, for example) will receive maximum points under this category. Points will also be awarded to those whose medical condition is less severe but where rehousing is likely to result in an alleviation of distress.

c) *Insecurity* This refers to people who have received an eviction warrant or a 'notice to quit' their homes and who therefore need urgent consideration. Fewer points will be granted to others who have no security of tenure (such as lodgers, who may be asked to leave at any moment) but where there is no pressure for them to leave at present.

d) *Social* A person's social circumstances are taken into account within this category. A range of points may be awarded where people are experiencing violence or fear of violence; harassment (racial or from neighbours or landlord); or relationship difficulties, including family separation and bereavement. Consideration will be made in this category for applicants wishing to move to smaller accommodation now that their children have grown up and left home and for those people who are isolated by distance from friends and relatives. The degree of social hardship and ability to cope will be taken into account.

e) *Property condition* Maximum points will be awarded to families whose home has been designated 'unfit for habitation' and a varying number of points will be awarded to others according to their house's general state of repair.

f) *Lacking or sharing amenities* People and families either lacking amenities (such as an inside toilet) or having to share resources (such as bathrooms and kitchens) will be awarded points related to the degree of inconvenience involved.

g) *Environment* This category relates to factors outside a person's dwelling – for example, where a family with children is living in an unmodernised pre-war block of flats. Environmental points are awarded for the presence of disruptive or distressing features as well as for the lack of essential or desirable facilities (such as play space or a grass area).

h) *Travelling* Applicants who have to travel long distances to work, to use public facilities or to receive or give support to relatives will be considered under this category.

i) *Multioccupancy* A multioccupied dwelling is defined by the Housing Act 1969 (section 58) as a 'house which is occupied by persons who do not form a single household'. Such dwellings include hostels, night shelters, guest houses and homes converted into bedsits where cooking, lavatory and bathroom facilities are shared. Some people in this category may have already been awarded points on other criteria (such as social, environmental or overcrowding), and the extra points they obtain under multioccupancy will emphasise their plight. This category in particular reflects the intention of some local authorities to phase out the inadequate hostels for single homeless people.

j) *Children at height* For reasons of safety and access to play space, children need to live at ground level. This category recognises the desirability for families with children to live in ground floor accommodation and awards points according to the number of children who live above ground level.

k) *Elderly* The age of an applicant does not necessarily represent housing need, but an elderly person is more likely to experience difficulties and an allowance on the points scale is made for this.

l) *Related issues* To be considered for rehousing, people must usually be residents of the council area, but exceptions are made for people living in 'overspill areas' beyond the local boundaries and for elderly or Forces personnel who wish to return to their area of origin.

m) *Time and housing need* The above categories combine to determine a person's or a family's housing priority – from them is calculated the applicant's position on a waiting list. Families who are classified as having only a 'medium need' to be rehoused would, under a static points system, have little chance of progressing towards the type of property they desire. However, consideration is also given to the length of time that families have spent waiting for accommodation – extra points are granted yearly on the anniversary of a family's original application for rehousing.

n) *Children leaving care* There is now a statutory duty on local authorities to provide accommodation for children who have been looked after by the local authority.

o) *A child in need* Section 20(1) of the Children Act 1989 places a duty on the local authority to provide accommodation to any child 'in need' including young people aged 16 and 17 who are 'in need' and whose welfare is likely to be 'seriously prejudiced' without the provision of services.

Homelessness

There are many reasons why an individual or family becomes homeless; a domestic dispute, a dispute with relatives, violence or accidents including fire or flood. In recent times an increased number of families have become homeless having had their homes repossessed by building societies as a result ot their inability to keep up with mortgage payments. Many families suffered from the vicissitudes of the employment and housing markets during the extended period of recession through the late 1980s and early 1990s.

Local authority housing departments took over the duty of providing for homeless people under the Housing (Homeless Persons) Act 1977. (This Act was incorporated under part 3 of the Housing Act 1985.) The legislation is not merely concerned with providing for people's immediate need for physical accommodation. It empowers local authorities to work in a preventive way and to make arrangements for families and individuals before they become homeless in order to lessen the trauma. Local authorities are obliged to provide help, but not necessarily permanent accommodation unless it can be established that the applicant has a 'priority housing need'.

Priority need

Under section 2 of the Housing Act 1977, certain categories of homeless people are regarded as having priority need for accommodation and they include the following:

a) those with a dependent child or children;
b) those made homeless through flood, fire or other disaster;
c) pregnant women;
d) anybody considered vulnerable or who is living with someone who is at risk because of physical disability, old age, learning disability or illness or 'any other reason'.

If any 'priority need' individuals or families are considered to have intentionally made themselves homeless the authority will not consider rehousing them permanently – but should offer temporary accommodation and give advice and assistance, over a reasonable length of time, aimed at enabling them to secure accommodation for themselves. If, however, the authority is convinced that a person or persons have become homeless unintentionally, then the local authority is obliged to make accommodation available to them. Help may initially be provided in the form of temporary accommodation until the family's or person's circumstances can be assessed and classified and their position on the housing list can be determined.

The homeless families section

Some local authorities provide support teams to help families who are homeless. Before such families are considered to be in 'priority need', they may be received into temporary hostel accommodation until a separate individual offer can be made. The length of stay in temporary accommodation may depend to some extent on their willingness to accept offers of accommodation made to them by the housing department which, for a variety of reasons, the homeless family may or may not consider suitable. Vacancies are more likely to occur in areas where nobody wants to live.

Housing problems are often inter-related with other difficulties. For example, a family made homeless by mortgage repossession or councilhouse eviction could experience related social difficulties in addition to financial hardship. For this reason, homeless family hostels are sometimes serviced by social work teams. Social workers may encourage involvement in groupwork and other activities aimed at building up a family's self-respect and confidence to counter the demoralising experience of being homeless.

Single homeless people

The code of guidance incorporated in part 3 of the Housing Act 1985 states that certain single people should be regarded as having priority housing need. This includes young women threatened with physical abuse and other young people exposed to financial or sexual exploitation. There is no legal requirement upon local authorities to provide accommodation for most other (able-bodied) single homeless people, although the code of practice recommends some help if it is possible. Some would argue that homeless single people are, by their very circumstances, vulnerable and that more should be done for them under the 'vulnerability' concept outlined in section 2 of the Act.

Housing officers will provide single homeless people with information about the resources available in the area. They may produce a list of recommended bed-and-breakfast hotels known to accept single homeless people and, for someone who is unemployed, provide information on the procedure for obtaining financial assistance from the DSS. They will also advise on the availability of housing benefit to applicants who are not unemployed as well as to those who are.

In 1985 the DSS introduced a contested ruling limiting the period that single people below the age of 26 could remain in hotel accommodation while receiving DSS benefit to eight weeks in a large city and four weeks in a smaller town. Hotel accommodation remains only a temporary solution to the problems of unemployed homeless young people.

The housing officer can also inform about *local authority hostels*, where they exist. These are usually single-sex establishments, often with dormitory accommodation. Where there are no local authority hostels, the housing officer can advise on the *voluntary provision* within the area (Church Army or Salvation Army establishments, for example) and comment on the vacancy situation and their charges for overnight or longstay accommodation.

Night shelters

These have come into existence in some major towns in response to the lack of provision for the single homeless. Most of these shelters – usually run by a church or other voluntary organisation with some local authority or DSS support – are extremely basic, providing just shelter, food and sleeping accommodation. Some shelters are mixed, but most have no provision for women. They may be based in a church crypt or even in a disused building. They tend not to refuse anybody who is homeless and they remain open for applicants up to a certain hour of the night or all night in a few cases. Such hostels are vacated early in the morning and a user is usually not allowed to return until the doors reopen at a specified time in the evening, although a growing number are remaining open for part of the day and some provide basic meals.

Teams working with single homeless people

Much of the accommodation for single homeless people is inadequate – it is often provided in large unadapted Victorian institutions which are inappropriate for the needs of the twentieth century. Some local authorities are committed to the closure of these institutions and to their replacement by smaller, more intimate units.

Innovative schemes to assist the institutionalised single homeless person to transfer to independent accommodation or smaller hostel accommodation within the community have been made possible where housing departments have set up single person strategy groups. Housing officers then have a home-making function, helping clients to obtain DSS assistance and to establish themselves in furnished or unfurnished accommodation within the community. This work is quite labour-intensive for the officer concerned, particularly when helping someone who has for many years been dependent on institutional settings.

Tenant participation

One thing that has been made clear by the experience of many housing departments from the 1950s onwards is that they failed to properly take into account the views of the people in need of housing and the communities within which they lived.

Partly as a consequence of housing departments' failure to consult tenants in the past and partly as a result of the growing recognition of the need for people to be more politically involved in their own lives, tenant participation is now actively encouraged.

Many local authority housing departments are engaged in improving the communication between housing staff and tenants. This involves the co-operation of housing officers, councillors, trade unions and tenants. To facilitate this, local authorities are obliged to display arrangements by which tenants can be consulted on major changes in housing policy. In the past, tenants' associations have been formed only to be disbanded after a particular issue has been fought. Today the aim is to encourage the development of a permanent tenants' association on every housing estate and to encourage communication between them.

Local authorities can provide individual tenant handbooks and can supply other information in local public display cases. Authorities may make accommodation available for tenants' associations and provide professional support staff and financial aid in the form of small starter grants. Typically, tenants may be involved in the vetting of repair schedules, gauging the needs of local interest groups (such as toddlers' clubs) and identifying community need. In this way, ordinary people will have more of a stake in where they live.

Local estate offices

Some local authority housing departments have decentralised and have relocated their offices within the community. Where this has happened, housing matters are dealt with by small management teams.

Local estate offices are concerned with the management and supervision of the council housing in their area – hence they are involved in rehousing assessments; allocation of properties; and the problems concerning disputes with neighbours, non-payment of rents, arrears and eviction of tenants.

Local authorities are usually reluctant to evict tenants, partly because they may have a responsibility to rehouse them. Instead, they will offer advice on income maximisation and may suggest helpful repayment schemes or offer limited practical counselling. If necessary, they will refer a family to the local social services department. In the past, some housing authorities have been guilty of reallocating ('dumping') families with large rent arrears into one specific area containing the less desirable properties and have so created 'ghetto' estates.

High rise living

Between the late 1950s and early 1970s, many housing authorities were engaged in the mass clearance of housing considered unfit for habitation. In the process, long established communities were destroyed and their homes were often replaced by high density architecturally innovative housing complexes. Although the buildings looked impressive on the drawing board, these high rise and deck access housing schemes are now acknowledged to have contributed to the social problems of the people obliged to live in them. Many buildings were poorly constructed – among their faults were thin walls and inefficient and costly heating systems. Furthermore, people living in deck access accommodation had little privacy and lacked an area outside their home which they could call their own.

In response to these problems, housing authorities have where possible rehoused families with children and other vulnerable groups and have used the high rise accommodation to meet the needs of single people and students. In extreme cases, some local authorities have pulled down high rise and deck access complexes, some of which were built less than 20 years ago. Some housing authorities have adapted and renovated existing accommodation to make it more appropriate to the needs of families. This has involved such alterations as removing the top floor of a three-tier block of flats and converting the building into a series of individual maisonette-type units. Such alterations are costly and different authorities have made varying progress with them.

When much of the high rise accommodation was being built, housing departments were under pressure to rehouse people from clearance areas quickly and central government threatened to withhold fundings if rehousing took too long. It is unlikely that housing authorities will repeat the mistakes they have made in the past.

Housing aid

Many local authorities run a separate housing aid service, normally from the city centre, which provides information on all housing matters, particularly those not related to council housing or public tenancies. In other areas, this type of service may be provided by independent voluntary bodies (such as Shelter or the Catholic Housing Aid Society).

Advice may be given on any of the following problems: excessive rent, overdue repairs, harassment, lack of supply services (gas and electricity) and evictions. Housing aid officers have access to a number of specialists within the authority, some of whom may be employed by social services – these include welfare rights advisors and housing benefit advisors. The housing aid officers themselves will be able to provide most information, but they will consult a specialist where the circumstances are more complex. Similarly, housing officers will themselves undertake basic debt counselling unless the situation requires greater expertise.

Community care

The need for housing services to be involved in joint planning has been recognised and representatives from the housing department are provided to the various joint planning teams for people with mental ill health, people with physical disabilities and elders. The housing department also provide staff to participate in the assessment panels for the development of care packages, so that any housing need can be addressed as an integral part of the care needed. The resources made available will depend on the service user's circumstances and present housing tenure. In some cases there will be a need for rehousing and in others the panel member will be able to recommend adaptations or to introduce other support for issues concerning housing benefit, repairs, heating or security of tenure.

The housing department may also make properties available for special schemes, such as supported living schemes for people with mental ill health; they may allocate a four bedroomed property to be developed as a 'cluster' for a 'core and cluster' scheme.

Community support for elders is often available through the area warden service. The warden supplies a form of minimal support and social contact to a large number of elders by calling regularly, perhaps once or twice daily. Service users may have access to a community alarm system and may therefore summon help in an emergency. This service has many of the advantages of sheltered housing schemes but enables people to remain in their own homes.

Conclusion

Housing services to both private and council tenants vary enormously throughout the country. Despite its legal obligations the local authority's role is diminishing: the demand for accommodation from all groups of people is rising, but the supply of available housing stock has been depleted over the years. Much has been sold and local authorities have as yet been unable to use the money from the sales for replacement housing. There are houses standing empty within the public sector but only in low demand areas. In densely populated areas demand for decent accommodation is high and waiting lists are long.

Housing associations are being encouraged to fulfil the provider role while local authority housing departments concentrate on monitoring standards and allocating funds to associations. Local authority housing departments and the housing associations have an enormous task facing them. In 1980 social housing stood at 107 000 new units, 86 000 of them built by councils, whereas in 1991 there were only 30 000 new units built, most of these by housing associations (*Guardian*, 1.6.93).

Community work

Community work is discussed separately in this chapter, although community workers are employed by the statutory agencies already mentioned. Community work has been defined as: 'A process through which people sharing a common concern or problem are enabled to identify the problem, and share in working towards solving the problem' (CCETSW 1991, p1). Hugh Butcher (1991) says similarly that:

> Community work involves working with people who have voluntarily come together in community groups and organisations to find answers to problems, and promote change, thus enabling them to achieve a greater degree of control over the conditions of their lives. (He adds) The focus of such work is common concerns, developing and sharing skills, knowledge, experience and awareness, and supporting collective responses. Priority is given to working with people and communities that characteristically experience little control over their lives – the powerless, the disadvantaged and the oppressed. (*Changing Social Work and Welfare*, Carter, Jeffs and Smith,
>
> Open University Press, 1992, p144)

The relationship between community work and social work is a source of some debate. Some community workers see their role as a branch of social work, others emphasise their independence from it. Essentially community workers focus on the needs of the community as a whole, rather than the needs of individuals. Community workers may be employed by a wide range of organisations in both the statutory and voluntary sectors. Their roles and tasks vary and whilst they are employed to undertake community work few of them are actually called 'community workers' – as Figure 4.3 shows.

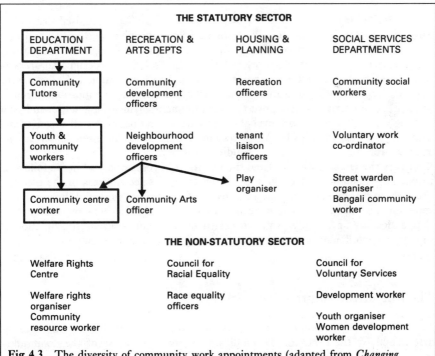

Fig 4.3 The diversity of community work appointments (adapted from *Changing Social Work and Welfare*, p 145).

The development of community work

The urban renewal programmes that started in the USA in the 1940s and 1950s did much to influence the development of community work in this country. The public became disillusioned with the bureaucratic nature of Government and the lack of public participation in matters affecting ordinary people. This coincided with the recognition, by the early 1960s, that the Welfare State had failed to protect everyone: that poverty and urban decay existed in many towns and cities. Furthermore, from the breakdown of many traditional communities, increased social mobility and problems experienced by new communities with mixed ethnic populations, it was clear that people were not sufficiently involved in determining changes in their own environment. For example, there were compulsory purchase orders on family homes to make way for new roads and office accommodation.

Community workers had been successfully employed by local authorities in new town developments in assessing need and encouraging community involvement. For example some new town corporations employed community workers *before* families moved in, to help the families settle in the new surroundings. Stemming from this innovation, the need to employ community workers in more established areas was recognised.

Official recognition of community need

The 1969 Skeffington Committee report *People and Planning* recognised that public participation 'can improve the quality of decisions by public authorities and give personal satisfaction to those affected by the decisions'. This opinion had already been made in the Seebohm Report (1968), which added that 'designated areas of special need should receive extra resources, comprehensively planned'. Following the Plowden Report (1967), education departments had introduced educational priority areas (EPAs) in regions where poverty owing to unemployment, low wages and poor housing was reflected in a low level of educational aspiration, high staff turnover and truancy problems in schools. More resources were to be invested in EPAs and teachers were to receive improved conditions of pay.

In 1969 the Home Office initiated the Urban Aid Programme and in the following year set up Community Development Projects in 12 selected areas of the country. From about this time, the volume and variety of community work and the number of appointments made within it were increasingly rapidly. In 1969 the Gulbenkian Foundation set up a study group to exchange ideas and examine the function of community work and its proper place in both practice and training.

The role of the community worker

The role of the community worker is not always clearly defined and will be determined by the needs of the employing agency and those of the community they serve. These needs may not always be compatible, therefore conflict is seen as an institutionalised aspect of the work – community workers may be involved in the dual

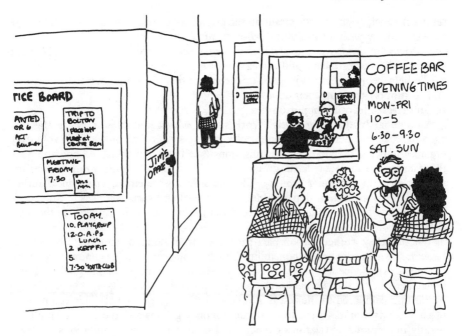

The community centre is often a focal point for a wide range of local groups and activities

task of assessing and developing community needs while pressing their own departments for the allocation of further resources. Some community workers will be concerned with the needs of a small area or neighbourhood and may be based in the local community centre; others will have a wider brief and may be involved in regional planning, new towns, expanded towns and decaying inner cities.

Whether they work from the 'ground level' or at an administrative regional level, community workers will share common aims:

a) To *encourage* people to act for themselves collectively – they are rarely concerned in helping people solve individual problems.

b) To *share* their knowledge and skills with groups within the community.

c) To *stimulate* neighbourhood interest in the development of self-help activities such as childminding and the running of community centres.

d) To *liaise* efficiently with other statutory and voluntary organisations.

e) To *establish priorities* in their aims to strengthen disadvantaged groups in disadvantaged areas who are seeking improvements in services and resources.

f) To *identify* and *assess* – looking at neighbourhoods and collating information with regard to the needs of people, organisations, services and building spaces.

g) To make *formal and informal contact* with local residents via newsletters, community newspapers, coffee mornings, sponsored fundraising and social events for the whole community.

h) To do *outreach work* which may include door-to-door visiting of local residents to encourage involvement and to determine need.

i) To offer encouragement to *existing groups* and to facilitate their development – to offer opinions and advice and back-up resources (such as typing and telephone services) which might relieve strain on the group. All of this is designed to encourage the community without inhibiting *self-determination*.

j) To seek to improve the *skills* and *confidence* of group members and their understanding of problems and issues.

k) To help people to *identify needs*, to encourage them to come together in a group and to support them in their action.

l) To increase learning opportunities.

A National Institute for Social Work survey of community workers in the UK showed that 59 percent of community workers were employed by voluntary organisations – either national organisations (such as Help the Aged and the Save the Children Fund) or local groups (such as citizens' rights groups, tenants' associations and consumer groups). The remainder were employed by local authorities – chiefly education departments (19 percent) and social services (11 percent). Many of the voluntary organisations received the bulk of their funding via the local authorities.

Whether they worked full- or part-time, the survey defined community workers as '*paid staff* whose primary responsibility is to develop groups in the community whose members experience and wish to tackle needs, disadvantages or inequality'. Forty seven percent of the workers were women and this represents an above average proportion compared to the rest of public social service personnel. Thirteen percent of community workers were from ethnic minority groups and these were employed mainly in community relations councils and other voluntary organisations. Overall, less than one third were professionally qualified in some way. (*A Survey of Community Workers in the UK*, Francis, Henderson and Thomas, NISW, London, 1984).

Social work, counselling and advisory groups

In addition to community work schemes such as neighbourhood and playgroup schemes, there are often specific social work and advisory projects funded by the State – either directly or via the local authority. These projects, run by non-statutory organisations, are set up to meet community needs that are not being properly catered for by existing services and are usually financed on a short term basis. This funding is periodically reviewed – it can be extended for a specific length of time or withdrawn altogether. Occasionally the work of some projects is taken over by statutory organisations and incorporated into their basic service.

The threat of withdrawal of funding makes working on temporary projects difficult in that future planning is restricted. Some projects are long established, so the workers may be confident that funding will be renewed (or extended). However it may still be difficult to tempt professional workers into an insecure job situation. The type of projects that are often experimental include those run for homeless or mentally ill young people, drug misuse centres and law centres.

Law centres

These operate from local offices and are part of the Law Centre Federation. Each centre is governed by a democratically elected management committee made up of local members of the community (which will include professional and ordinary working people). The aim is to provide a legal advice service to local people on matters that are not covered by Legal Aid. Under the Legal Aid scheme, anybody on a low income (calculated on disposable capital and disposable income) can receive initial services from a solicitor up to £50 free before contributing towards full legal costs according to calculations made on their income. Not all matters may be dealt with by Legal Aid, so recourse to advice centres is essential.

Law centres employ qualified solicitors, advice workers and sometimes barristers. They deal with a wide range of problems, including matters involving industrial disputes, unfair dismissal, industrial accidents, low pay and welfare benefits. The law centre representative may act as an advocate for someone attending a DSS appeals tribunal. Workers may be involved in helping people with their debt problems or negotiating with gas and electricity boards in order to prevent disconnection of supply. Additionally, the centre may be engaged in running a 'take-up campaign' by publicising information in order to encourage people to claim welfare benefits they are entitled to.

Community drug teams

These have developed in response to the growing problem of drug misuse and the absence of specialised help for people with drug problems. They deal with all forms of drug abuse – both legal and illegal – ranging from reliance on prescribed sedatives to dependence on heroin and other 'hard' drugs.

Structured therapeutic communities exist for people with serious drug problems and, as a preparation for these, people may receive some induction at the local drugs project centre to prepare them for involvement in a residential setting. It is important to realise that the desire to change one's lifestyle has to come from the individual and cannot be imposed externally. Local drug project centres and therapeutic communities may enable people to achieve their desired goals.

Community drug teams work with members of the community who have drug problems, engaging them in groupwork, counselling and support. Work is also done with relatives of drug misusers, outlining facts related to drug abuse and encouraging support and understanding. However, the focus of their work is on the individual – they are encouraged to consider the options and alternatives open to them, but without inner commitment there can be no change. Community drug teams employ workers who are experienced in counselling and groupwork. Former drug users may also be employed.

Some problems of community work

Community workers are not free agents – they are bound by the limits imposed by the organisation for which they work. This provides constraints for the community worker. Another dilemma frequently experienced by some workers occurs when they are seen by local people merely as 'paid professionals' from outside the community who have no personal investment within the area. This may lead to feelings of resentment. Lack of proper resources is another problem – for example in the field of education, where high fees and inadequate grants act as a barrier to formal education.

This will sometimes hamper the efforts of community workers who want to encourage people to further their learning.

There is a tendency for the more motivated, more able members of the community to take up leadership roles in groups and organisations, and it is important that the community worker encourages this. At the same time, it is also important for them to get in touch with the less articulate, more isolated members of the community so that they too may be enabled to influence what happens around them.

Community workers are often funded by local authorities whose policies and practices have traditionally been targets for change for community organisations. Consequently, 'Community workers increasingly find themselves in the paradoxical position of working with local campaigns to defend public services . . . including their own jobs' (ibid., p154).

The growth of marketplace thinking and its concern with outcome measures and performance indicators has meant that there are fewer openings for generalist community work. Funding has become tighter and more emphasis is placed on short term, time-limited activities.

As mentioned earlier community workers work mainly with disadvantaged people. Not everybody gained from the increased affluence generated during the 1980s: 'What's happened over the last ten years to material standards is that, broadly speaking, the bottom third of the population have in terms of income, become more and more detached from the top two thirds and the top two thirds have generally done allright. Community workers tend to work with the one third at the bottom of the pile' (ibid.). Consequently much of the activity of community workers is directed at supporting 'the reintegration of casualties of current public policies into mainstream society . . . Employment training, housing and industrial co-operatives, community care, and other initiatives represent, in a sense, the community worker's contribution to the development of the enterprise culture' (ibid., p155).

Community police work

The police are primarily concerned with law enforcement and crime prevention; however, there is also a strong community relations aspect to their work. During the 1960s and early 1970s, for reasons of efficiency and expediency in response to manpower shortages, much police work was done by officers in 'panda' cars. The sight of the 'bobby on the beat' became less common and the day-to-day contact between the police and the public was lost. Police officers became distanced from the communities they served. Since the early 1980s, however, there has been a move to re-establish local policing and foot patrolling. This has been made possible by increased recruitment.

Although community relations is a part of every police officer's general duties, it is often also a specialist function of police work which is carried out by a separate community contact department. This department, headed by an inspector, will be engaged in the two-way process of ascertaining community feelings and transmitting these to other police officers.

Community contact

The inspector, or an officer, will endeavour to make contact with the various community leaders, youth workers and heads of religious organisations and other community groups. Members of this department may also go into schools – both junior and secondary – and local colleges to talk about the history and practice of policing. The idea is to inform about the role of the police, to attempt to break down barriers and to challenge the stereotype images that tend to develop about their activities – indeed, to present the human element of those involved in police work.

Missing persons

The police are involved in trying to trace people who are reported missing for various reasons. The police may try to find someone in response to a request from a family member who is concerned for that person's safety. Once the police have located someone who is listed as a 'missing' person and are satisfied that they are safe and well and are not being coerced to remain in their present situation, they will report this to the friend or relative who instigated the inquiry and take the reported name off the missing persons list. The police are not obliged to reveal the whereabouts of any adult who wishes this to be kept secret.

Juvenile offenders

The police are generally reluctant to bring a child before the court, particularly if they have not been in trouble before. First offences are therefore often dealt with by a caution in the presence of the child's parents. There have been occasions, though, when even a series of cautions has not had the required effect and so a court appearance has become unavoidable. In all cases of juvenile crime, the police aim to obtain an indepth appreciation of the child's social setting, schooling and family circumstances and these will be taken into account before any decisions are made.

Child abuse

Cases involving child abuse are dealt with by police officers, the majority of whom are women working in a specialist team. A representative of the police will be present at all case conferences to provide relevant and confidential information about the family involved.

Like social workers, the police have a statutory power to remove a child from home to a 'place of safety' if necessary (the placement of the child is usually arranged in consultation with the social services department). An emergency protection order taken out by the police expires after 72 hours, but it does not have to be granted by a magistrate, as is the case with a social services application.

It is becoming standard practice to videotape interviews with children who are the victims of sexual and/or physical abuse. These may later be used as evidence in court.

Rape crisis/domestic violence units

Specialist police officers, again principally women, are involved in interviewing and counselling women who are the victims of violent and or sexual attacks, including rape. They will have received training intended to enable them to deal sensitively and supportively with this particular client group.

Domestic violence units were first introduced in June 1987 in Tottenham by Colette Paul and Annette O'Reilly. This practice has spread throughout the UK. Wherever possible police officers will work from neutral, informal settings, often ordinary housing, in order to reduce undue anxiety and put people as much as possible at their ease.

Interagency co-operation

Countless reports and enquiries over the past 20 or so years have stressed the need for and value of interagency co-operation. These recommendations have met with some success; today, in some areas, specific procedures are in place to ensure that interventions are co-ordinated. However, we are still a long way from the establishment of a fully integrated, co-operative, multidisciplinary interagency system of providing care.

In 1973 the tragedy of Maria Colwell – the seven year old girl who died as a result of sustained maltreatment by her stepfather while in the care of the local authority – drew the attention of the general public to the harsh realities of the problem of child abuse. It also highlighted the inadequacy of the collective response of the caring agencies. The public inquiry which followed criticised the professional agencies involved with the family, not only for some of the decisions reached but also for the lack of communication between them. As a result, all local authorities have now published guidelines for those who may be involved in the investigation of, or working with, families in which non-accidental injury has occurred or is considered likely to occur. Liaison with other agencies is built into the procedure. Non-accidental injury refers to psychological cruelty, physical harm and sexual abuse.

Child Protection Register (CPR)

The names of all children who have been, or are suspected of having been, abused by those in charge of them are placed on the child protection register (formerly known as the non-accidental injury register). Once their names are on the 'at risk' register, as it is generally called, the cases are reviewed at regular intervals, initially after three months and then six monthly, until such time as all the agencies concerned in working with the family are convinced that the child is no longer in danger. This register will be kept in a named place (such as a children's ward in a hospital, civic centre or in an NSPCC special unit, where this exists,) and will be accessible at all hours of the day and night, every day, to all professionals who are dealing with the family. Parents have a right to know that their child is on the register; they are invited to the case conference and given written details of its outcome and recommendations.

Other reports

It is not only in the field of child protection that interagency collaboration has been consistently urged and recommended. In 1974 a DHSS circular outlined the need for the newly reorganised health service to work more closely with local authorities. Statutory joint planning was introduced for health authorities and social services departments in 1977 (DHSS Circular 1977/HC4 on the Health Services Act 1976.) The Barclay Report 1982 stated that: 'Dealing with a vulnerable person with a complex problem often entails the development of a network of collaborative relationships between social worker, client, family, the local community, others who may be concerned and one or more of the public, or voluntary agencies that have relevant interests or resources' (8; 2 p113). The 1984 DHSS Health Circular (HC84/9 Health Services Development) extended collaboration between the NHS and local authorities to voluntary organisations. The Disabled Persons' (Services Consultation and Representation) Act 1986 made provision for the disabled person to be personally involved in the joint assessment. Later the reports *Agenda for Action* (1988) and *Working for Patients* (DOH, 1989) and the White Paper *Caring for People* (1989) all stressed the need for collaboration and this has been echoed in subsequent legislation, notably the National Health Service and Community Care Act 1990 and the Children Act 1989.

Barriers to collaboration

There is no great tradition of collaboration between the different agencies because of a number of factors:

1. Various public services developed separately from one another. 'Some, for example, medical and educational services, have roots that reach deep into the past and have developed a high degree of professional self-confidence, other services are more recent' (Barclay Report, 8.2).
2. Organisational structures differ, so that doctors, for example, are generally more autonomous within the health service than social workers working in local authorities.
3. Except in the whole of Wales, much of Scotland and in parts of England, health authority boundaries are not the same as those of the local authority and this has led to administrative confusion and practical difficulties.
4. Professional rivalry and mistrust of other organisations owing to differences in backgrounds and training experiences.

5. Lack of proper structures for interdepartmental collaboration. In a recent survey of social services departments in London carried out by Centre Point, '60 percent of SSDs felt existing structures were ineffective and 53 percent felt structures for collaboration with other agencies were not working properly' (*Community Care*, 18.3.93).
6. Bad feelings when 'troublesome exceptions' have been referred on. 'The fact that another service has difficulty in dealing with a problem does not necessarily make it a social problem to which a social worker is the right person to respond' (Barclay Report, 1982).
7. Ignorance of another person's role. For example, a medical social worker who recently sought fellow colleagues' knowledge and awareness of social work commented: 'Many of our colleagues viewed us, basically, as (just) arrangers of domiciliary help, meals on wheels, and residential care' (*Community Care*, 4.3.93, p25).
8. Pressure of work and lack of time to meet and discuss service users' circumstances as frequently as desired.

Advantages of collaboration

The advantages of interagency co-operation are quite obvious: information can be passed; links can be made; and checks can be more easily carried out. Ultimately it leads to a better service for the client because it lessens confusion; it facilitates a unified approach to planning; and it adds to the worker's overall understanding. This last point is particularly important with regard to the stipulations of the Children Act 1989: according to section 17 (10) of the Act, 'Services should be provided for children who cannot achieve or maintain a reasonable standard of physical, intellectual, social and behavioural development and physical and mental health without the provision of those services'. Social workers are unlikely to be sufficiently knowledgeable in all these areas to be able, alone or in teams, to fully assess a child's health and development. They are therefore urged by the guidelines accompanying the Act to consult a broad range of professionals in order to obtain the necessary information.

Collaboration is further emphasised by the demands made by the NHS and Community Care Act 1990. For instance, all local authority community care plans must include contingencies for joint working between the local authority, the health authority, voluntary organisations, 'not-for-profit' and private organisations. Additionally the service user and their carer need to be informed and involved in service planning and delivery. Similarly the Children Act 1989, as well as hastening the development of joint working between the agencies, has extended the idea of partnership to parents and young children.

Case conferences

Case conferences may be called for reasons other than suspected child abuse – for example, to discuss an elderly person who is at risk in order to decide whether or not they need permanent residential care. Similarly, an establishment for adults with

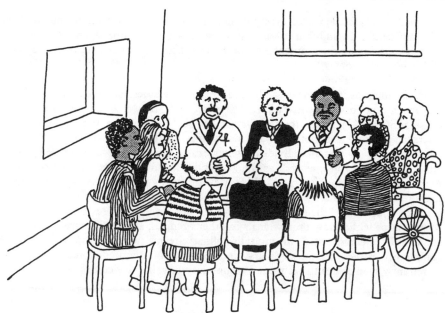

Case conferences enable representatives of various agencies to share knowledge and assess
and plan future involvement

learning difficulties may arrange a case conference to see whether or not a person is
ready to move on to a more independent form of living. In each case all the
professional workers involved from the various agencies and the staff of the
establishment concerned will be invited to attend to offer interpretations and
observations of the person's circumstances as seen from their perspective. It is
appropriate to invite parents or relatives to listen to what is said and to invite them to
contribute to the decision that is made.

Other agencies who may call a case conference include the education department
and the health authority.

Case conferences are sometimes held when another agency becomes involved or
takes over responsibility – for example, when the Probation Service assumes
responsibility for a young person from social services when they have offended
and have been brought before the court; also, when a family whose name is on the
child protection register in one area moves to another area.

Case conferences should not be confused with reviews, which are usually carried out
internally within establishments or area offices without necessarily involving outside
agencies. (Child protection case reviews however, involve all agencies.) It is a statutory
requirement that children who are accommodated should be officially reviewed at least
once every six months (after the initial series of reviews) but some are reviewed more
often. This procedure gives the main social worker involved (the residential social
worker, if the child is in a home; the fieldworker if the child is in the community) an
opportunity to outline work done, consider any existing difficulties and determine plans
for the future. Written care plans must be made with the parents and the child. A report
will be presented and discussed with senior management and other interested parties.

Although there is not always a legal obligation to do so, other clients are sometimes reviewed in this fashion – for example, older people, mentally ill adults and families with difficulties. In addition to social services departments, other agencies carry out reviews in the same way; for instance, probation officers may consider their progress with clients at reviews.

Interagency working, as we have seen, is very necessary for the achievement of good, harmonious care. However, there are many difficulties yet to be overcome. The Department of Health investigation *Child Abuse – A Study of Inquiry Reports 1980– 89* (HMSO, 1991) states that: 'A lesson to be learned from the 1980s is that interagency working is not easy, and not self-evidently useful'. (p 41) It goes on: 'That is not to say that an individual agency can go it alone, but separate viewpoints and confusion of roles, as well as the availability of multiple settings for communication, are a recipe for muddle'. However, the more proactive agencies have managed to overcome some of the obstacles and now work together to provide service. Individuals themselves have struck up beneficial, reciprocal working relationships with fellow professionals in other agencies; and collaboration has been successfully demonstrated in multidisciplinary teams within hospitals, and in community based, multidisciplinary, interagency, jointly funded teams such as community mental health teams and community learning difficulties teams.

Conclusion

This chapter has dealt with the caring services of the statutory agencies other than the Probation Service and the social services authorities. Each agency has its own primary function, too detailed to describe here and beyond the scope of this book. Instead we have sought to outline the social care functions of these organisations.

As has been mentioned, the statutory agencies developed independently and at different times concerned with their individual spheres of responsibility; consequently even the geographical boundaries of local authority and non-local authorities often cut across one another. However, in recent years co-operation and joint planning have increased. This is evident in many fields: community care plans; homeless family projects combining personnel from local authority housing, education and social services departments; and the interagency involvement required to ascertain a child's educational special needs.

The statutory sector is in the process of relinquishing its provider role in favour of one incorporating the functions of assessment, purchasing and inspection. Local authorities and health authorities are performing their roles within a mixed economy of care which, in addition to the statutory sector, is made up of voluntary, not-for-profit and private agencies. It is to this independent sector we now turn.

Appendix 1 – example of a problem presented to the head of the third year in a secondary school

Barry Shoefield is a 13 year old twin whose brother Michael is also at the school. They have three older sisters who are either still attending or have left the same school. Barry has a history of sporadic attendance, whereas Michael (who is in a different class) works well and enjoys school. The difference in attitude to work and to school has been most clearly marked since their transition from lower to upper school three months ago.

Monday

Barry is absent from school all day. His twin brother is unable to offer any reason for this.

Tuesday

Mrs Shoefield, the boys' mother, who has expressed an 'anti-school' attitude in the past, calls to see the year tutor, bringing barry with her. She begins with an explanation. The previous day, Barry met his 18 year old friend in the twon centre at 9.00 a.m. and did not return to the family home until 11.00 p.m. When he arrived home, he claimed to have been kidnapped by two men on his way to school. The uniformed branch of the police became involved, and later Barry was interviewed by the CID. Eventually, at 2.40 p.m, Barry broke down and admitted that he had made up the story in an attempt to avoid being punished for what he had done.

Response

The head of year appreciates the mother's concern, particularly in view of her previous unco-operative attitude towards the school. As a short term measure he suggests that Barry be placed 'on report'. This means that he is given a report card which is to be signed by teachers detailing attendance for morning and afternoon sessions, conduct and effort made. This card is then stamped daily by the head of year and taken home by Barry and signed by his parents. Thus a detailed up-to-date record of attendance and attitude is obtained. Meanwhile, Barry is referred to the educational psychologist.

Mrs Shoefield is informed that the social services department could be involved if she would find this useful, perhaps to explore Barry's relationship with other family members.

At the same time, the year tutor makes himself available to Barry, saying that he would be happy to see Barry any time he feels like making an appointment. At present, Barry is not very forthcoming about why he stays away from school.

Comment

In this case it can be seen that the year tutor does all he can to try to solve the problem within the school. Problems are often brought into school from outside – from within the family or community – and teachers are restricted in the type of help they can offer.

Appendix 2 – typical duties for a head of year

8.20–8.45   Arrive at school. Check mail, notes, letters, court reports, telephone messages, etc. See staff about any outstanding problems. Check staff absences to see if I need to substitute for anyone.

8.45–9.00   Pupils arrive.

   8.50   Registration. See as many pupils as possible about chasing up problems/ truants. For more difficult problems, tell pupils to come back when I am free.

   9.00   Assembly:
   Monday – full school assembly.
   Tuesday – third-year assembly, led by year tutor.
   Wednesday – third- and fourth-year assembly, led by head of upper school. Tutors come to see me.
   Thursday and *Friday* – tutor period: pupils see their own tutors. As head of year, same as 8.45–9.00.

	Mon	Tues	Weds	Thurs	Fri
9.15–10.25	Free*	3rd yr games	Free*	5th yr community project	Support†
10.25–10.40			Break		
10.40–11.50	5th yr links with FE	3rd yr PSE	Support†	5th yr skills programme	Free*
11.50–12.45			Lunch		
12.45–12.55			Registration		
12.55–14.05	See Education Social Worker	4th yr history	5th yr AC	5th yr PSE	3rd yr history
14.10–15.20	3rd yr history	Free*	Free*	4th yr PSE	5th yr careers

* Free from teaching. Time spent on phone calls, meetings with parents, social workers, probation officers. See pupils. Write letters. Sometimes called to classroom to deal with pupils' misbehaviour. Do all my own filing; write up records; do all the jobs I've been putting off for weeks, write reports for courts or social services.

† Teacher may book me to go into a class to help with less able pupils, enabling her to work with a smaller group on a specialist topic.

PSE = personal and social education

15.20 onwards See as many pupils as possible. Some arrive with report cards checking behaviour/attendance/work. Others arrive with notes from teachers concerning problems related to the day's lessons – behaviour, work, 'no pen', etc. Make phone calls. See parents. See available staff about pupils. Attend meetings (average two or three a week on personal issues, curriculum, etc.). Try to go to watch my year's teams – cricket, netball, hockey, football, etc. Occasionally make home visits, usually as an emergency – injuries, long term truancy, both parents working (now quite rare) or parents genuinely unable to get to school.

17.15 Go home – provided there is no union meeting, staff development course or parents' evening.

Exercise 1 – role play – an example of a case presented to a head of year

8.50 Mrs Hallam and her daughter Liz (aged 15) arrive at the head of year's office without an appointment. Mrs Hallam slams down a tin of glue, saying that last night she went into her daughter's room and found Liz semiconscious. Mrs Hallam would like to know, 'Is the school going to do anything about this?'.

Roles

1. Liz   This was the first time you had used solvents at home, but you have sniffed glue outside the home several times.
2. Liz's *mother*   Angry and desperate, expecting the school to be able to provide a solution.
3. *Head of year*   You decide on the head of year's response.

Task

Role play the scene (ten minutes).

Exercise 2 – role play – an example of a problem presented to a form tutor

Jenny Best is 16 years old and in the fifth form of a comprehensive school. During the second year she had attendance problems for a few weeks, around the time that her mother remarried. Since then she has worked well and she is now preparing to take her GCSEs.

She has always been overweight and, since she broke her leg four weeks ago, has recently depended on her stepfather to bring her to and pick her up from school.

One morning when he brings her to school, her stepfather rather angrily points out to the form teacher, Ms Martin, in front of Jenny that he has had 'enough of Jenny's behaviour at home', which is rapidly deteriorating. Mr Best is asking for some kind of help from the teacher.

As soon as her stepfather leaves, Jenny breaks down and starts to cry.

Roles

1. *Jenny*

a) You are anxious about your forthcoming exams. Your teachers expect you to pass them, but you feel that you will not be able to do enough work in time.

b) You are worried about your weight. Being immobile with a broken leg is adding to your problem.

c) You have recently discovered that your stepfather is having an affair with another woman. Your mother is aware of this.

d) You are the oldest of three children, but your brother and sister are too young to talk seriously with. Since you have been studying for your GCSE's, you have lost contact with your best friend and do not really know who to talk to.

e) You like Ms. Martin and have done so since she taught you English in the second year.

2. *Ms Martin*

a) You like Jenny and feel that she is a good student, capable of doing very well provided she continues to work hard.

b) You have other teaching duties (a class in ten minutes).

c) You could see her for some time after school.

Task

Role play the talk between Jenny and Ms Martin.

Exercise 3A – a points system for housing allocation

Devise your own points system for housing allocation, based on the categories already outlined in this chapter. You can decide on which category should be allocated the highest number of points – for example, start with 100 points and apportion them between the categories you decide upon.

Exercise 3B – allocation of a one-bedroomed dwelling

Apply your points system to the following applicants for a one-bedroomed dwelling and establish a priority waiting list:

a) *Mrs Silcock* (49) lives alone in a bedsitter. She has no separate kitchen and shares the bathroom with six other people. The bedsitter is damp and in poor condition. Mrs Silcock has recently had a stroke and would like to move nearer to the hospital where she attends regularly for physiotherapy.

b) *Mr Worrell* (35) is single and currently in prison. He would like accommodation on his release in four weeks' time. He has the prospect of fulltime work locally.

c) *Mr Jarvis* (32) is single and living at home with his mother and father in a three-bedroomed flat. He would like to move nearer to the city centre, where he works as a shop manager. At the moment it takes him an hour and a half to get to work each morning by public transport.

d) *Ms Flynn* (46) is a voluntary patient in a psychiatric hospital where she has been staying for three months. She is being encouraged by nursing staff. She would like self-contained accommodation near to her parents, who live in a small council flat.

e) *Mr Akram* (27) is unmarried and a tenant in a one-bedroomed multistorey flat. He has a fulltime job and is studying for A-levels at night school. He would like eventually to go to university. He finds the noise and music from the surrounding flats distracting and would like to be transferred to a quieter area.

f) *Mr Grogan* (28) is legally separated from his wife but is still living in the three-bedroomed family home with her and their three children. He sleeps on the sofa in the living room and shares all the facilities of the home. Mrs Grogan is distressed and has repeatedly asked him to leave, but he claims that he has nowhere else to go.

g) *Mrs Hutchins* (59) is a divorcee who lives in a three-bedroomed house. This is now too big for her needs, as all her children have left home. She would like a smaller dwelling – preferably a ground-floor flat, as she has arthritis and climbing stairs is difficult for her.

Exercise 3C – allocation of a three-bedroomed dwelling

Apply your points system to the following applicants for a two- or three-bedroomed dwelling and establish a priority waiting list:

a) *Mr and Mrs Connelly* own their own three-bedroomed house. Their daughter is physically disabled and now too heavy to be carried upstairs. They would like ground-floor accommodation with bathroom facilities at ground level.

b) *Mr and Mrs Lynch* and their two sons and daughter are tenants of a three-bedroomed house. The family is the victim of racial harassment, and recently youths physically assaulted their home, breaking a window and damaging the front door. They would like to move away from the area, particularly because the children are becoming distressed.

c) *Mrs Hanson* is a young single mother who cares for her six year old daughter in their two-bedroomed council flat. Mrs Hanson has recently been violently attacked by the child's father and fears further violence. She feels that the only way she can be safe is to move out of the area altogether.

d) *Richard Lord and Dianne Turner* are a young couple lodging with Richard's parents. Dianne is expecting a baby within the next two months and they have been asked to leave before the baby arrives.

e) *Mrs Carroll* is a single parent and lives with her young twin sons in a two-bedroomed council flat. The neighbour below keeps complaining unduly about noise from their flat. She writes abusive letters and shouts foul language along the corridor. Mrs Carroll is very anxious and has been prescribed sedatives by her doctor. She would like to move to another area.

f) *Mrs Eduh* is a widow who, together with her adult daughter, lodges in a one-bedroomed flat. Mrs Eduh has arthritis and finds the stairs difficult. They are sharing facilities with the landlord, who now would like them to leave as he intends selling his house.

g) *Mrs Thompson* has been living in another part of the country in army accommodation with her husband and two children. The couple's marriage has now broken down and she would like to return to her city of origin and obtain two-bedroomed accommodation for herself and two children.

Exercise 4 – interview with a service provider

Either provide a brief report or detailed notes on which to base a short talk to others in your group. You may find it useful to cover the following questions.

1. Why did the incumbent choose to do the job?
2. What training did they have?
3. What does the job involve?
4. How much power do they have within the organisation?
5. How much autonomy does the person have?
6. Do they enjoy the work?
7. Are there any constraints on their role?
8. What is the person's view on the agency's equal opportunities policy?

Remember to ask permission to take notes or to use a tape recorder during the interview with the service provider. You need to assure the interviewer that the material will only be used in the confidential setting of the teaching seminar for learning purposes.

Questions for discussion

1. There is often much 'stigma' attached to people who experience mental illness. Why do you think society feels so differently about physical and mental illness?
2. Compared with other EEC countries, preschool provision in the UK is low. In countries like France and Belgium, 90 percent of three to five year olds have fulltime places in nursery schools or their equivalent. What advantages –

particularly to the socially disadvantaged child – can be had from nursery provision?

3. There are very few black police officers in this country. Why do you think this is so and what can be done to improve recruitment from ethnic minority members of society?

4. Some people argue that it is important for professional carers – social workers, teachers and community workers – to actually live in the area in which they work, in order to more fully understand the families whom they are seeking to help and to identify with the needs of the community. Consider the advantages or disadvantages of this proposition.

5. Consider the statement, 'All single homeless people are vulnerable by their very circumstances and should be offered support'.

6. The statutory sector should be expanded because it is more likely to produce a cohesive service than one which is made up predominantly of voluntary and private agencies.

Further reading

1. *Give me Shelter*, Michael Rosen (Bodley Head, 1991). An anthology of poems, stories and illustrations about the lives of people who are or have been homeless.

2. *Opting Out – Choice and the Future of Schools* Martin Rogers (Lawrence and Wishart, 1992). A clear and factual guide to what 'opting out' means for teachers, parents, students, governors and local authorities.

3. *Coming out of the Blue*, – Marc Burke (Cassell, 1993). British police officers talk about their lives in 'the job' as lesbians, gays and bisexuals.

4. *The NHS Under New Management*, Philip Strong and Jane Robinson (Open University, 1990). An up to date, readable guide to the changes made to the NHS.

5. *The Hidden Struggle*, Amina Mama (London Race and Housing Research Unit, c/o The Runnymede Trust, 1989). A detailed and interesting account of the experiences of homeless black women who are fleeing violence and the discrimination they are faced with at the hands of statutory agencies.

6. *Young, Gifted and Black – Student-Teacher Relations in the Schooling of Black Youth*, Mairtin MacanGhaill (Open University Press, 1988). A very detailed account of the relationship between young black people, their teachers, the school system and the effects of racism.

5

The Independent Sector – The Voluntary Sector in a Mixed Economy of Care

Introduction

The voluntary sector is sometimes called the 'third sector' (statutory and private organisations are the first and second, respectively). It consists of an estimated 400 000 voluntary organisations in the UK, many of which are concerned with social care. Following the restructuring of the Welfare State over the past 15 years, voluntary bodies form an important part of today's mixed economy of welfare. This mixed economy is made up of:

1. *Statutory services*, e.g. Social Services Departments, the Probation Service and the Education Welfare Service;
2. *Voluntary organisations*, e.g. Gingerbread and the National Schizophrenia Fellowship and specific local community organisations;
3. *Private companies*, particularly in the field of residential care, less well-established, as yet, in domiciliary services.
4. *Not-for-profit (or 'non-profit') organisations*, made up mainly of a growing number of 'trusts', set up to manage former local authority residential homes.

The last three categories, voluntary, private and not-for-profit organisations, make up the *independent sector*, i.e. bodies that are 'non-statutory', that is, independent from the state. The extent of this independence will vary, depending on the particular relationship the organisation has with the local authority (the 'local state') or central Government. Government funding, for example, may bring with it a certain amount of state control.

This chapter concentrates on the voluntary sector because it has been established for a long time and is of considerable importance as a provider of social care. The voluntary sector is by far the largest provider within the independent sector. The chapter also deals with the growing private and not-for-profit sectors; these are having an increasing impact on care provision.

What is a voluntary organisation?

Finding an acceptable definition of a voluntary organisation is a complex matter. The boundaries between the voluntary and other sectors are becoming increasingly blurred. *The Voluntary Agencies Directory* provides a broad definition: 'A self-governing body of people who have joined together voluntarily to take action for the betterment (as they perceive it) of the community, and are established otherwise than for financial gain' (p xi). Voluntary organisations should not be linked to any political party. Some are registered as charities.

Currently, over 170 000 voluntary bodies (less than half) are officially registered as charities. Charitable status is granted by the Charity Commission in England and Wales, or the Inland Revenue in Scotland and Northern Ireland. The authorities must be satisfied that the purpose or object of the organisation is exclusively charitable and that it benefits the community in some way. Examples of 'benefit' are the relief of poverty or the advancement of education or religion.

The word 'charity' is derived from the Latin word *caritas*, meaning 'regard, esteem, affection, love'. In the mid-nineteenth century, when the first voluntary organisations were founded, they were literally known as 'charities'.

Registered charities gain the following advantages: they may claim tax and rate relief and they are allowed to receive money in the form of covenants. Each year some 4 000 new charities are registered and some, of course, cease to exist.

It is important not to confuse voluntary organisations with *voluntary work* performed by *volunteers*. A voluntary organisation is a non-statutory body. Some happen to be staffed by unpaid volunteers, but others use no volunteers at all – they employ only salaried staff; only their management committees give their services free. It is the status of an organisation that makes it voluntary, not the status of the staff working within it. Many statutory agencies use volunteers too; the Probation Service utilises volunteers for such tasks as providing transport (expenses paid) for relatives to visit a prison.

Having said this, most voluntary bodies do rely on volunteers to perform a wide variety of tasks. Two examples may make the situation clearer:

1. Age Concern employs salaried staff at its central office and elsewhere, but recruits volunteers to work with elderly people in its local branches.
2. MIND (the National Association for Mental Health) employs salaried staff for its national organisation functions, but volunteers are used at local level to counsel distressed people who seek help.

A national survey of voluntary activity in the UK, carried out in 1991 by the Volunteer Centre, provides some interesting data about 'working for free'. Over 23 million adults were found to be involved in some form of voluntary work each year. According to the survey, fundraising was the most common type of voluntary activity. People aged between 35 and 44 were the most likely to volunteer and women were slightly more likely to volunteer than men.

Many voluntary organisations employ professionally qualified workers in salaried posts, just as statutory services do. Two examples are social work staff working for the NSPCC or Family Service Units (both voluntary bodies) and trained nursery nurses working in voluntary sector playgroups.

Origins of the voluntary sector

The process of industrialisation and the establishment of cities and large urban conurbations in the late eighteenth century and through into the nineteenth century

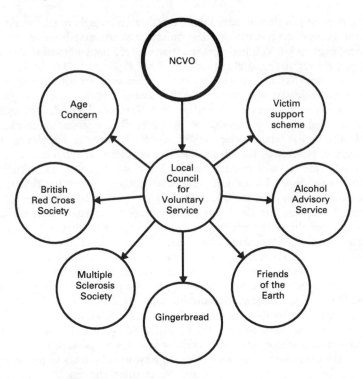

Fig 5.1   The NCVO co-ordinates local Councils for Voluntary Service, and these in turn co-ordinate the activities of a wide range of different groups.

brought with it a range of problems and social pressures: overcrowding, poverty, squalor, drunkenness and child labour became commonplace. By about the mid-nineteenth century there had developed a strong feeling, particularly among sections of the middle class, that some form of relief must be found. Various 'philanthropic organisations' were formed by people of altruistic concern, very often professing the Christian faith. Many of these organisations are still with us today and remain within the voluntary sector. For example, Dr Barnardo's was founded in 1866; the Church of England Children's Society in 1881; and the NSPCC in 1889.

But charity organisation got out of hand; there was such a proliferation of charities, and such a confusion and overlapping of services, that in 1869 the Charity Organisation Society (COS) or, to give it its full title, the Society for Organising Charity and Repressing Mendicity was formed, to conserve efforts and plan more rationally.

Later, in the twentieth century, the COS became the Family Welfare Association and moved from its role as a co-ordinating body to become more directly involved in the relief of poverty and the promotion of mental health. Its umbrella role was taken on by local and national Councils for Voluntary Service and by the National Council for Voluntary Organisations, which was established in 1919 as the National Council for Social Services, describing itself as 'the representative body for the voluntary sector'.

During the period of the two world wars and the economic depression of the 1930s, the State moved increasingly to provide welfare services directly, but the creation of the Welfare State did not do away with the need for voluntary organisations. The Second World War years, in particular, saw very close co-operation between the State and voluntary effort; many voluntary groups including women's groups, citizens' advice bureaux and the Red Cross played an important part in the war effort.

Since 1945 various voluntary bodies have evolved to meet particular needs as they arose or as public concern highlighted need. To give a few prominent examples: in 1946, MIND (the National Association for Mental Health) was formed; in 1965 the APEX Trust was formed to help people with a criminal record find employment; in 1970 Gingerbread was formed to support lone parents; and in 1986, London Lighthouse was formed to help people with the HIV virus and/or AIDS.

The great strengths of the voluntary sector continue to be its variety, its flexibility and its predilection for keeping in step with the times. Because of the economic and political move towards a unified Europe, a European Council for Voluntary Organisations has been established; it held its first General Assembly in June 1990.

The range of activity

The range of interests and activities of voluntary organisations is wide and diverse. This may be illustrated by looking at some of the differing roles of voluntary bodies and some specific examples:

1. *Self-help* bodies provide mutual aid or support centred on a common need or interest, e.g. Alcoholics Anonymous (AA);
2. Some voluntary organisations have a *pressure group* function; they campaign or press for a particular cause or interest, e.g. Child Poverty Action Group (CPAG);
3. Others have an *advocacy* function; they speak for, or represent, the views and/or interests of particular groups of people, e.g. *Release* works with drug users and will arrange legal representation for those in trouble with the law;
4. There are bodies that have a *co-ordinating* function; they act as an umbrella organisation for a number of other agencies, e.g. the Organisation Development Unit; this recently became independent of the NCVO and acts as a development agency for black voluntary groups;
5. Finally, some groups have a *service-providing function*; they provide a direct service to people in a variety of ways, in kind or in the form of information, advice and support; for example, the Spastics Society (soon to be renamed) provides a whole range of services, including residential care for people with cerebral palsy and related disabilities.

It would be erroneous to try and pigeonhole all voluntary organisations into the above five categories. In fact, most would consider themselves to be multifunctional, incorporating several of the above roles, in addition to providing information, carrying out research, educating the public, monitoring other, perhaps statutory, services and attempting to innovate and bring new ideas or practices into social care and welfare.

The past 30 years have seen a phenomenal growth in the voluntary sector, with more new groups being formed than at any other time. The estimated total income of the sector is currently running at £17 billion per year, which represents over 4 percent of the gross national product (GNP). There are some 250 000 paid employees, 1.5 million employees if volunteers are included. Central Government funding for voluntary bodies has been cut in recent years and with the announcement in November 1992 of the phasing out of the Urban Programme (cut from £240 million in 1992–3 to £176 million in 1993–4 and to £91 million in 1994–5), is set to decrease further.

Local authority funding for the voluntary sector is also decreasing. An NCVO survey published in 1992 showed a drop of £29.4 million in the financial year 1991–2 over the previous year, with a further cut of 13 million in 1992–3. At the same time, contributions from private, profit-making businesses (sometimes referred to as the 'corporate sector') are decreasing, as are contributions from the public. The former stands at £100 million per year, the latter at £5 billion. The overall picture is therefore one of a growing number of voluntary groups competing for a decreasing amount of money.

The changing nature of the voluntary sector

The Beveridge Report of 1942, which led to the consolidation of the Welfare State during and after the Second World War, referred to voluntary groups as being 'society's conscience'. Such groups keep in touch with changing needs in society and respond to them as they arise. Because they are moderate in size and have flexibility of organisation and management, they are often better placed to defend and champion the interests of minorities in society than are the statutory services.

However, many people believe that the future of some voluntary organisations may be under threat because of changes brought about by the recent community care legislation. In particular, local authority social services departments in England and Wales, and social work departments in Scotland, are being transformed from direct providers of services (residential, domiciliary, day care, etc.) to purchasers of services from other agencies. Financing for nursing and residential care has been transferred from the Department of Social Security to local authorities and 85 percent of the total sum a local authority spends on these services has, as from 1st April 1993, to be spent in the independent sector which, of course, includes the voluntary sector.

As a result of these changes some voluntary organisations have begun to have a different relationship with the statutory sector. They are now providing services under contract to local councils and consequently their relationship with the statutory sector is more formalised than in the past. The last few years have seen the emergence of what has been called a 'contract culture' and a move away from the simple grant aid that local authorities provided for voluntary groups. This has thrust voluntary bodies into the world of business, with much talk of 'financial management', 'markets' and the 'marketing of services', 'budgetary control' and 'returns'. Some voluntary organisations' contracts with the local authority are having agreements tied to the continuation of their general grants. Therefore, if their contract is not renewed, their financial security and future existence could be placed in jeopardy.

In turn, local authorities are having to be more stringent about how they distribute grants and award contracts, as the relationship between the local authority and the voluntary sector becomes more businesslike. They are more demanding, less amenable and more critical of services provided.

Fears concerning these developments have been openly expressed by key people and groups in the voluntary sector. The 1991–2 Annual Review of the NCVO stated:

> The main fear about the contract culture is that it will force voluntary organisations to become more commercial and competitive and less charitable. Critics also say that contracts will squeeze out smaller community groups, ethnic minority groups and those who do work that isn't about providing measurable services.'(p 11)

Lynne Berry, director of the Family Welfare Association (FWA) writes: 'Many voluntary bodies are concerned about this trend (towards becoming "businesses") and are weighing up the need for financial viability against a loss of independence and self-direction' (Social Work Today, 28.1.93) In referring to the more formalised link with the statutory sector, she continues, in the same article: 'Moreover, the subsidising of public services is a highly questionable use of charitable funds'.

The private sector

The private sector has a tradition of providing care. For example, people who have been able to afford to pay have lond had the choice of being able to buy their own care from private nursing and social care organisations.

In recent years, notably since 1980 when the Government, via the Department of Health and Social Security, undertook to meet residential care costs of individuals who did not have private means, there has been a proliferation in the number of privately run establishments. The growth in the number of private care homes can be traced to this initiative.

The subsequent rising cost to the Government of residential care for older people who had not even been assessed to establish whether or not they needed residential care caused great concern and was a primary reason behind the introduction of community care legislation. Only those residents who were in homes before April 1993 will continue to be supported directly through the DSS. From this date the local authority has been responsible for assessing whether someone needs to go into residential care and for purchasing that care.

It is not only care and nursing homes for older people that are being supplied by private organisations; other client groups are also being serviced. Encouraged by the Government's push towards diversity of choice, privately run homes for young children, teenagers and young people, and adults with learning difficulties have opened. Of course private day nurseries and independent childminders have a long history of providing a child care service alongside a depleted and specialised public sector service. The local authority social service provision has been targetted on the needs of particularly deprived children including those at risk of harm or those failing to thrive in the home environment. In 1991 there were over four times as many registered private day nurseries as there were local authority day nurseries (National Children's Bureau Statistics, 1991).

Domiciliary services such as meals on wheels or home care, respite care and supported accommodation have been contracted out in some areas. Social services authorities have become more rationalised into discrete provider sections such as the training and research section, the juvenile justice team, and the home care team. All these can be 'hived off' to allow the service to be provided by private operators, where this can be done at a lower cost to the local authority.

Diversity, flexibility and adaptability are the reputed characteristics of private organisations. They can quickly respond to felt needs in the market. Unencumbered by the weight of a statutory bureaucracy, private providers are in a position to respond to developments, to make innovations and introduce improvements to practice. Many private organisations have contributed to developments of good care practice. Against this it has to be argued that private companies, by definition, will only be interested in providing services which make a profit, so residential homes, for example, will only be established in 'profitable' areas, not necessarily within the communities where need exists. They will be provided for clients out of whom they can make money and not necessarily for those people whose need for care is the greatest. With regard to residential provision it would appear that the local authority will have a residual role in providing for those people that the private and voluntary sectors are unwilling or unable to cater for, i.e. 'when other forms of service provision are unforthcoming or unsuitable' (Caring for People, para 3.4.11).

Not-for-profit organisations

The first acquaintance of the above, rather strange term for many people in social care would have come from a careful reading of the White Paper *Caring for People: Community Care in the next Decade and Beyond*, published on 16 November 1989. A sentence in the middle of paragraph 3.4.1 reads: 'The Government will expect local authorities to make use wherever possible of services from voluntary, 'not-for-profit' and private providers insofar as this represents a cost effective care choice' (p 22). It goes on to say that: 'Social services authorities . . . will be expected to take all reasonable steps to secure diversity of provision'.

Four years on, there is a growing number of these not-for-profit or non-profit 'trusts'. Some are staffed by ex-local authority workers and provide services under contract to social services departments; others are staffed by workers seconded by the local authority and others operate completely independently.

It is not easy to provide a clear definition of what a not-for-profit organisation is. The term 'not-for-profit' is American in origin. In the USA the term 'voluntary sector' is not used; instead the 'not-for-profit' sector signifies a grouping of all bodies that are neither statutory nor private profit-making businesses. For this reason, some people in Britain have dismissed the term as jargon, but it *is* being used increasingly to describe newly constituted providers of social care.

A number of not-for-profit trusts in the UK have been set up to run residential care homes, mostly for elderly people. The principal incentives for hard pressed, cut back, local authorities to set up such trusts were financial. Under the proposals for community care, local authorities were to be responsible in full, after 1 April 1993, for the cost of residents in local authority homes. In contrast, residents of non-local authority homes before that date had their benefit entitlements preserved; they had what was known as 'protected status'. There was therefore a clear financial incentive for local authorities to increase the number of residents in the 'protected' category, in order to avoid having to bear their financial responsibility. Many local authorities rushed to transfer their own homes to the 'non-profit' sector.

In doing so, social services authorities reduced their own revenue costs and, from the sales of homes, obtained capital funds; some of them used this capital to upgrade remaining homes in order to meet the more rigorous registration standards introduced by the 1984 Registered Homes Act.

Two important features help to differentiate not-for-profit organisations from voluntary bodies: firstly, unlike voluntary organisations, the boards that run them consist of salaried members; secondly, they do not involve the giving of voluntary effort either in time or money.

The pattern of these hybrid bodies varies across the country; sometimes their operations overlap with the domain of statutory, voluntary and private agencies. They differ in pattern throughout the country in organisation, status, legal structure, staffing and size. It is too early to accurately gauge their impact on the long term provision of social care but the expectation is that not-for-profit organisations will continue to grow.

Some examples of voluntary organisations

The voluntary sector and its relationship with the other sectors is changing continually. For this reason we cannot provide a comprehensive review of it in this chapter. That which follows is a look in more detail at a small number of voluntary organisations. Clearly, voluntary bodies vary in their structure and coverage. Some function at a national level; they campaign as a pressure group; they usually disseminate information in order to reach a wider audience and educate the public. The Terrence Higgins Trust fits this category.

Others have a national office and operate a national structure and profile, but also have a network of local groups or units. Both the Carers National Association and the NSPCC fall into this category. Finally, some voluntary bodies are purely local and small-scale, engaged in, say, 'grass roots' activity. The Pepper Pot Club and the Yemeni Community Association are two examples of such groups.

Of the five voluntary organisations featured, the NSPCC is the oldest, the others are more recent arrivals on the voluntary scene.

Carers National Association (Carers)

'Often you will acquire this post overnight, and therefore have no opportunity to train for this very demanding role, or to consider the great responsibility entailed. Not a job for the squeamish – you will carry out tasks you would never have thought you could do, which often require the expertise of a nurse, doctor, psychiatrist or accountant. (You need great skill in making ends meet, as many extra expenses occur.)' (*The Carer*, November 1990, p13)

In the above passage, a carer writes of the experience of being a carer and outlines some of the pressures and demands involved. In the UK today, there are an estimated six million individual carers. These are people who look after a family member, a relative or a friend who cannot manage at home without some form of help because of illness, frailty, disability or the effects of the ageing process. A carer may be caring for more than one person. The time involved in caring will vary a great deal according to a number of factors but most commonly, the degree of dependency of the person being cared for. 1.4 million of the six million carers spend more than 20 hours per week in caring for a person, or persons, in the person's own home.

Over the years, a variety of organisations have arisen, both at a national and local level, to cater for the needs of carers. But on 14th May 1988, two existing national voluntary organisations – the 'Association of Carers' and the 'National Council for Carers and their Elderly Dependents' – amalgamated and out of the merger was formed the 'Carers National Association' (CNA) or 'Carers' for short. This has now become an important support organisation for representing the interests of *all* carers.

The Association has four aims: 'to encourage carers to recognise their own needs; to develop appropriate support for carers; to provide information and advice for carers; and to bring the needs of carers to the attention of government and other policy-makers.' It has highlighted a number of problems that beset carers: social isolation; financial hardship and deterioration in mental and physical health.

In the financial year 1990–91, the total funds handled by the Association went over the £1 million mark for the first time. Funding comes from a number of sources including membership subscriptions, donations, fundraising, legacies and central and local Government grants. In addition, a large number of corporate sector businessess provide sponsorship.

Carers is a membership organisation, the membership of which has been constantly rising since its inception. Any individual carer can join, as well as others who wish to support the organisation, as individuals, as groups or as separate organisations that support the above aims. The Association is a member of the National Council for Voluntary Organisations (NCVO) and the Disability Alliance and it works very closely with a number of other voluntary organisations, e.g. Age Concern, the Alzheimer's Disease Society and the Parkinson's Disease Society. With a few other bodies, it has more formalised links: it has run a joint training project with Contact a Family which supports the parents of children with special needs; it has paid for two workers for Caring Costs, a coalition of national, regional and local voluntary organisations whose aim is to achieve an adequate income for all carers.

The Carers National Association is managed by a National Committee, made up of 16 elected carers and one co-opted member. Approximately 10 000 members meet either in one of the national network of local branches, of which there are about 100, or in smaller local groups. The size and activities of branches vary a good deal and just as there is no typical carer, so there is no typical branch. The branches represent the true 'lifeblood' of Carers. Meetings are held fortnightly or monthly and are of crucial importance. They allow carers to keep in touch, support each other, pass on information and skills, socialise and, very importantly, take a break from caring.

A representative sample of branch activities may include fundraising; setting up helplines; organising sitting schemes, publishing a newsletter and running a mobile clinic that visits shopping centres to give information, advice and support to carers, while at the same time campaigning to draw the public's attention to the needs of carers. A member of the Havering Branch in Essex is quoted as saying: 'We have a

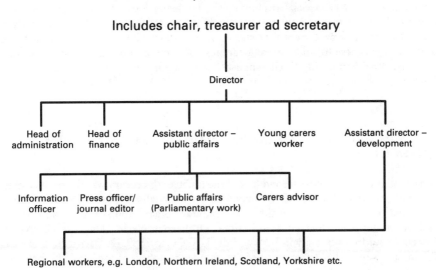

National Committee of Management
(16 elected by members, 1 co-opted)

Includes chair, treasurer ad secretary

Director

Head of administration | Head of finance | Assistant director – public affairs | Young carers worker | Assistant director – development

Information officer | Press officer/ journal editor | Public affairs (Parliamentary work) | Carers advisor

Regional workers, e.g. London, Northern Ireland, Scotland, Yorkshire etc.

Fig 5.2 Simplified organisational structure of the Carers National Association.

wonderful spirit of friendship in the group. Members feel they belong; it is their club where they meet friends' (Annual Report 1990–91, p7).

Apart from the central office in Barbican, London, which is the national co-ordinating centre, there are offices in Scotland, Wales and Northern Ireland, Yorkshire and London. Working from these bases are a growing number of paid workers who work to a high professional standard. Based at the central office is a public affairs team, consisting of an information officer, press officer, carers advisor and a public affairs team leader. The press officer also edits the Association's bimonthly journal *The Carer*. Branches are supported by salaried workers who help to co-ordinate activities and start new initiatives.

Carers has become increasingly skilled at using the media, including television, radio and press, both nationally and locally. The Department of Health has recently increased its grant and many social services departments consult the Association on community care arrangements. Carers has a growing public profile, but as Jill Pitkeathley, the Director, recently wrote, there must 'be no lessening of (the Association's) efforts – on the contrary, we must build on the firm base we have now established, to ensure that carers are recognised by the reality as well as by the rhetoric of social and political policy' (Annual Report 1990–91, p3). In addition, the 1990–91 Annual Report contained the optimistic statement: 'At long last, the word "carer" seems to mean something to journalists, policy-makers and the public' (p10).

Recently, the Association turned its attention to two groups of carers who are often overlooked and who need more support: rural carers and black and minority ethnic carers. Within the latter group, young people who act as carers are thought to need particular help, suffering as they do from 'double discrimination'. Carers, along with the King's Fund Centre, jointly organised a national conference in 1991 on the theme 'Young Carers in Black and Minority Ethnic Communities'. Delegates discussed issues such as poor financial resources, the inadequate supply of interpreters and translated information and the need for more advocates for carers. It is a strength of organisations such as Carers that they can operate flexibly and speedily to bring issues such as these to fuller social awareness. For more information contact Carers National Association, 20–25 Glasshouse Yard, London EC1A 4JS. Tel: 071–490–8818.

The National Society for the Prevention of Cruelty to Children (NSPCC)

A particular concern in the second half of the nineteenth century was the predicament of many children who were either exploited for their labour potential or mistreated, neglected or abused. Three of the large voluntary organisations which still care for children today were formed at this time: Dr Barnardo's in 1866, the Church of England Children's Society in 1881 and the NSPCC in 1889. Dr Barnardo, as well as founding his own charity, was one of the founder members of the NSPCC. From its origins in Liverpool in 1883, it started work in London and its organisation soon spread to provide national coverage for England, Wales and Northern Ireland. (In Scotland its sister group is the Royal Scottish Society for the Prevention of Cruelty to Children.)

The role of the NSPCC has changed considerably over the years. In its earlier days it was an investigative and prosecuting organisation which frequently resorted to the courts to get protection for children. Today, it is a much wider, larger and more complex organisation. It summarises its role as a 'strong, national, independent and challenging voice for children' (p3, *Strategy for the 90s*). It is in a unique position for a voluntary body – it has the authority to take legal action on behalf of a child and it also has access to the child protection register (or 'at-risk' register) which contains details of families who have children who have either been abused or are at high risk of being abused. This involves a close working relationship with other agencies such as social services, health services and the police. Many of its staff are professionally qualified, having a Certificate in Social Service (CSS), a Certificate of Qualification in Social Work (CQSW) or a Diploma in Social Work (Dip.SW).

The NSPCC is part of a multiagency network that sets out to protect children and young people aged 0–17 years. Its Statement of Values reflects the United Nations Convention on the Rights of the Child (1989). To quote the first of the three points of the Statement:

All children, whatever their race, sex, beliefs, and physical and mental abilities, have the right to grow up unharmed, to have the opportunity to develop fully and to have their basic needs met. They should be respected in body and mind, their safety and well-being ensured, and their personal dignity guaranteed. (*Strategy*, p4)

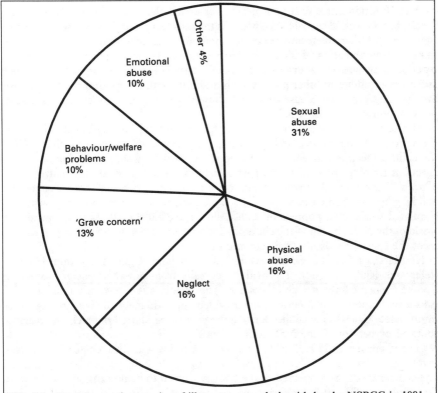

Fig 5.3 Breakdown of categories of ill treatment as dealt with by the NSPCC in 1991 (Annual Report 1991, p 7).

The aims of the Society are:

'To prevent children suffering from significant harm (as defined in the Children Act 1989) as a result of ill treatment; to help and protect children who are at risk from such harm; to help abused children to overcome the effects of such harm; and to work to protect abused children from further harm; whether this occurs through the acts, or failure to act, of individuals or institutions or as a result of social, political or economic policies. (Strategy, p5)

The Society is organised into eight regions: Eastern, Home Counties, London, North West, Northern, Northern Ireland, South West, and Wales and the West Midlands. Each region has a regional director and develops a local plan which is in line with national strategy, but which has the flexibility to respond to particular local needs and problems. For example, inner-city Manchester (in the North West region) has developed a black children and young persons' counselling and advice service, in conjunction with the Black and in Care Group; the Eastern region has set up a special Helpline for young people who have been abused in residential care; and the Home Counties region has created specialised services for children with special needs who have suffered sexual abuse.

Over 80 different teams and projects exist within the NSPCC; 64 of them have a special focus on child sexual abuse which is the most common problem dealt with (see Figure 5.3). Others concentrate on treatment services, assessment work, investigations or a combination of all three. An NSPCC child sexual abuse consultancy is based in Manchester and provides a specialist national resource for both the Society and a large number of other professionals and organisations. Within the Society, the average length of time a case of sexual abuse is kept open is six months, a case of physical abuse three and a half months.

The heart of the work of the NSPCC, which has a total paid staff of about 1400, is the network of over 40 *child protection teams* staffed by child protection officers. All of the child protection officers are qualified social workers who, in addition, are given specialist training by the Society, particularly in investigative and preventive work. They will use the full range of their social work skills to bring about change in a child's situation. Some examples of the skills used are role play, life story work and simulated work using puppets or dolls. All of these aid the officer to get inside the world of the child. Seven of the child protection teams are now developing services to meet the special needs of ethnic communities.

In March 1991, the Society launched a 24-hour Child Protection Helpline (telephone 0800 800 500); it provides free calls from anywhere, at any time, for anyone concerned about a child's safety. The Helpline is receiving around 120 000 calls a year (about 10 000 per month) of which approximately 100 000 are dealt with immediately by Helpline counsellors. In the year it was started the Helpline received some 53 percent of all the NSPCC's referrals.

On any one day in 1991, NSPCC staff were working with an average of 1962 cases, involving 4300 children. One third of these were on the child protection register; and one quarter of all cases referred to the Society proved to be no cause for concern. In the whole of 1991, 20 384 referrals proved to be of a 'serious' nature and involved 38 034 children. The sources of referrals were as follows:

38 percent from the general public
19 percent from the parent in charge of a child or children
11 percent from another relative
10 percent were anonymous
8 percent from social services departments
7 percent from the child personally
7 percent from 'other officials'

The NSPCC also employs family care staff who work with children and their families either in the home or at NSPCC family care centres. These workers are professionally trained nursery and child care workers and they liaise closely with child protection officers. They use counselling and play therapy and they help family members with a wide range of practical household tasks.

The Society performs a number of other important roles: it conducts public campaigns to promote children's rights; it presses for changes in child care law and was an important contributor to the formulation of the Children Act 1989; it conducts research into the ill treatment of children; it administers an emergency relief and welfare fund for cases of particular hardship; it provides a great deal of training for other organisations and professionals; and it operates an internal inspection unit which encourages and supports good practice within the Society.

Almost 90 percent of the NSPCC's income in 1991 (£31 592 000) was provided by the public in a variety of forms, e.g. donations, fundraising events and legacies. The Society claims that 79 pence of every £1 given is spent directly on services to children. Individuals can become a Friend of the NSPCC; there are some 12 000 who, in addition to other activities, have volunteered to raise funds. Young NSPCC, a 'club that helps children', mainly by fundraising, celebrated its centenary in 1991.

Although the economic recession has meant recent staff cuts, the NSPCC faces the future with confidence and optimism. For more information, contact the NSPCC, 67 Saffron Hill, London, EC1N 8RS. Tel: 071-242-1626.

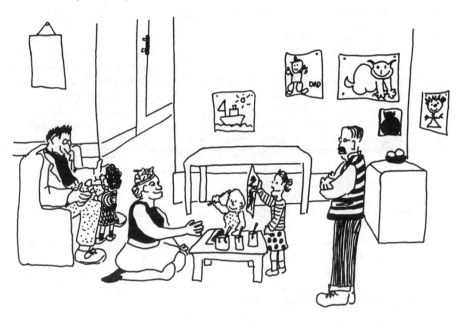

NSPCC Special Units encourage the whole family to relate freely in an informal atmosphere while staff offer support

Locally based organisations

Locally based voluntary organisations often develop to meet specific needs within the community that have not been met by existing services. Since they are not statutory and since many of them do not have charitable status, they have the immediate problem of financing their organisation. They may have to raise their own funds from service users and others within their local community. Apart from these sources, their major source of funding will be the local authority, to whom they will apply periodically, usually annually. Local authorities' resources are diminishing so local organisations are having to vie with each other for sponsorship.

The 'contract culture' we increasingly find ourselves in has added to the uncertainty of local groups; few are sure of financial support beyond the short term future. This inhibits planning and uses up a good deal of management time because managers have to spend a disproportionate amount of time seeking funds. Black voluntary organisations, existing as they do in a culture in which racism leads to discriminatory treatment and support, often have particularly acute problems in securing funding. This in turn frequently hampers potential development.

This section now looks in some detail at two well-established local community voluntary organisations. Both have developed from very humble beginnings in response to particular needs within the community. They represent different sections of the black community.

The Pepper Pot Club, Kensington, West London

The Pepper Pot Club is now in its twelfth year. It began as an informal drop-in centre for displaced and isolated Afro-Caribbean elders who had initially presented themselves at the local Citizen's Advice Bureau. As one of them says, of this time: 'In the country you share so many things. Those were good days, man. You feel lonely when you come here. When we come here we thought it would go on the same' (*Nice Tastin*, p56).

The club still predominantly serves Afro-Caribbean pensioners, but it also caters for some 'younger members of the community who may be unemployed, redundant, on early retirement or incapacitated through ill health, for example, early users of wheelchairs, and those in the community who have suffered some mental illness or depression' (*Profile of the Club*, p3).

The objectives of the club are:

1. 'To enhance the quality of life of club members by providing a setting where they can meet their friends and make new ones; read the books and papers provided; take part in the varied recreational activities; and eat a nutritious, balanced midday meal (taking account of dietary needs, e.g. diabetes or hypertension);
2. To provide a support service to the elderly members of the Caribbean community, monitoring their needs and liaising with the statutory services so as to enable them to remain at home.' (ibid.)

The club relies on an annually renewable grant from the local authority for its main source of funding and obtains additional support from charities and trusts. The club also derives income from those members who pay for lunches at the club or for the meals on wheels that they receive at home. Each year the club earns proceeds from its craft exhibitions and from the sales of its book, *Nice Tastin' – Life and Food in the Caribbean* produced by some of its members. The book details exciting recipes, herbal remedies and aspects of life in the West Indies.

Pepper Pot now has six fulltime staff including a co-ordinator, care assistant, cook, assistant cook and a cleaner. There are three part-time staff comprising two craft teachers and a social worker; the latter runs a regular reminiscence class. A driver is available for the club's minibus which has disabled access and is used to transport service users from and return them to their individual homes. The minibus is also used to take members to various places of interest, for example to the theatre, to exhibitions or on day trips. The club itself hosts events. It has received visits from parties of foreign students and representatives of local radio stations and has regularly held its own bring and buy sales and dominoes tournaments.

Up to 35 members attend each day; some come each day of the week, others attend on only one or two days. Not everyone has a midday meal, although most do. They may choose to take part in the planned activities: craft classes, including batik; dressmaking; keep fit; theatre trips; music; bingo or carpet bowls, or they may visit places of interest or sit around, read, talk to others or watch television.

There are now over 130 registered members of the club, two of whom are Portuguese and some others are of Scottish, Irish and German origin. They enjoy the relaxed, friendly atmosphere and the wide range of facilities offered by the club.

Like so many other voluntary organisations, the Pepper Pot Club seeks to expand in order to fully meet community demand. The club would like 'larger, purpose-built premises for kitchens and dining rooms large enough for our needs; and rooms to provide health services, laundry facilities, hairdressing and other activities' (*Profile of the Club*, p10). But such an expensive development remains, for the present, an ideal for the club. In the meantime it will aim to build on its success and continue to fight for additional funding in a competitive market place.

The Yemeni Community Association, Sheffield

In common with many other post-Second World War migrants from poorer countries, many Yemeni men left their largely impoverished agrarian communities and travelled 4000 miles to Britain in search of better work prospects. A large proportion of these men settled in the 'steel city' of Sheffield, which today has the second largest Yemeni community in this country, approximately 3000 people, including the women and children who have subsequently come to join their menfolk.

The work they found in the steel industry was often poorly paid, dangerous and carried out in noisy, dirty conditions. The jobs they had were not to last long, because the recession in steel that began in the late 1970s came to a head in 1985 with widespread closures; the subsequent redundancies fell mainly on unskilled or semiskilled workers. In that year, unemployment among Yemeni men in Sheffield approached 90 per cent. It was this depressing situation and the accompanying hardship of poverty that brought about the creation of what is now known as the Yemeni Community Association, based in the north Sheffield inner-city district of Pitsmoor.

Rather than despair in the face of great odds, the Yemeni men displayed great resourcefulness and, between themselves, created a self-help group. They collected donations from Yemenis over a period of years and eventually acquired enough capital to purchase a Victorian house which became both the hub of the Yemeni community and the official base of the Association.

In the early days the Association's work focused on issues around unemployment benefits, industrial accidents and industrial related diseases and disabilities, particularly deafness. Today, interests and activities are very much wider; they have the overall aim of uniting the city's entire Yemeni community and catering for as many needs as possible.

With its base in the Association's community house, the Yemeni welfare advice centre provides information on benefits and welfare entitlements and information on civil and legal rights. Help is offered in matters concerning social security, housing, social services, social care, immigration, local education classes, interpreters, translation services and any other welfare problems that arise. The Association liaises with statutory services and sometimes seeks the expertise of lawyers and other professionals. The advice centre is open five days a week, from 8.30 a.m. to 5 p.m. and, in addition, workers are available at weekends for home visits to people who require help.

Literacy classes in Arabic and English are run at the centre, as well as a number of other educational classes, including subjects such as numeracy, information technology and health. There is a library covering a diversity of subjects, e.g. Yemeni history, cultural and religious festivals, literacy skills and computing. A well-equipped kitchen serves a range of Yemeni food and luncheon clubs are run for elderly people. A creche is available, staffed by volunteers, and women's groups meet regularly. In addition to all these activities, the centre also provides an essential meeting place where Yemenis may meet friends and chat in a friendly atmosphere. Trips out are planned and the Association's two minibuses enable groups to travel together. A youth club is run in the evenings.

The management committee, made up of seven elected members, relies on volunteers to maintain the continuance of the Association's and Centre's activities. There are a few paid workers, both fulltime and part-time, an advice worker, a seconded community worker (salary paid by the local social services department) and three literacy teachers, who are funded by the local authority education department. Virtually all other activities depend on voluntary effort.

Apart from the financial contributions of the Yemenis themselves, funding comes from a variety of sources: for example, the local authority, the Urban Programme (now being cut back by central Government) and the local development corporation, which has recently been set up with the aim of rejuvenating inner-city areas. Sufficient funding is a constant problem and takes up a great deal of time and effort.

Despite this ever-present difficulty and the humble origins of the organisation, ambitious plans for the setting up of a Yemeni economic and training centre have been going ahead and are nearing practical realisation. The lease is to be purchased on a nearby local authority 'vestry hall', a large building which will allow activities and facilities to expand.

It is envisaged that four fulltime staff will be employed initially at the Centre: a centre co-ordinator, enterprise development officer, information administrator and a caretaker. The main aim of the centre will be to provide education and training for Yemenis of all ages, to enable them to diversify and prepare for new jobs, careers and economic activity, to counter the poverty and deprivation that high unemployment has brought. Some examples of the skills to be taught are: woodwork, craft, pottery, hairdressing, retailing skills and information technology. Fully equipped workshops will be available, a commercial cafe open to the public is planned and access for disabled people will be ensured. In addition to the practical help provided by the centre, it is also hoped that this new development will further unite the local Yemeni community.

The Terrence Higgins Trust (THT)

Terrence Higgins died with AIDS in 1982; he was one of the first people to be diagnosed in the UK. His friends, shocked and saddened by the intolerance and discrimination he had suffered and dismayed by the lack of support and reliable information available, founded the Terrence Higgins Trust in 1983. It was Britain and Europe's first AIDS service organisation. Ten years later it has a salaried staff of about 60 and over 1600 volunteers. The Trust is now deemed by the World Health Organisation (WHO) to be one of the leading AIDS agencies in the world.

Since 1983, when the Trust was created, some 7000 people have developed AIDS in the UK and of these 4300 have died. At present in this country it is estimated that about 50 000 women and men are infected with HIV, the virus that lead to AIDS. It is thought that approximately 12 million adults are HIV infected worldwide, 500 000 of them in Europe. The WHO calculates that between 30 and 40 million people will be HIV-positive by the end of this century.

The aims of the Terrence Higgins Trust are:

to inform, advise and help on AIDS and HIV infection; to provide welfare, legal and counselling help and support to all people affected by AIDS and HIV infection and to their partners, friends and families; to disseminate accurate information about AIDS and HIV; and to provide health education. (Annual Report 1991, p 2)

Staff of the THT feel that they still have to struggle against a great deal of misinformation, ignorance, indifference and discrimination in furthering their work. Much media and press reporting, particularly of the 'tabloid' or 'popular' variety, is extremely unhelpful. It is often polarised; it either denies there is a problem (at least for the heterosexual population) or it spreads panic about the issue. AIDS-related items are frequently presented in a sensational manner. To counter this the Trust places great emphasis on education and information. In 1991, 1.1 million leaflets and posters were distributed in the UK.

The THT's education and information division aims to spread educative information as widely as possible; the general public are reached by the Roadshow which tours pubs, clubs, colleges, workplaces, shopping centres, cinemas and sports centres, as well as special events such as the Notting Hill Carnival, held in West London every August Bank Holiday weekend, gay men are reached by a volunteer gay men's health education group, which emphasises HIV prevention; women are reached by the women's HIV/AIDS network (WHAN), which stimulates discussion and debate amongst women's groups and researches the gaps in the health education needs of women and seeks ways of meeting them. World AIDS Day on December 1st each year disemminates educative AIDS information internationally.

Great emphasis is placed on the Trust's work in providing practical care and support. This is done in a number of ways. An advice centre deals with hundreds of welfare rights enquiries every year, giving reliable information on benefits and entitlements. Housing matters are dealt with by a separate service and legal advice is available, backed up by 'Legal Line' a telephone line, available on Wednesdays from 7 p.m to 9 p.m. A general Helpline is also provided, available on a daily basis from 3 p.m. until 10 p.m. In 1991, 60 percent of calls were from men, and the majority of all calls were from heterosexuals (65 percent). Most enquiries were from the London area and 30 percent came from other parts of the UK.

The 'buddy' programme is a befriending service in which HIV-positive women and men are provided with a 'buddy', introduced by the Trust. One third of buddies are female. Buddies offer practical and emotional support. They are by far the largest group of volunteers within the THT – 700 of the 1600 available. They take on virtually any task the person they are caring for wants them to. The buddy is a kind of companion, but the relationship is more complex than friendship. Many volunteer to be a buddy because they have lost friends through AIDS. One volunteer said of the role: 'Buddying can be very demanding but it's also very rewarding. It's totally altered my life – I've reassessed how I treat other people' (*Guardian Weekend*, 17.4.93, p 19).

The 'helper cell' service represents the second largest group of Trust volunteers. Helper cell volunteers provide practical support, for example, decorating, DIY, housework, plumbing in a washing machine or simply walking the dog. However, by far the greatest number of requests for help are for daytime driving to hospitals and clinics. The health of someone with HIV can change quickly and unpredictably so this is an extremely useful service. A minibus has been donated and has been adapted for wheelchairs. The helper cell service became an autonomous group within the Trust in 1991 and it now has a fulltime paid co-ordinator.

The THT does a lot of work in prisons, both of an educational and practical nature. Recently a 'prison buddy' service was set up. Much education and advice on drug misuse and its links with HIV infection takes place, both in prison and in the community. Volunteers are offered training on this subject. The Trust is also closely involved in pioneering research into the medical use of drugs for the treatment of AIDS.

Face-to-face counselling is offered by 30 volunteer counsellors who provide short term focused work on issues concerning HIV. Sessions usually last one hour and are on an appointment and a drop-in basis. The largest category of people counselled (32 percent of the total) are, in fact, the carers of women or men with HIV. For them, counselling will often incorporate the effects of bereavement and grief and prebereavement work.

A family support network exists to support families through the complete process, from the time of an AIDS diagnosis through periods of ill health to death and bereavement. A hospitality scheme run in conjunction with London Lighthouse offers five days free bed and breakfast to family members who are visiting hospitalised relatives; volunteer host families provide the service.

The Trust works closely with a number of other agencies from all sectors both in the UK and abroad; it lobbies central Government on relevant issues, particularly on welfare benefits. It has a very well-equipped library, provides speakers and produces numerous publications, including *The Trust*, a bimonthly newsletter.

Over half of the Trust's income currently comes from voluntary contributions. With regard to its other funding, a bitter blow was dealt the THT in April 1993, when it was announced that the Department of Health was cutting its grant by two thirds, form £450 000 per year to £150 000. This cut, which represents 10 percent of its current budget, is to be spread over three years. Nick Partridge, the chief executive, said at the time: 'We now face the immensely difficult task of maintaining our vital services with progressively less support from the Government'. He went on: 'this news comes just three days after the preliminary results of the AZT drug trial, which highlighted the absence of effective drugs for people who are currently well and living with HIV, sadly confirming the continued need for our services for many years to come' (*The Independent*, 6.4. 93).

For more information contact The Terrence Higgins Trust, 52–54, Grays Inn Road, London, WC1X 8JU. Tel: 071-831-0331.

Conclusion – what is the independent sector's future?

As we have already said, these are important yet uncertain times for the independent sector. Change within and between the voluntary, private and not-for-profit sectors is constant and at the present time, is occurring at an intense and speedy rate. As Jeremy Kendall and Martin Knapp point out: 'Organisations can migrate from one sector to another over time, and also alter their function and type as a result of changing relationships with the other sectors' (*Defining the Nonprofit Sector: The United Kingdom*. Jeremy Kendall and Martin Knapp, University of Kent, 1993, p 22). This has clearly led to a blurring of sector territories.

Central to current uncertainties are the recent arrangements for community care. The future of all sectors in regard to this, including local authority services, is far from predictable. The private sector may continue to grow, but we should remember that it is always especially vulnerable to the economic health, or otherwise, of the country owing to the profit motive. The new not-for-profit sector demonstrates a wide variety of organisational structures, legal status, management and financial arrangements. Relationships between trusts and local authorities also varies across the country. Currently, much innovation in regard to trusts is taking place, but we will have to wait to see whether or not they will prove economically viable and whether they will move towards a greater independence from social services authorities.

The greatest future uncertainty, however, appears to involve the voluntary sector. Income from all four of its main sources of support – central and local Government, businesses and the public – is dropping. Although dependent partly on the state of the economy, it seems likely that funding from both levels of Government will continue to decrease. The NCVO has calculated that the phasing out of the Urban Programme alone could lead to the loss of 34 000 paid jobs and the closure of 10 000 community projects, most of them voluntary organisations. In addition, the decision by central Government not to 'ring-fence' funding for the 140 or so voluntary drug and alcohol units has led to broad-based predictions that many of them will close by the end of 1994.

The 'contract culture' we are now in may mean more financial security for some bodies, if they are successful in delivering contracted services. This may include some of the smaller, community-based voluntary organisations that have emerged in response to local felt needs. However, some bodies will fail. Many others are kept on short term contracts by local authorities; this makes future planning extremely difficult and this in turn breeds insecurity. We should remember that quite a number of voluntary organisations are entirely dependent for their survival on local authority funding.

Localised groups, including those that represent the interests of black people, may also be vulnerable. In *Home from Home*, a report commissioned by the Race Equality Unit of the NISW, we read: 'Black projects have a history and continuing reality of uncertainty surrounding their funding situation. They are often on short term or minimal funding, which hampers potential developments' (p42). The report writers believe that funding bodies lack awareness of the changing needs of black communities. Financial insecurity also means that managers have to spend a disproportionate amount of time seeking funding and this keeps them from their other management and development functions.

As we move from a Welfare State to a mixed economy of welfare, the independent sector will have a higher profile and an increasingly dominant role. We must hope that despite all the uncertainty that presently abounds, it will have an assured, secure future. Most particularly, we should trust in the continuance of that which has made the voluntary sector so special and important – its independence, its spontaneity and what is true of so many of its workers, the simple desire to give energy and time without wanting any material reward.

Appendix – a typical working day for an NSPCC child protection officer

9.00   Arrive at office and read through mail. This includes an anonymous letter making allegations of a child being neglected. (This kind of letter is commonly received. It contains only an address – the name of the family is not mentioned.) In response to this, check through case files, the 'at-risk' register, and with other agencies (social services department and health visitors) to see if the family is known. It is known, so decide to visit the home tomorrow to assess what risk there may be to the children.
Read through case conference minutes from the previous week.
Receive four phone calls from clients already being worked with, requesting help with such matters as housing and financial assistance from the DSS. Time spent between calls in getting up to date with case recording.

10.30   Child protection team meeting. Case discussions and a good deal of mutual support! The latter is particularly pertinent at this time, as two of the team were recently the victims of violent attacks by angry parents.

12.00   Lunch.

1.00   Office interview with a rather isolated couple who have two children. The wife is worried that she may injure her baby of six months. This child has spent three periods in hospital and there appears to be a poor bonding relationship between the child and mother. The family has large financial debts of some £3000, despite the husband being employed (on a low wage). The result of the discussion is that I agree to contact a health visitor in order to find out what parent-and-toddler groups there are in their area and I also agree to visit the family in two weeks' time to assess what progress has been made.

2.30   Case discussion with a social worker, health visitor and probation officer. We all work with the same family and we discuss co-operation and the family's progress. We agree on a joint strategy.

3.30   Contact a health visitor about a recent case referral. She will contact me after she has visited the family home again.

3.45   Telephone referral received about a two year old boy with a badly bruised eye. Check out the case and find that the social services department is officially involved. In fact the boy is in hospital under the terms of an emergency protection order, so it is unnecessary for us to become involved.

4.15   Telephone call from a neighbour making allegations that two children aged ten and 12 are being left alone for long periods. Write out referral and pass to the team leader for allocation to a member of our staff.

4.30   Administration and report writing.

Exercise 1 – local voluntary organisations

a) Select a local voluntary organisation. (Do not choose the local branch of a national organisation.) It may be worth scanning local newspapers to see if they carry any stories about its work.
b) Arrange to visit its office and interview one or more people working for it.
c) Write up an account of what it does and how it is organised and financed.
d) Interview a number of local residents to find out whether they know of its work. If they have had some contact with it, what is their impression of how well it functions and the services it provides?
e) Finally, write up your assessment of the organisation.

Exercise 2 – national voluntary organisations

a) Select a national voluntary organisation and write a report about its activities. This will involve making direct contact and asking for information to be sent to you. (Be sure to enclose a stamped addressed envelope when you write to any voluntary organisation for information.)
b) Find out how it is organised and funded.
c) Find out if there is a local branch or office in your area and contact people who work for it. Has it set up any projects locally? What does it do in your area? How is it organised and funded?

Exercise 3 – the Citizens Advice Bureau

The Citizens Advice Bureau (CAB) has been described as 'the GP [general practitioner] of the voluntary sector'. Imagine that you are a volunteer at your local CAB. Today (a Tuesday) is an average day and ten people come in with a variety of queries, as below. Some of them may have to be referred to other agencies, either statutory or voluntary; others you may be able to offer advice to yourself. Work out what you would do in each case.

a) A man with what he describes as 'shoddy goods' – a pair of shoes he bought two weeks ago, which have split and are unwearable. He had his receipt for them and returned to the shop to complain, but was told they could not replace them or refund him.
b) A married man who says that he and his wife have experienced substantial problems in their relationship over the past few months. He now feels desperate and realises that they need some help and advice urgently.
c) A young woman who has been living in a private rented flat and was told last night that she must be out of it, removing all her property, by the end of the week. She has no formal agreement with the landlord and no rent book.
d) A married man with three children has recently lost his job as a computer engineer. The family now face repossession of their house as they cannot keep up

with the high mortgage payments. They have almost exhausted their savings.

e) A couple with a 14 year old son are convinced he is 'glue sniffing' – they are extremely worried about him – but their angry confrontations are met by adamant denials. He behaves oddly at times, his mood fluctuates rapidly and he has appeared as if drunk but without the smell of alcohol on his breath. They are desperate for some kind of advice and assistance.

f) A man (about 40) has been denied access to his two young children (aged four and seven) on the past two weekends. His ex-wife is refusing to communicate with him and he wants to know quickly what he should do.

g) A very agitated single mother with one child complains that she has not received her latest girocheque from the DSS. A visit and phone call to the local office have not helped – she feels that she has been 'fobbed off' when told her money will arrive by the weekend. She has no money, not even for food, and no friends or relations who are able to help.

h) An Asian couple who have just moved into town are keen to receive help with speaking English. They feel that poor English has limited their social life and they want to improve the situation.

i) A single man of 28 has just arrived in the area, having heard that there is work to be found here. He does not have any address to go to, has no friends or relations near and is asking for help in finding accommodation.

j) A woman with two children whose partner recently left the home has just lost her job through stress-related absences. She says she has entered a 'debt spiral'. Her telephone has been cut off and she has outstanding gas and electricity bills. She has been borrowing a lot of money from family and friends, but is now panicking about her situation. She feels 'desperate'.

Exercise 4 – training

Increasingly, volunteers in the caring services receive some form of training. Choose two of the following and explain what kind of training you think volunteers working with them should receive:

a) People with learning disabilities;
b) Young people in a playgroup;
c) People with physical disabilities;
d) Elders;
e) Offenders.

Questions for discussion

1. The real cost of care could never be fully borne by the State – it would be too expensive.
2. 'Contract culture' is not really about diversity of provision and increased choice for service users, it merely disguises the Government's true purpose, which is to dismantle the Welfare State.

3. What advantages does the volunteer have over the professional in the caring services?
4. Private and not-for-profit organisations are less directly accountable and less democratic than statutory or voluntary agencies. Is this true? If it is true, what are the consequences?
5. The statutory services have failed to cater sensitively to the needs of black and minority ethnic communities. Is this true? What are some of these needs?
6. With the development of the Welfare State after the Second World War, some thought that all voluntary activity would be taken over by paid professionals working for statutory caring agencies. This has not happened. Why do you think voluntary effort is still very much in evidence?

Further reading

1. *Charities Digest* (Family Welfare Association, 1994). Published annually, it provides a comprehensive guide to charities in the United Kingdom.
2. *Snapshots of the Voluntary Sector Today*, Perri 6 and J. Fieldgrass (NCVO Publications, 1992). Information about the voluntary sector today against background details of the wider social setting.
3. *Inform, Advise and Support – 50 years of the Citizen's Advice Bureau*, Jean Richards (Lutterworth Press, 1989). Traces the history of the CAB and details the kinds of enquiries it deals with today.
4. *The Voluntary Agencies Directory, 1993/4* (NCVO Publications, 1993). The standard reference work, listing about 2000 voluntary organisations, with details of their activities and aims.
5. *Voluntary Action Research – The 1991 National Survey of Voluntary Activity in the UK*, (Volunteer Centre, 1991). Detailed research about volunteering in the UK – who does it and what they do.
6. *Social Care in a Mixed Economy*, Gerald Wistow *et al.* (Open University Press, 1993). Based on extensive research, this book traces developments towards a mixed economy of welfare.

Note: Most voluntary organisations publish material about their work. It is a good idea to enclose a stamped addressed envelope if you write for information.

6

Good Practice – Client Rights and Choices

So far in this book we have looked at the provision of caring services and examined the roles and responsibilities of those who are involved in delivering them. This chapter alters the focus and examines the standard and quality of care. It aims to explore the component parts of good practice and the ideals and values upon which it is based.

In recent years much has been said about good practice. This has stemmed from a growing awareness about the need to make services more responsive and accessible to all service users; the extent of oppression and the damaging effects of prejudice and discrimination; and the need to safeguard the rights of individuals, both as citizens and service users. Documentation in the form of reports, codes of practice, charters and statements of purpose have been produced in the last decade, especially in the past five years, in a fashion which suggests that good practice and the rights of clients are something entirely new. The statements, codes and charters are new but the notion of good practice has always been present in the caring relationship where clients are treated as whole persons. Furthermore, service users' rights are rooted in the history of social care, health care and social work: in theories and philosophies and in the practices of the Welfare State, particularly since its consolidation in the immediate post-war years.

Influential Reports, Codes of Practice and Charters

In 1984, *Home Life: A Code of Practice for Residential Care* (Centre for Policy on Ageing) sponsored by the DHSS, was produced mainly to provide guidelines for a minimum standard of care for the benefit of the growing number of voluntary and private care homes. The Registration of Homes Act followed in the same year. Later in 1990 *Community Life: A Code of Practice for Community Care* was published, again by the Centre for Policy on Ageing, in response to changing forms of service delivery. It made a number of recommendations about the practice and delivery of community care for the 1990s and into the twenty first century.

In 1988, a full independent review of residential care was chaired by Lady Wagner and reported in two volumes: *The Research Reviewed* which looked at the historical development and current practices in residential care for a range of service users, and *A Positive Choice* which further analysed the role of residential care and made recommendations to ensure that in future, 'No-one should be required to change their permanent accommodation in order to receive services which could be made available to them in their own homes' and that 'People who move into a residential establishment should do so by a *positive choice*' (Wagner Report, p114).

The Wagner Report was acclaimed for its substance and recommendations but was criticised for its failure to address the crucial issue of black people's rights to a 'positive choice' with regard to residential care. The National Institute of Social Work's Race Equality Unit (REU) established the black perspectives group which formed a subgroup of the Wagner Development Group. Its report, '*A Home from Home – The Experiences of Black Residential Projects as a Focus of Good Practice*, was published in 1992 (Race Equality Unit/Wagner Development Group) It produced 11 recommendations relating to residential homes and a further five for local authorities and funding bodies.

Together with the Griffiths Report '*Community Care – An Agenda for Action*' of the same year, the Wagner Report contributed to ideas contained in the White Paper *Caring for People* (1989) which in turn formed the basis of the National Health Service and Community Care Act 1990.

In the same year that the White Paper came out, the Social Services Inspectorate (SSI), along with other individuals and agencies concerned with providing and regulating residential care, produced *Homes are for Living In* (HMSO, 1989) as a model for evaluating the quality of life experience of care residents. Since then the SSI has also produced other models of care practice specific to different client groups; for example, *Guidance on Standards for Residential Homes for People with a Physical Disability* (HMSO, 1990).

The Social Care Association (SCA) published its *Code of Practice for Social Care* in 1987. It included the Principles of Clients' Rights. This was followed in 1990 by the SCA's *Action Checklist for Antiracist Practice in Social Care*. More recently, in response to developments in community care, the National Association of Race Equality Advisers (NAREA) produced the *Black Community Care Charter* (1992). This outlines individual users' and carers' rights and provides guidelines on assessment, care packages, contracts, quality issues, monitoring and complaints procedures.

Other health, social care and social work bodies have provided statements of good practice. The British Association of Social Workers (BASW) declared its Twelve Principles of Social Work Practice in 1988. More recently the Care Sector Consortium (now the Occupational Standards Council) outlined the nine Principles of Good Practice (1992) upon which 'all workers should act'.

During the period that these reports were being produced the Government published its own Citizen's Charter (1991) which was a comprehensive, general statement of citizen rights. Related to this, in the field of health, the Patient's Charter' had been introduced in 1991. It asserted seven basic rights of patients which included the right to 'receive health care on the basis of clinical need, regardless of the ability to pay'. Nine National Charter Standards were added which are aimed at ensuring that 'proper personal consideration is shown to users of the NHS'.

The Probation Service and the Prison Service, along with other public services, have produced mission statements. In the case of probation, the service has made a statement of purpose (1992) which briefly states the aims of the organisation and outlines what service users and the public can expect from the service. It states that offenders have the right to read a copy of any presentence report concerning them (*National Standards for the Supervision of Offenders in the Community*, Home Office, 1992, p18) and to be involved in the drawing up of their supervision plan.

In addition many local authorities have issued their own discrete statements on standards of care practice and clients' rights. This has been encouraged by the recent requirements of the NHS and Community Care Act 1990 now that local authorities have to publish their own community care plans annually (since 1991). These provide details of service provision and the complaints procedure. Hammersmith and Fulham SSD's 1993–4 community care plan, for example, identifies seven key principles for the delivery of community care and states that: 'People's religious and cultural needs will be properly identified during the needs assessment and properly provided for within the care package' (p50).

There have been some disturbing instances of bad practice in residential care within both the public and private sectors. Rather predictably, the media has given disproportionate attention to these events; the more general, higher standards of care practice tend to be taken for granted and are therefore not considered newsworthy. However, there has been a renewed emphasis on rights and practice and this has led to a number of developments including a substantial push towards the establishment of full citizenship, culminating in the Citizen's Charter (1991). Linked to the need to preserve standards is the continued call for control and accountability. There has been some pressure for the establishment of a General Social Services Council (GSSC) which would contain the names of all carers who, in turn, would need to be registered in order to practice. It is proposed that such a body would have the power to remove a negligent or an abusive carer's name from the register and so prevent their access to the caring profession.

There has been concern, too, that welfare agencies in Britain have become overbureaucratic and insensitive to individual need and that this has often led to impersonal service delivery. Attention has been drawn to issues such as quality of service; accountability of organisations and their employees; greater public awareness of services; knowledge of clients' rights and clear complaints procedures. This focus is to be welcomed but there is some anxiety that any changes made with these issues in mind may only be superficial and that glossy manuals and procedures may provide a polished front to a service that is ultimately unable to deliver owing to inadequate funding and resourcing.

Some people point out that many of the rights and principles mentioned in the above codes and charters are not new. They point out that rights are located, in essence at least, in the Universal Declaration of Human Rights. When it was published after the Second World War, this charter reaffirmed 'fundamental human rights, the dignity and worth of the "human person" and equal rights for men and women'. It has been further claimed that the principles of good practice and clients' rights, as we have already mentioned, can be found outlined in many of the established social, health care and social work texts.

Notwithstanding the above, social and health care and social work have learned much from the experience of recent years. In particular, more is known about the effects of racism and how public services have generally failed to meet the needs of black people; the damaging effects of institutionalisation and the need for people to live in ordinary settings so far as this is possible; the need for people to remain in their own communities, again, where this is feasible; the value of residential or nursing home care which increases a person's independence and is provided in response to client choice; the benefit of respite and short term care; and the normalisation inherent in the provision of foster care for both children and adults. There is greater awareness, too, about the special needs of different user groups which has stemmed in part from the increased participation of users in service delivery and from demands made by them. The contribution and value of work carried out by the many informal carers in their own homes and the homes of others has at least been acknowledged:

'The greater part of care has been, is and always will be, provided by families and friends' (White Paper foreword, para 2), even if it has not always been formally supported.

Statements of clients' rights and the various codes of practice have reaffirmed basic principles at a time when there is growing concern about standards of social and health care practice. It is felt that there is a danger of these being eroded following the decline of the democratically accountable public provision of services, in favour of the expansion of private, 'not-for-profit' and voluntary agencies within the mixed economy of care. It is to be hoped that service users' rights and the principles of good practice can be properly safeguarded in contracts and service agreements. The idea of purchasing services through contracts is not new. For example, it is estimated that at least 11 percent of social services department expenditure in 1978–9 was devoted to purchasing services, mainly from the voluntary sector (*Practice with Care*, p12). Now, however, private, not-for-profit, community and voluntary organisations are set to become the principal care providers and there exists the fear that care standards may not always be compatible with the profit motive.

It should be remembered that a person's rights are not absolute: they exist only in so far as they are respected and tolerated by others. In the world of care this is determined by the care regime and the practice of committed care staff. However, by being written down and incorporated into procedures they strengthen a person's recourse to redress. Written statements may also raise the consciousness of carers and service users who, separately or together, may work towards their fulfilment.

The following outline of the principles of clients' rights has been clustered into groupings consistent with the elements of the National Vocational Qualifications (NVQ) and Scottish Vocational Qualifications (SVQ) Value Base Unit 'O': *Promote Equality for All Individuals* (Care Sector Consortium, *National Standards for Care*, HMSO 1992):

a) The right to receive antidiscriminatory/antioppressive care;
b) The right to confidentiality and privacy;
c) The right to have individual rights and personal choices respected;
d) The right to have personal beliefs and identity acknowledged and acted upon;
e) The right to support through effective communication.

The right to receive anti-discriminatory|anti-oppressive care

All clients have the right to receive a service which does not unfairly discriminate against them in any way. It is already illegal to discriminate against people on the grounds of race, religion or sex following legislation in the 1970s (Race Relations Act 1975; Fair Employment Act Northern Ireland 1989; Sex Discrimination Act 1975). Overt instances of discrimination may be easy to identify and act upon, but more subtle forms of indirect or covert discrimination, whether performed by individuals or organisations, consciously or otherwise, are less easy to prevent. Discrimination may be seen to occur where people are treated differently and either do not receive a service or it is delivered to them in an inappropriate way. Unfair discrimination can

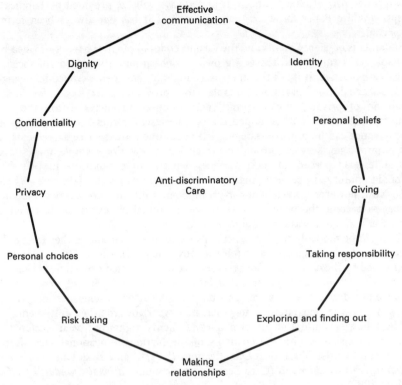

Fig 6.1   Elements of antidiscrimatory care.

occur on grounds of age, class, caste, colour, creed, culture, gender, health status, HIV status, lifestyle, marital status, mental ability, mental health, offending background, physical ability, place of origin, political beliefs, race, religion, responsibility for dependents, sensory ability, sexuality or other specific factors.

There is much evidence of communities and client groups failing to receive an adequate or appropriate service. The introduction to *A Home from Home* (REU, 1992) begins: 'It is a truism that social services and related mainstream agencies have not adequately fulfilled their responsibilities in providing sensitive social care to black families and their communities' (p1). It goes on to point out:

> On the one hand, those members of the black community who have received mainstream residential care have experienced prejudice and racism which has denied them their cultural reality, racial pride, self dignity and black identity. On the other hand, myths and stereotypes of black families, such as 'they look after their own' and 'residential care is not part of their culture' have worked against the interests and welfare of their members in need of residential care.
>
> (Ibid.)

Evidence of discriminatory treatment of black people is provided by the 'disproportionate number of black children and black persons with mental illness in residential care, and little or no presence of black elders, disabled and black persons with learning difficulties in residential care' (p3). This, the report suggests, is not accidental: 'There is a direct connection between the over-representation of certain members of black communities in residential settings and *control*, and the under-representation of other members of black communities and *welfare*'. (ibid)

There is now generally much more awareness of the need to make services available to all communities and greater efforts are being made by statutory, voluntary and private organisations alike to achieve this. Amongst the 12 recommendations for good practice made by the study are that in future, 'All residential homes have a black perspective fully integrated into all policies and practices'; that 'recruitment of staff reflects the community reality and the needs of residents' and 'that residents' physical needs are met, including health, skin care, food and language' (p49). Some of this emphasis is reiterated in the Black Community Care Charter which stresses the need to recognise the long tradition of providing care within black communities and the skills and expertise represented within it. The Charter stipulates that, 'Care managers should reflect the composition of the population in terms of race, class, gender, sexuality and disability' and insists that 'All contractual agreements should be provided in an antiracist, antidiscriminatory ethnically sensitive manner' (p8).

Some of these principles have been incorporated in new policies. For example, the Hammersmith and Fulham 1993–4 Community Care Plan states: 'Independent sector provision will not be commissioned if there is any evidence that the home or organisation discriminates against people because of their race, gender, or sexual preference' (p50) and that 'racism from service users or providers will not be accepted, and if it occurs it will be quickly and properly investigated and acted upon' (ibid). Further, the authority pledges to support people's right to complain through its complaints procedure if principles are not fulfilled. Other statutory and voluntary organisations have similarly committed themselves to antioppressive practice.

Service users are discriminated against on grounds other than race. For example, many female carers have been denied support from social services because of the implicit assumption that they 'should' provide care. In similar circumstances male carers have been granted services to enable them to cope. Within the health service older people have not always had equivalent access to services such as psychotherapy as younger people. It may be felt that mental stress is inevitable and synonymous with growing older and therefore untreatable. Disabled people and people with special needs continue to be unfairly discriminated against when the physical environment remains inaccessible to them or they do not have the same independent access to resources enjoyed by ordinary people. The National Charter Standards have acknowledged the right of everyone, including people with special needs, to use health services. It states: 'The Charter Standard is that all health authorities should ensure that the services they arrange can be used by everyone, including children and people with special needs such as those with physical and mental disabilities, for example, by ensuring that buildings can be used by people in wheelchairs.'

Gay service users have not always found it easy to express their sexuality in care regimes which may be hostile. Where the assumption is that heterosexuality is the only model for human relationships it is difficult for all service users to feel valued and respected. Very little is explicitly stated about the needs of lesbian and gay people in charters and codes of practice other than the recognition of their disadvantaged status alongside other groups. Perhaps this itself can be taken as a sign of the marginality of gay people. However, their needs are generally recognised within the principle that 'antidiscriminatory practice should be developed and promoted so that each individual is guaranteed the same quality of service' (*Principles of Good Practice*, Care Sector Consortium).

Discrimination can be the result of organisational practices and procedures or the result of individual action. Either way, codes of practice and declarations of service users' rights give a recourse for clients or their advocates to fight instances of discrimination. They also help to remind carers of the need to be permanently mindful to eliminate prejudice and discrimination from their own practice.

The right to confidentiality and privacy

The right to confidentiality

Confidentiality is an essential principle of good care practice. The relationship between carer and service user is built upon mutual respect and trust and it is important that this is not violated. There are times, though, when information given in confidence may need to be passed on to others, either for the protection of the service user or the protection of another. When this occurs reasons for the breach need to be fully explained and justified. The establishment of absolute confidentiality is often a prerequisite for disclosure and carers entering into such an agreement need to be fully aware of their own responsibilities. Paid carers are, after all, employed by organisations who need to be fully informed about the clients in their care if they are to provide an effective service.

Indeed, for the sake of planning, accountability and service delivery, confidential records are maintained on clients detailing personal information, health, personal circumstances and social and welfare particulars. Under certain Acts of Parliament (Data Protection Act; Access to Medical Reports Act 1988) clients are entitled to access to their own records (except in exceptional circumstances). Indeed it is now regarded as a creative aspect of social work practice to share recordings with the service user so that progress and direction can be clarified and the integrity of the worker's involvement can be demonstrated.

The impact of HIV and AIDS and its implication for service provision and delivery has heightened the significance of confidentiality within a caring relationship. Owing to the social stigma attached to the condition, people who learn of their positive HIV status may be forced to conceal this information even from close friends and their own families who normally would be potential providers of support. Carers need to be aware of certain information about people with HIV in order to respond to issues of health and safety. Foster carers, for example, would need to know the HIV status of children being fostered and of their parents in order to be able to act responsibly in their role as substitute parents. The ignorance and uncertainty surrounding the virus has meant that services have sometimes been insensitive and judgemental and this has had the effect of undermining the confidence of service users.

Confidentiality should be distinguished from secrecy, which is concerned with withholding information for its own sake or for some other purpose. Confidentiality is concerned with the restricted sharing of information with appropriate people and withholding it from others in respect of the wishes of the information giver. The privileged information which we receive about the lives of others has to be treated with responsibility and integrity. One of BASW's 12 principles of social work practice refers to the absolute 'confidentiality of information and divulgence only by consent or exceptionally, in evidence of serious danger'.

Related to confidentiality is the individual right to privacy.

The right to privacy

It is important that people have their own private space, over which they have some degree of control regarding how it is arranged, who else may be permitted to use that space and the times when they may be alone.

Until relatively recently it was not uncommon for residents of care homes and nursing homes to have to share a bedroom with another person or persons and this is still the case in many of the older establishments. A recommendation of the Wagner Report was 'that no one should be required to share a bedroom with another person as a condition of residence' although some may choose to do so (para 4.12). The report added that the possession of 'a personal key carries with it the power to withdraw to the privacy of one's own room' and recommends that' each person in a residential establishment shall be entitled to a personal key' (subject to certain safeguards including staff holding a master key and a regular review of the policy).

Home Life stresses that residents should be encouraged to 'personalise their private space with the addition of soft furnishings, pictures, photographs and personal possessions.' It further suggests that 'residents should be able to meet whom they wish in private, either in their own room, or in other comfortable accommodation'.

A service user's right to privacy may not always be granted in circumstances where it may be unsafe to leave that person unsupervised for any length of time; for example, young children or children or adults who may be a danger to themselves.

The right to have individual rights and personal choices respected

The right to make choices

Acknowledged good care practice involves the service user as fully as possible in their care. In the case of residential care this should involve a positive choice, where somebody freely elects to enter a home, having had the implications of fulltime residential care fully explained and having had the opportunity of a trial period of residence. The Wagner Report further stresses that residents should also have choices over their daily lives and that this should be respected.

It is important that people within residential and day care settings should be able to make equivalent choices to those they would be able to make in their own homes. For instance, to be able to make decisions about the food they eat, the recreational activities they take part in and the times they get up in the morning and retire at night.

Service users have a right to express their views about the running of the establishment and regular members' meetings are a mechanism for ensuring that such involvement in the decision-making process takes place. The community care proposals place service users centrally with regard to their own care plans. It is intended that, in conjunction with their care manager, they should be able to decide on appropriate services. Similarly, the essence of the Children Act 1989 is to serve the interests of the child and to involve the young person as much as possible in their own care programme.

It is administratively easier for care staff to make decisions on behalf of residents – to decide what activities should take place, at what time and who should take part. By doing this, some establishments can ensure a smoother running of the home, but this is achieved at the cost of the residents' independence. Order and routine are necessary in any group living situation, but people should be allowed to contribute as much as possible to decisions affecting their own lives. Mass bingo sessions, constant television and everybody rising at a certain hour of the morning for communal breakfast will suit some people but not everyone. It is far better that people should be able to opt out of group activities that they are not keen on, decide on their own meal times and bed times and instigate activities that are of personal interest to individuals and to small groups.

The right to take risks

Linked to the need to make decisions is the need to take risks. It is all too easy for residential care establishments to create dependence within the first few hours following admission. If people have things done for them from the moment they become members of a home they learn to rely on, and expect, help at all times. Where staff patiently encourage residents to manage by themselves whenever possible, the sense of achievement created – however small – can be built upon. It may be convenient or tempting to agree to a resident's request for a wheelchair but time spent encouraging the client to move on their own with the use of handrails or a Zimmer frame will enable the resident to maximise their own resources and be ambulant longer.

There are, of course, risks attached to allowing mentally confused people to wander into the community and for this reason some homes keep their front door permanently locked. The erection of secure fencing would overcome this problem and allow all residents more freedom of movement between the home and the grounds. David and Althea Brandon point out that 'In the past, people with disabilities have been protected against all sorts of real and imagined risks. They have often lived in isolated settings being kept safe from the ordinary world. Sometimes they have been almost suffocated by a bizarre combination of care and control' (*Staff Practice Handbook*, p12). They go on to suggest, 'We need to give people more opportunities for more rich experiences – travelling on buses; going to fairs; dancing in discos; going abroad on holidays; eating in restaurants . . . All of these new experiences involve some sort of risk or danger'. *Home Life* advises that 'Responsible risk-taking should be regarded as normal and residents should not be discouraged from undertaking certain activities solely on the grounds that there is an element of risk. Excessive paternalism and concern with safety may lead to infringements of personal rights. Those who are competent to judge the risk to themselves should be free to make their own decisions so long as they do not threaten the safety of others' (1:2:8, p17).

The right to make relationships

This right applies to relationships not only with the staff and other residents within the home but also outside the home as well. Residential homes for adults, or hospitals that encourage community involvement with, say, local children from schools or youth groups via open days and garden fetes, enable residents to form relationships with people from the community. This is further encouraged when residents themselves are involved in community activities outside the home. As *A Home from Home* declares: 'Churches, temples and mosques play a vital role in the lives of many black people and entering residential care does not mean that this has to change' (p27). One of the principles of the Wagner Report is that residential care should be seen to be a 'part of community care' and not distinctly separate from it. The report recommends that people who move into a residential establishment should continue to have access to community support services and to have access to leisure, education and other facilities offered by the local community. The Children Act 1989 recognises the value of preserving family relationships and directs that links between young people and their families should be maintained wherever possible; that siblings should be placed together when accommodated by the local authority and that children should be placed with the extended family rather than with strangers, wherever this is appropriate.

Group living itself and the interdependence it fosters helps people to form deeper relationships with one another, based on trust, respect and mutual support. Naturally, people in residential homes have the same need to develop intimate relationships as people living in the community and this should be facilitated as far as possible but care should be taken to protect anyone who may be vulnerable. All residents, regardless of age, disability or mental health have an inner need to express themselves physically, emotionally, sexually and spiritually and to form significant relationships with others.

The right to explore and find out

Society often views older people and people with disabilities as being somehow less interested in being involved in the world around them, particularly if they are living in a residential or nursing home. Rather narrowly, they are defined by their reduced physical capacity alone; their need for stimulation and their capacity to develop new or maintain old interests is ignored. Music, painting, embroidery, reading, chess and dominoes are just a few of the many interests people in residential care may easily take part in. Raised garden beds and the provision of special implements can make gardening accessible to most residents. Similarly special facilities could provide access for all people to swimming pools and leisure centres.

Residents who are neglected by relatives or visitors may have little opportunity of getting out of the home in order to attend a meeting, to visit shops or places of interest or

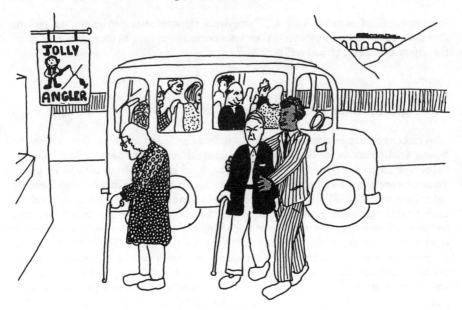

New surroundings are often a sufficient stimulus in themselves and can act as an antidote to residential living

simply to have a change of scenery and a chance to breathe in fresh air. Establishments that have their own transport are able to take residents to local centres of interest, perhaps the nearest community college, in order that they may take part in available activities or on longer journeys, say on day trips to the sea or countryside.

People with learning difficulties increasingly make use of community resources as part of social and lifeskills training; they may attend leisure centres and use cafes and restaurants, transport systems and local shops in order to develop their independence. Physically disabled people are still hampered by physical barriers to access at such places as cinemas, theatres and restaurants and thay are often required to make elaborate prior arrangements in order to enjoy a social evening out.

The right to take responsibility

People have a right to be allowed to take responsibility for their own actions. Living with other people enables individuals not only to take responsibility for themselves – to manage tasks such as preparing light meals, making cups of tea, washing up and table setting – but also involves them in the support of other residents. Living in groups means that roles need to be allocated and responsibilities shared. Even people with restricted physical ability or reduced mental capacity can cope with a fair range of tasks, including collecting meals, serving out, clearing away and returning used crockery and so contribute in some way towards their own care. Residents can meaningfully increase their involvement in the running of the home if they can contribute to policy issues and the type of activities planned, say, through the forum of a staff/residents' meeting. They may also comment on the establishment of any rules and procedures and make suggestions on ways of improving the home.

Learning to take responsibility is a vital part of a person's development, so children's homes will encourage young people to take on responsibility commensurate with their age. After all, this is what would be expected to happen in ordinary household settings. But it is particularly important that young people living in children's homes should acquire skills and take on responsibilities, because they have to prepare themselves for the time when they will no longer be looked after by the local authority.

The right to give

Where residents are always the recipients of caring and have no opportunity to return help, they are more likely to feel that they are a burden to others. To be denied the chance to assist others is to be diminished in terms of personal human capacity. Group living, with shared interdependent roles, enables residents to give and receive help from others. The simple achievement of making refreshments for oneself and another group member may take a little time but it can nevertheless be a satisfying process for the person responsible. The opportunities for this type of practice will be facilitated in homes where, for each small group of residents, there is a raised electric socket and an automatic kettle, established on a firm base, close to a small fridge which should be easily available and accessible. Where group living is practised and residents are involved in mutual daily care, the therapeutic effect of an active life can be observed in the interested attitudes of service users and confidence they display in coping.

System-induced old age

Residential care homes run along traditional lines have often been criticised for the unimaginative way they are run and the lack of stimulation they provide for residents. These 'routinised' establishments, with their preoccupation with order and administrative convenience, neglect the development of the individual. This poor quality care can lead to institutionalisation.

Figure 6.2 illustrates how the philosophy of the home determines the various practices which in turn can be seen to hasten an older person's physical and mental decline. This process is referred to as *system-induced old age*. The institutionalised process is not confined to older people; it can occur with any client group in any care setting.

The right to have personal beliefs and identity acknowledged and acted upon

The right to beliefs and identity

In order for service users to be cared for holistically, their identity, beliefs and practices need to be recognised and valued. It is not enough to acknowledge, for example, that a resident is of the Christian faith and merely organise transport to

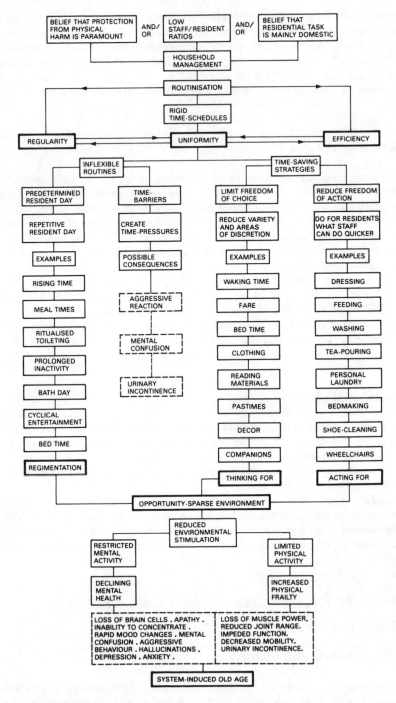

Fig 6.2   Traditional residential care – a benign guardianship (reproduced by kind permission of Bob Browne).

church each Sunday. The client's whole life may revolve around their religion and so its meaning to the individual, needs to be explored and accommodated where possible. In their Community Care Plan 1993–4, Hammersmith and Fulham SSD state that the department will ensure that in its own directly managed establishments, residents are able to:

a) eat food with which they are familiar and have this prepared in accordance with their religious beliefs;
b) have available suitable hair and skin products and ensure that these are properly used;
c) actively enable people to follow their religious practices in life and for appropriate rites to be administered at death;
d) assist the person to maintain links with their own community;
e) celebrate their major religious and cultural festivals;
f) ensure that an elder who does not speak English is admitted to a home where there are staff who speak their language.

The importance of the last point is reiterated in *A Home From Home* which emphasises the value of having care staff of a similar cultural background, not simply for communication purposes but because, according to their findings, 'racial and cultural identity, although expressed visually in some places, was mainly created by staff having the commonality of cultural traditions'. The report adds, 'It is not enough to have Bob Marley pictures on the wall or curry on the menu to make black residents feel valued.' Instead there needs to be a 'holistic approach which is evident in the feel and smell of the establishment, and the sense of belonging and peace which is created'.

The right to dignity

The right to dignity is central to the caring relationship and underlies the whole value base of social and health care including the right to 'have beliefs and identity acknowledged'. Dignity is defined as 'Recognition of the intrinsic value of people regardless of circumstances by respecting their uniqueness and their personal needs: treating with respect' (*Homes are for Living In*, HMSO, p18). It can be expressed in many ways: in the environment by 'the privacy of sanitary facilities or the availability of personal space'; within care practice by 'the admission process and care given to cleanliness and the appearance of residents' accommodation and clothing'; by the staff 'as depicted by adequacy of numbers, continuity of staff/resident contact and the extent to which staff enjoy being with residents' (ibid.).

Dignity is further indicated by the 'existence of formal qualifications amongst staff and the extent to which staff appraisal and supervision arrangements focus on dignity of residents and the training of volunteers'. It is evident, too, 'in the manner in which letters or cash are given to residents and visiting procedures' (ibid.). 'Dignity is also inherent in the way in which case records and documentation are held and the extent to which residents' files contain information which helps staff to provide care in a manner which is sensitive to residents' backgrounds, problems and preferences' (ibid.). Meals and mealtimes also provide opportunities for staff to ensure a client's dignity, by assisting those who have difficulties in eating to do so more easily and by allowing residents a choice to eat by themselves.

The right to support through effective communication

Communication is a two-way process. It involves the client's right to information about services and the right to be involved in service delivery through collaboration and consultation. Ultimately service users have the right of complaint and to appeal when they feel redress is due.

As we have already stated, not all members of the community have always been aware of the range of service provision available to them. Language has been one barrier. Hopefully this will be mitigated to some extent by the stipulation that community care plans have to be published in all community languages. It is important that residents and their families are able to communicate in a language which they feel comfortable with. The 1992 Patient's Charter was made available in nine languages. It states directly to every citizen that they have the 'right to be given a clear explanation of any treatment proposed, including any risks and any alternatives before you decide whether you will agree to treatment'.

Some people who are in need of services may require an interpreter to ensure that all questions can be asked and that the range and implications of services are properly understood. The use of interpreters from local communities is to be supported but care should be taken that they are not exploited. For instance, the Black Community Care Charter urges that 'interpreters should be properly remunerated'.

The system of community care is one which 'allows people to live to their full potential in the way they choose. It is a system of services tailored to meet individual needs'. For this to be the case, service users need to express their own views from the initial consultation. The use of British Sign Language, Makaton and other forms of communication will need to be offered by service providers.

Similarly, access to advocacy is a right of all individuals and service users may wish to make their own comments or make group representations (self, peer or group advocacy) or have a friend or expert make out their case on their behalf (citizen's advocacy). Either way it is important that the client's wishes are fully and accurately transmitted.

Service users may wish to complain about a service and they are entitled to do so; straightforward, detailed procedures accompany each local authority care plan. This right is similarly respected in the Patient's Charter. In the *Staff Practice Handbook – a Guide to Practice in Services for People with Learning Difficulties*, the authors state 'Any resident, relative, visitor or friend has the right to complain about anything. All staff have a responsibility to see that everyone understands how to make a complaint. This organisation welcomes complaints. They can improve the services' (p 16).

Conclusion

Many of the principles of good practice and clients' rights outlined above have been illustrated with reference to residential care. Social and health care and social work are practised in a number of settings – hospitals, nursing homes, residential care homes, hostels, day centres, luncheon clubs, youth clubs, community centres, foster homes, nurseries, childminders' homes and ordinary family homes, where the majority of caring takes place. Whatever the setting and whatever the client group, service users' rights remain fundamentally the same. It is the carer's task to ensure that these are acknowledged and respected and that this is evident in their own good care practice.

Exercise 1 – good practice – priorities exercise

Read the following case study.

You are a specialist social worker for people with physical disabilities. You have a client, Anil, who due to circumstances lives in a residential home for elders. The establishment is an old converted building with 34 residents who mainly occupy single rooms. There is no lift in the building. It is Friday afternoon and you are on office duty in your area.

Anil rings you from the public telephone box inside the residential home. He is 28 years old and was born of Indian parents. He is paralysed from the waist down following a motoring accident in which both his parents were killed. On discharge from hospital, he was 'temporarily' placed in the care home until more suitable accommodation could be found for him. He has been in the establishment for nine months now. He remains very bitter about his condition and regularly complains about staff and other residents. He is not always well liked. There is still no purpose-built accommodation because of cuts in the local authority housing budget. A previous attempt to find temporary accommodation within the private sector was vetoed as 'too costly'.

Since being in the home, Anil has received no mobility allowance and is frustrated by the fact that his electric wheelchair has been in for repairs for the past six weeks. He has no family locally and has had only one visitor since leaving hospital.

Anil says that he has had yet another row with 'that cow' the care officer whom he accuses of making racist remarks. He also claims she has hit him and he wants to make an official complaint. He would like you to get up there and 'sort things out, now'.

What will you do?

Exercise 2 – support a client in transition due to their care requirements

You are a home carer attending to Hilda who is 84 years old and has been living alone in her own home for over 55 years. She bought her small terraced house, having been a sitting tenant for several years. She is well known in the neighbourhood.

Hilda suffers from arthritis and oedema, is partially sighted and forgetful. She has recently bruised herself, having fallen over in the house on occasions. She is very fond of pets and has a 14 year old labrador dog, two ageing cats, a goldfish, two gerbils and a hamster. She does not have much money and spends a good deal of her income on her animals. Two local teenagers take it in turns to walk the dog each day.

The house is unsafe and due for complete modernisation. Hilda is loath to leave the house and her animals for a short period in order to allow builders to get on with the necessary repair work which includes underpinning, reflooring, replastering and rewiring. Once the work has been done the house will be safer, there will be no open fires and an electric cooker will be installed in place of the gas cooker which Hilda sometimes leaves on.

Hilda is at risk in terms of health and safety. She cannot remain in the house while such extensive work is being undertaken. Your task, as her key worker, is to try to persuade Hilda to leave her home for a period of four weeks in order that it can be made safe. You will need to ensure that all of Hilda's concerns are allayed. (You may structure your answer against NVQ Level 3 Unit W3 Element a and use this as a guideline. Be sure, too, to refer to the elements of the NVQ Value Base Unit 'O'.)

Exercise 3 – a difficulty in a home for people with learning difficulties

Tony Barton is a resident in a hostel for people with learning difficulties. He is in his early thirties and suffers from epilepsy. Most of his life has been spent in residential care. He does not cut his own toenails nor does he like anybody else doing this for him – he has to be held down by staff when it becomes necessary to perform this task. Recently, a member of staff accidentally nicked Tony's cheek with a razor while she was shaving him. Since the incident Tony has refused to allow any member of staff to go near enough to shave him. He now sports a stubbly beard.

It is anticipated that it will eventually be dangerous to trim Tony's beard without his co-operation when this task becomes necessary. Tony does not seem to be very happy with his appearance.

What should the members of the care team do to regain Tony's confidence?

Exercise 4 – a difficulty in a residential home for elders

Mr Graham is 75 and a resident of a care home. Over the past few months he has developed a special friendship with another resident, Miss Burgess (72). They spend a good deal of time in each other's company and sometimes hold hands when sitting together in the lounge. Staff have noticed that Miss Burgess tends to encourage Mr Graham's affections but does not always return them.

During one particular evening it is noticed that Mr Graham is not in the lounge and neither is he in his own room. Mr Graham is located in the bedroom of one of the more confused female residents, who is partially undressed.

How do the staff team deal with the difficulty of encouraging personal expression while safeguarding the rights of other residents?

Exercise 5 – client's needs on discharge from care

Imagine you are a client about to be discharged from residential care. Write down what you consider would be your needs and outline the preparations you would like to be made in order to feel confident to make the change.

Produce a list of headings with an accompanying brief rationale for each.

Exercise 6 – cultural and religious awareness

Select one cultural or religious group and research and record the cultural characteristics of this group. You may find it useful to use the following headings: festivals and celebrations; personal hygiene; food and diet; religious observances; fasting; clothes and fashion; death and dying; family traditions and roles; pastimes.

Questions for discussion

1. What do you understand by the term 'institutionalisation'? How can establishments combat this and encourage individuals to participate more fully in day-to-day events?
2. With reference to any adult client group, consider the ways in which individuals can be encouraged to form relationships and express their sexuality.
3. Charters, mission statements and codes of good practice are merely rhetorical statements of good intentions and rarely bring about real changes in practice and service delivery. Discuss.
4. Some people argue that service users have the right to a carer who is of the same background regarding gender, class, race and sexual orientation. Others say that this is irrelevant and that a professional carer will maintain a constant standard of care regardless of these factors. Discuss.
5. Service users' rights are not absolute, they exist only in so far as these are respected and tolerated by others. What can care workers do to ensure that they are upheld?
6. The establishment of confidentiality is a prerequisite for disclosure by service users. What kinds of issues might warrant a breach of this?

Further reading

1. *A Home From Home – The Experiences of Black Residential Projects as a Focus of Good Practice*, Adele Jones *et al.* (Race Equality Unit/Wagner Development Group NISW, 1992). A report emphasising the black perspective in relation to good practice in residential care.
2. *Assessing Elderly People for Residential Care – A Practical Guide*, June Neill

(NISW, 1989). Based on a study of older people. It is a practical guide to assessing their needs.

3. *Social Issues for Carers – A Community Care Perspective*, Richard Webb and David Tossell (Edward Arnold, 1991). An accessible account of discrimination and structural inequality in relation to social care and social work.

4. *Living Well Into Old Age – Applying Principles of Good Practice to Services for People with Dementia*, Kings Fund Centre Project Paper No.63 (Kings Fund Centre, 1986). An outline of good practice for those working with older people, including elders with dementia.

5. *Ceremony of Innocence – Tears, Power and Protest*, Kay Carmichael (Macmillan, 1991). A sensitive book on the value of tears and the expression of emotions.

6. *Promoting Equality in Care Practice – Preparation for the NVQ Unit 'O'* Waterside Education and Training, (The Association for Social Care Training 1993). An education and training pack designed to prepare candidates for assessment at level 2 and 3 in Social and Health Care. This pack is full of relevant excercises drawn from a variety of care settings.

7

Qualities of an Effective Carer

There are no 'golden rules' to learn in order to become an effective carer – we each do the job differently according to our own personalities. However, for the purpose of analysis it is useful to break down the task of caring into a number of basic elements. Each aspect of the carer's role can then be examined separately and its independent value appreciated.

Let us start by examining some of the important characteristics present in a good caring relationship. While reading through this chapter, try to consider the relative value of each quality, whether it is present within yourself and whether you feel you would want to work towards developing it.

Some of these qualities will seem to be similar, while others may overlap to some extent and the list below is by no means exhaustive.

Anti-oppression

Anti-oppression relates to the individual carer's attitudes, values and qualities that are evident in the way they approach and carry out their work. Whatever attributes and qualities a carer may possess, they only have validity if they are expressed in an antioppressive way. This means treating everybody as an individual while establishing and respecting the aspects of their status and background which have significance for them.

We must not assume, for example, that British-born Afro-Caribbean or Asian young people will always want to identify with their traditional cultural heritage; that all women will automatically wish to care for dependants and that men will only do so reluctantly; and that group games, music and pastimes will be equally appreciated by all the residents of care and nursing homes.

Developing antioppressive practice is an ongoing process and will involve carers regularly checking with service users to ascertain their preferences, choices and idiosyncrasies. Carers need to build up their knowledge about the lifestyles and cultural background of the people with whom they work.

Personal qualities

Empathy

Empathy means appreciating a person's feelings from that person's own point of view and life situation. It requires understanding and an ability 'to stand in someone else's shoes.' Of course, total empathy remains an ideal which cannot be fully achieved because of differences in class, culture, disability, gender, race and sexuality.

'Empathy' should not be confused with 'sympathy', which also implies understanding but is coupled with feelings of pity. Action inspired by pity, however well-intentioned, can be harmful – for example, a parent may be overprotective of a fragile child and prevent their growth towards independence or a carer may perform tasks for an elderly person that the client may well be able to do for themselves.

Some people feel that empathy can be heightened by practical experience: by spending a day in a wheelchair or being toileted by another member of staff, a carer may appreciate what it feels like to have a disability and be dependent on others. However, not all conditions can be experienced in this way.

Others argue that it is not necessary to undergo artificial experiences at all. They say that simulation exercises of this kind provide a trivialised distraction and are not always serious learning experiences. Instead, people should be able to rely on their intellectual capacity to put themselves in another's place.

Love

Love is an impossible word to define accurately; we all have our own individual interpretations. However, for the purpose of this analysis it means having a warm affection, a strong fellow feeling towards other human beings. It is likely that all social carers and social workers are attracted to the job initially because they feel a generalised love for other people – particularly for those less able to help themselves. Does this mean that all individuals cared for are loved by those who provide care? Or is it possible for a professional carer to attend to people's needs without necessarily loving them? This dilemma is perhaps highlighted if the people being cared for are unco-operative.

Sensitivity

In this context, sensitivity refers to someone's ability to be aware of and responsive to the intimate feelings of another person. People are different and may express themselves in a number of different ways. Some people are unused to giving expression to their personal requirements and they may therefore conceal their true needs. A sensitive carer will often pick these up without their having to be made explicit. For instance, having one's intimate personal needs attended to by a stranger can be embarrassing for some people. Others, who may be more used to the situation, may be less concerned. It is therefore necessary to treat each person accordingly.

Being sensitive also requires a carer to anticipate a person's feelings; for example, they should be aware of the bewilderment and confusion often experienced by children who are undergoing their first experience of being looked after by foster carers or by carers in a children's home, especially in emergency circumstances; and they should be aware of the grief and despair felt by people who have recently been bereaved.

Basic courtesies

Being respectful

Being respectful means a carer must have an awareness of an individual's personal rights, dignity and privacy and must show this awareness at all times. It is particularly important to be respectful to clients when performing intimate personal tasks (such as feeding, dressing and toileting); the service users are the ones who know best how these tasks can be performed and it is essential that they retain as much control over the situation as possible.

Care and nursing homes are, in many cases, the permanent homes of residents and the way an establishment is run should reflect its respect for the people who live there. Residents should be able to influence the way the home is run and they should be encouraged to participate and make decisions wherever possible.

Politeness

Politeness is the means by which we are able to demonstrate our respect for someone and before we undertake to care for people it is important that we should be aware of the value of good manners. This does not mean that caring relationships should be formal, only that there should be consideration on both sides. For example, it is important for carers to knock on the door of a person's room before entering. They also need to ask service users how they wish to be addressed – do they prefer to be called 'Mr', 'Mrs' 'Ms' or by their forename?

Communication and interpersonal skills

To be an effective carer, it is important that one is able to communicate. This means that one needs to be able to receive and review information and express oneself accurately. A caring relationship is a two-way process. English is not the first language of some service users and so it may be necessary to draw on the skills of an interpreter or the translation service. Carers may aid basic communication by learning some rudimentary words and phrases of the service user's own language. Similarly some clients will have special hearing and speech difficulties so carers will need to develop such skills as using Makaton or signing with British Sign Language (BSL) and be able to operate a range of technological aids where this is necessary.

The ability to listen

The ability to listen goes beyond simply listening to what a person is saying. There is a distinction to be made between listening and hearing. We all listen but we do not always hear. Often this is because we are too preoccupied with our own affairs and things that are currently concerning us. Communication is further complicated by clients who, through shyness, embarrassment or any other reason, are not always direct in expressing their needs, who instead tend to obscure or hide them. Carers too may also be embarrassed or shy on occasions; they will need to work towards overcoming this in order to communicate effectively.

Sometime a person's real needs are communicated not by what is said but by what is left unsaid. For example, a child who is accommodated by the local authority may be reluctant to talk about their family because it brings back painful memories. It is important that the social carer or social worker should try to create an atmosphere of trust and security so that direct expression may be encouraged.

Facial expressions, posture and other forms of body language all give clues to a person's feelings. A good carer will be aware of these forms of *non-verbal communication*. It is thought that non-verbal messages reflect a person's mood or true desires far more accurately than does immediate verbal communication.

Being assertive

Carers should strive to be assertive in order to express themselves clearly and to understand others more fully. This involves being more honest about our own wishes, rights and needs and respecting those of others. Part of the process of being assertive lies in setting boundaries; for example, by not allowing ourselves to be overloaded by colleagues or managers or by being prepared to say 'no' when this is appropriate. Saying 'no' will often be harder or more uncomfortable than saying 'yes' but it is a valid response nonetheless. If a carer is assertive from the beginning of the relationship and maintains this assertiveness throughout, it leads to more clarity concerning expectations and responsibilities and service users can be clearer about the worker's role. Furthermore, assertiveness, owing to its direct and honest nature, can be seen as one of a number of coping mechanisms which deal with stress.

Liking people and showing it

Liking people we care for is important and there are various ways in which this can be demonstrated. Smiling and touching are both simple reminders to people that we like and care for them. Obviously, touching can sometimes be inappropriate – it is very personal and we should not offend people. For example, the touching by a carer of an adolescent of the opposite sex would usually not be acceptable. Of course, it is much easier to like people who are pleasant and co-operative than those who are not, but the carer must make the effort to see the human being beyond difficult personality traits.

Warmth, friendliness and cheerfulness

Warmth and friendliness are vital ingredients of a caring relationship because they help create a positive atmosphere.

Nobody wants to wake up to or be touched by a reluctant carer. It is important to be cheerful as you undertake routine tasks, but this should not be taken too far – superficial pleasantries can soon be seen through, so one's cheerfulness should be genuine.

Naturalness

Bearing in mind that the most valuable asset we bring to the job is ourselves, a good carer should allow their natural personality to come through.

Naturalness reflects in ease of manner, relaxation and trust; this is often contagious and can encourage the service user to be natural too, which helps to eliminate any barriers that may exist. So, be yourself as much as possible.

Practical ability

Whatever the social, health care or social work setting, it is important that carers demonstrate competence in their work and encourage the service user to feel confident about their practical abilities. If, say, a social worker is taking a group of children on an outdoor pursuits weekend it is essential that the children trust in the worker's ability to lead and care for them. Similarly, the severely physically disabled person needs to have complete faith in the person lifting them into and out of the bath. These practical tasks need to be carried out assertively in order to make the client feel safe and confident.

Attitudes

A carer's attitudes are not always voiced but they are nearly always conveyed. That is to say, a service user will pick up how a carer thinks of them. Consequently, carers should strive to develop positive attitudes.

Acceptance

Acceptance involves recognising the human being in a person and taking the person as they are. It may be difficult for someone to inwardly warm to, say, a bad tempered older person whose face is badly disfigured or to a severely disabled child who persistently coughs up food, but acceptance requires the carer to look beyond a person's physical condition or any behavioural problems and care for the person as a person.

Being non-judgemental

Related to the notion of acceptance is the principle of being non-judgemental. This means being open-minded and resisting the tendency to blame a person for their circumstances. Blame can only hinder an enabling process. For example, in a case of child abuse it may be difficult to accept, in an unbiased manner, the parents responsible for injuring the child, but how is the nursery officer, teacher, health visitor or social worker going to be of any help to the child's parents and ultimately the child without non-judgemental acceptance?

Tolerance and patience

One requirement of a social carer or social worker is that they may at times have to be prepared to 'soak up' other people's anger and frustration. This is not to say that the relationship is one-way and that a social carer or social worker can legitimately reject inappropriate anger.

At other times a social carer or social worker may see a way out of a client's difficulties but the service user may not initially be receptive to any outside direction. The social carer or social worker should be patient and move at the client's own self-determined pace.

Knowledge

Knowledge derived from various sources is an essential component of an effective carer's resources. As we have stated earlier, knowledge about cultures, traditions and lifestyles is an integral part of anti-oppressive practice.

Academic knowledge

It is important that carers have a basic knowledge of psychology, sociology, race and class and human growth and development in order that they may be more aware of a person's needs and the influence of their social environment. This means that the service user will be viewed not in isolation but more comprehensively in their family and social setting. This fuller information will, hopefully, lead to the person being cared for more sensitively and their needs being more responsively catered for.

The carer should also have some knowledge of the differing theories contained in helping strategies (this is dealt with more fully in Chapter 8).

Awareness of other agencies

Part of a carer's duty is to be familiar with the role of other caring agencies and the way in which service users can benefit from the resources offered – for example, those who work with people with learning difficulties need to be aware of what is offered at the local college of further education, both during the day and in the evening, to see if their clients could benefit from the courses or other facilities provided.

It is very important that all social workers have an up-to-date knowledge of the social security benefits available to clients. It is also necessary to know whom to contact at the DSS if difficulties arise in relation to this.

In addition, a carer needs to be aware of what is happening in the community that may be of interest to service users; for example, jumble sales, furniture auctions and social and leisure events which may add to the enjoyment and enrichment of people's lives. Most of these events will be organised by informal or voluntary groups and organisations.

Life experience

Many people believe that life's experience is the best teacher. However, a great deal depends on how effectively and intelligently we use the experience that life offers us. In our caring for others, we will often gain insights from past experiences which increase our understanding and empathy. We also learn a great deal from our own unhappiness and sorrow and this should help us to identify with other people who are going through difficult or testing times. Similarly our joy can help and inform the way we work.

Mature entrants into social care, health care and social work often bring with them much varied and valuable life experience: this may include being a parent, caring for a dependent relative, voluntary work in the local community or the experiences of coping with their own disability or ill health.

Political awareness

We could also call this 'political consciousness'. A great deal of what we do in our private or working lives is limited or controlled by constraints. These may stem from financial, social or political factors or from all three. Caring for others can be political activity in two ways. Firstly, our making decisions about other people's lives and how they will live is a political activity – with a small 'p'. Caring for others often means that we are in a powerful position with regard to our clients. It is up to us not to abuse this power, but to use it in a loving and sensitive way in the best interests of the service user. We will need to recognise the potential for service users to act on their own behalf and devise their own solutions and should be mindful that our own need to care for others does not get in the way of this process.

Secondly, the social and other caring services in our society receive a financial slice of a much larger cake – the total resources which central and local Government decide will be spent on provision for defence, housing, education and other services. This necessarily involves the caring services in a struggle for more resources and this again can involve us in political debate and activity.

A knowledge of political, social and financial issues and questions is necessary because such knowledge helps to inform the way in which we work and enhances our knowledge of the world about us.

Conclusion

It is important to point out that the above qualities should be balanced as well as inter-related. For instance, a brilliant academic knowledge without empathy or basic courtesies will be of no use. The ideal is a well-rounded or 'whole' person who has several areas of strength upon which to draw when caring for others. One area will complement another and lead to a situation of overall competence if not excellence.

A note of caution which may be of some encouragement – the ability to be an effective carer does not depend on passing written examinations or obtaining paper qualifications. Research conducted into the effectiveness of social work tends to point to three factors as being of over-riding importance: empathy, non-possessive warmth and genuineness. It is these qualities that produce positive results.

Leisure

What is this life if, full of care,
We have no time to stand and stare.
No time to stand beneath the boughs
And stare as long as sheep or cows.
No time to see, when woods we pass,
Where squirrels hide their nuts in grass.
No time to see, in broad daylight,
Streams full of stars, like skies at night.
No time to turn at Beauty's glance,
And watch her feet, how they can dance.
No time to wait till her mouth can
Enrich that smile her eyes began.
A poor life this if, full of care,
We have no time to stand and stare.

William Henry Davies, 1871–1940

One final point needs to be stressed – caring for others effectively in a fulltime capacity requires energy. This means that you *must* find time and space for yourself – time to relax, enjoy yourself and 'lose yourself' in an activity which is completely different from work. Obviously your friends and family are a tremendously valuable resource in this regard. If you do not 'recharge your batteries', then you will become depleted and will be of little help to either yourself or others. You may even begin to suffer from stress, which at its most acute may lead to 'professional burn-out'. This is a serious state of affairs, but sadly many people in the caring professions experience it. The result is that the carer's relationships, partnerships, marriage and quality of life will suffer.

In order to help others we must help ourselves. There will be times when job satisfaction and appreciation from clients will not be there, yet the job must still be done. It is therefore very important that we look after our own physical, mental and emotional needs. We will each find our own particular ways of doing this. Generally, however, good food, regular exercise and relaxing and interesting leisure activities will be of great benefit. Having fun and enjoying a sense of humour – whether our own or others' – will have a restorative effect. In the end, not only we ourselves but also our service users will reap the benefits.

Exercise 1 – your personal qualities

Read through the chapter, write down the qualities you feel you already possess and consider the areas you need to improve upon.

Exercise 2 – someone else's personal qualities

Choose someone you know well and may have observed in a caring situation. Write down what you think their caring qualities are and assess which qualities you feel they need to develop.

Exercise 3 – investigating personal feelings

Divide into pairs and complete the following set of sentences as spontaneously as possible. Discuss your answers with each other. Finally, assess whether you think that this has been a useful way of investigating personal feelings.

1. One thing I really like about myself is . . .
2. I dislike people who . . .
3. When people ignore me, I . . .
4. When someone praises me I . . .
5. When I relate to people, I . . .
6. Those who really know me . . .
7. My moods . . .
8. I am at my very best with people when . . .
9. When I am in a group of strangers I . . .
10. I feel lonely when . . .
11. I envy . . .
12. I think I have hurt others by . . .

13. Those who don't know me well . . .
14. What I am looking for in a relationship is . . .
15. I get hurt when . . .
16. I am at my best with people when . . .
17. I like people who . . .
18. What I feel most guilty about in relationships is . . .
19. Few people know that I . . .
20. When I think about intimacy, I . . .
21. One thing I really dislike about myself is . . .
22. I get angry with . . .
23. One thing that makes me nervous with people is . . .
24. When I really feel good about myself, I . . .
25. When others put me down, I . . .
26. I feel awkward with others when . . .
27. I feel let down when . . .
28. In relationships, what I run away from most is . . .
29. I hate people to see that I am . . .
30. I feel most embarrassed when . . .
31. I . . .

Exercise 4 – guiding

a) To be performed in pairs. One of the partners in each pair has their eyes covered by a scarf or towel. Half the group then lead their unsighted partners around the room, giving verbal prompts and taking care to avoid contact with any other couples in the group. After five minutes the roles can then be reversed.

   Consider how it feels to be totally reliant on somebody else. Did you feel secure and able to trust your partner? Conversely, did you feel confident as a guide?

b) The above exercise is repeated, this time with non – verbal instructions only.

Exercise 5 – feeding

To be carried out in pairs. If it is possible, arrange with your workplace catering staff to be served meals at two separate sittings. At the first sitting one partner assumes that they are disabled and unable to feed themselves and is fed by the other partner. The roles are then reversed.

The aim of the exercise is to experience the dependency of having to be fed by someone else. How does it feel? At the same time, you might comment on the kind of feelings you experienced while feeding someone else.

Exercise 6 – role play – an incident in a children's home

Roles

Terry: You are 14 and living in a children's home which is preparing you for a permanency foster or adoption placement. You have been at the home since first being accommodated by the local authority ten months ago. Your parents divorced three years ago and you have had minimal contact with either of them. You experienced an unhappy family background characterised by much violence, particularly between your parents.

Earlier this afternoon, during a game of football, you were fouled badly as you were nearing the goal. You got up and hit the boy in the face. The boy you hit was your closest friend and you haven't seen him since.

Nine months ago you were placed with foster carers, but they were too bossy, you think. They felt they were unable to control you. New foster carers have now been found for you and, having met them twice, you think you'll like them. You want to live in a family home and don't want to remain in a children's home, although you get on with the staff and some of the children.

You are concerned about your outbreak of temper and resorting to physical violence, which you thought you had learned to control. You are also sorry that you hit your friend and feel that he will now withdraw his friendship. You are concerned too that your behaviour might jeopardise your chances of being placed with new foster carers.

Key worker: You are disappointed to learn that Terry has been in a fight but consider it to have been a spontaneous reaction rather than premeditated. You have talked to the other boy involved, who has returned from hospital with very bad bruising around the nose and eyes. He is still angry and resentful towards Terry.

You like Terry and feel that he desperately needs to be part of a family. He was disappointed that his other foster placement broke down and sometimes despairs of being able to be placed with a family. You have high hopes that the current foster placement being considered for Terry could be successful – the new carers are younger than the previous ones, understanding and have said that they like what they have seen of Terry. They have a son of their own, 18 months younger than Terry, and two younger daughters aged seven and six. The family also like animals and have a dog and three cats. Terry is very fond of animals.

Since he returned from playing football at 5.30 p.m. Terry has been in his room and missed the evening meal. It is now 8 o'clock and you have called into his room half an hour ago to let him know that you would like to see him shortly. He mumbled that he did not want to see anyone.

Task

Role play the key worker visiting Terry in his room to talk out the events of the day.

Questions for discussion

1. Working as a professional carer, how do you unwind and prevent stress and its harmful effects?
2. What respective contributions are made by the following to a carer's competence:

   a) life experience;
   b) academic knowledge;
   c) personality?

3. What sources of information would you use in order to find out more about cultures other than your own? Plan and carry out research into one minority culture of your choice.
4. Empathy is 'putting yourself in another's situation'. Think of someone you perceive as having some kind of difficulty and concentrate on viewing the world as that person sees it. Write an account of a 'day in the life' of the person you have chosen, describing it from their perspective.
5. Should carers love the people they care for or is it possible to look after someone whom you do not particularly like?
6. All societies have rules and taboos about physical contact between people. Consider the situations where it might be appropriate for a carer to touch a client and how this might be done in an acceptable way.

Further reading

1. *Ordinary Magic – A Handbook for Counselling people with Learning Difficulties*, David Brandon (Tao, 1992). An imaginative book that stresses the value of all individuals and draws on spirituality as a motivating force.
2. *Race and Child Protection – A Code of Practice* (REU Black and White Alliance, 1989–90). Good practice in relation to child protection focusing on issues of race and ethnicity.
3. *A Woman in Your Own Right*, Anne Dickinson (Quartet, 1989). A positive book about assertiveness written for women.
4. *Living, Loving and Ageing – Sexual Relationships in Later Life*, Wendy and Sally Greengross (Age Concern England, 1992) A book which challenges stereotypes and offers practical suggestions for promoting rewarding and loving relationships.
5. *Taking Good Care – A Handbook for Care Assistants*, Jenyth Worsley (Age Concern England, 1989). A very accessible basic guide to caring, whether in a residential home or in the community.
6. *Working in Residential Homes for Elderly People*, Paul Brearley (Routledge, 1990). A very concise and detailed book which describes good quality care practice in residential homes for elders. Very readable and highly practical.

8

Strategies for Helping

Introduction

This chapter looks at the wide range of strategies for helping available to those who work in the caring services. The strategies are dealt with in three sections: some are discussed in this Introduction, along with an indication of their historical origins; three case studies follow, each of which has three different strategies attached to them; a final section examines other approaches not yet dealt with and the chapter ends with an analytical tool, by which we can examine our practice and approach to caring. In the Appendix there is an intervention checklist, which asks basic, relevant questions about the helping process.

It is not possible for this chapter to be fully comprehensive because there are too many approaches to be considered. However, although limited in number, as wide a variety as possible is presented in a condensed, simplified form. The reader who wishes to know more should consult the 'further reading' section at the close of the chapter. We advise readers to examine as many strategies as possible because we believe, as practitioners, one should pick and choose and not get stuck with one approach. The three case studies are an attempt to show that each of the strategies used has something to offer; very rarely is there only one way of working with people.

Terminology can be a problem; often a particular strategy will be called by a different name by different people. Taken as a whole, those we deal with may be given more formal titles such as 'social work theory', 'social care practice' or 'methods of social work intervention' by some writers and practitioners. The problem with such terms is that they can imply an elitism, sometimes a professional elitism; the debate about the difference and demarcation between 'social care' and 'social work' is illustrative of this (see the Introduction to *Social Issues for Carers*, p.xi, by Webb and Tossell for an exploration of this).

The phrase 'strategies for helping' is preferred because it is general; no one kind of worker and no one kind of work setting has a monopoly over this particular phrasing.

Social carers and social workers use different strategies for helping as do all therapists, psychologists and health care workers. They are utilised within a wide range of settings: residential, institutional, fieldwork, domiciliary and day care. They are also used with all client groups, e.g. children and young people, elderly people, offenders and people with disabilities or mental ill health.

The origins of helping strategies

Most available strategies used in the caring services have been borrowed and/or adapted from such disciplines as psychology, psychiatry, sociology and criminology.

The three major schools of psychology – *psychoanalysis*, as originated by Freud and later developed by others, *behavioural* psychology, most notably associated with B.F. Skinner and *humanistic* psychology, whose best known proponent is Carl Rogers – have had the most significant influence on caring strategies.

In particular, psychoanalysis has been of great historical importance, mostly in social work. From the 1950s on, Florence Hollis and others working in the USA developed what they called 'psychosocial casework' from Freud's body of work. More recently known as 'psychodynamic casework', 'social casework' or simply 'casework', their work, which started to influence social work in Britain in the 1960s, became *the* model of professional one-to-one working for about 20 years, losing ground only when counselling and a range of other, more recently developed approaches came to the fore.

Often accused, even from its earliest days, of being a form of 'amateur psychoanalysis', casework focused on the internal stress of and the external pressures on an individual. The casework relationship was key to the process which happened between carer and client. Within this relationship the social worker would use two main procedures to help the client; sustaining procedures which offered support and affirmation while the relationship was being formed and maintained, thus reducing stress; and modifying procedures which aimed to reduce outside pressure, whether familial, interpersonal or societal, by helping the client to gain insight into their situation. Although rather outmoded and unfashionable, particularly in regard to the language used, casework remains a very important influence today.

Behavioural and humanistic psychology have been responsible for the development of a range of techniques within caring. Behaviourism or behaviour modification tends to focus on externally observable behaviour of a problematic nature with the purpose of devising ways of changing or modifying that behaviour, either because it causes problems for the individual client or because it causes problems for others; both could be involved, of course. The approach studies how people become conditioned in their behaviour (through a process of *stimulus, response* and *reinforcement*) and how it might be changed by punishment or reward. The 'token system', often used in social care with people with learning disabilities – a way of withholding or giving rewards for unacceptable or acceptable behaviour – is an example of this approach.

In humanistic psychology, perhaps the best known approach is Carl Rogers' 'client-centred therapy', described in present day terms as 'person-centred therapy'. For Rogers, there were two especially important ways in which therapy was 'person-centred'; firstly, the carer must be empathic, to gain an understanding of how the individual sees and feels about the situation they are in; secondly, to recognise that the client has the key to the healing process already within their personal being; that the carer merely helps the client to move this process on. Rogers believed that all people 'are potentially competent'.

The humanistic school of psychology has a positive and optimistic attitude to life and the world. However, it puts great onus on the carer to have high standards of practice; they should be 'congruent', i.e. genuine and 'integrated' (or whole), should hold the client in 'unconditional positive regard' as a valued and valuable human being, and should always have 'empathic understanding' of the individual they are caring for.

Humanistic psychology has given birth to a wide range of helping strategies or 'therapies' (to use its own terminology) and many of them have found their way into, or have at least informed, mainstream caring. Some examples are gestalt therapy, co-

counselling, encounter groups, transactional analysis (TA) and primal therapy. In the psychoanalytic and behavioural traditions the therapist/practitioner tends to have a very powerful position; the psychoanalyst is frequently interpreting past events and their effect on past or current behaviour; the behaviourist has a powerful array of techniques to draw on, the client's understanding of which may be only incidental. In contrast, humanistic psychology faces up to the question of power in the caring relationship, admits that it is an important and significant issue and addresses how it might be dealt with, to the satisfaction of all parties. We owe it a debt for the influence it has had on bringing empowerment, user involvement and self-advocacy to the fore.

Power in the caring relationship

This chapter is entitled 'Strategies for *helping*'. Some comments need to be made about this. Coulshed has written: 'All forms of helping are really forms of power' (*Social Work Practice – An Introduction*, 2nd edition, p 111). In more detail Thompson has written: 'Social work is a *political* activity; that is, it operates within the context of sets of power relations – the power of law and the state, the power inherent in social divisions such as class, race and gender, and the micro-level power of personal interactions.' He goes on to give an instance of the sort of issue carers deal with: 'Also, many of the problems social workers tackle have their roots in the abuse of power – child abuse, for example' (*Antidiscriminatory practice*, p 150).

Whatever job we do, in whatever setting and with whatever client group, we should be as aware as possible of what power we have and how it affects the way we work. Good care practice will help clients as much as possible *to help themselves*. Only rarely is good practice about doing things *for* people. For example, when someone is in deep shock following a bereavement, we may have to be more directive and take over for a while, but only for as short a time as is practicable. And if someone has no money, no food and no shelter, we have to provide what might be called direct help, either in kind or financial. Generally, though, good care practice is concerned with interaction, a dynamic, two-way process involving both client and carer. In other words, 'strategies for helping' are ways of intervening in people's lives, working with or alongside them in co-operation, to facilitate positive change.

But we may go further than this: many of the people we care for may be powerless and marginalised, discriminated against, stigmatised or experiencing a combination of all of these processes. Perhaps the most helpful and acceptable strategy we can adopt with oppressed clients is to empower them. For Payne, 'empowerment aims to use specific strategies to reduce, eliminate, combat and reverse negative valuations by powerful groups in society affecting certain individuals and social groups' (*Modern Social Work Theory*, p229). Empowerment is two things – it is both a process and a goal. It is closely involved with two other processes:

1. User – or citizen – involvement, which aims to involve clients as much as possible in the planning, administration and delivery of services – to actively ensure they have a part in decision-making;
2. Self-advocacy, which aims at encouraging people to speak for themselves and assert their rights, both as individuals and as groups of people sharing similar experiences or beliefs. Within groups a form of self-help and mutual support can

develop to cater for people's personal and political needs and members are also able to pass on skills to each other. We should differentiate self-advocacy from advocacy, which means a process whereby someone actively supports or speaks on behalf of another. A very long established example of an advocate would be a lawyer or legal advisor.

Some recently completed research by Parsloe and Stevenson has stressed a significant fact concerning empowerment: often the very agencies or settings in which carers work, and in which they attempt to empower clients, have the effect of disempowering them as workers. For example, carers may not themselves be involved in decision-making or work allocation. The two writers stress that there is a need for agencies to change throughout each unit. They assert: 'The attempt at empowerment will fail if it is seen as simple, or as requiring change only in frontline staff' (Community Care. 18.2.93).

Anti-oppressive/anti-discriminatory practice

Empowerment is a powerful way of breaking down oppression and discrimination. In fact, as Thompson states: 'A practice which does not take account of oppression and discrimination cannot be seen as good practice, no matter how high its standards may be in other respects' (*Anti-discriminatory Practice*, pp10–11). As carers we are not in the business of helping people to adjust to unsatisfactory situations; antidiscriminatory practice requires that we enable people as much as possible to change situations in a positive way. Otherwise we could stand accused of being agents of social control.

The principle and practice of normalisation may also be considered as an integral part of antioppressive practice. Normalisation, as used with people in institutions or residential care and with people with learning disabilities, aims to counter stigma and marginalisation and provide people instead with valued lifestyles and opportunities in common with the majority of people in the community.

Oppression and discrimination are often unintended or unconscious. Many people find charitable giving perfectly acceptable. At the present time the State fully encourages it. And yet a large number of people with disabilities have empowered themselves and exercised self-advocacy and formed a pressure group under the title 'Block Telethon'. They have used and still use the slogan 'Piss on Pity' to protest against 'Telethon', the annual television fundraising event. They claim it is patronising and oppressive and in place of charity they demand rights, justice and decent, State-provided services.

The 'process' of helping

The helping relationship usually begins with an assessment of the needs, difficulties or problems that the client presents. All strategies for helping have some kind of inbuilt facility for assessment. Some, for example task-centred work are stronger on assessment than other approaches. Assessment procedure is usually based upon interviewing a number of people, including the client and any other professionals involved. The process requires gathering a great deal of information. Sometimes a more formal event will be part of assessment, such as a case conference, reflecting a multidisciplinary or multiagency approach, or an internal review, made up of key staff and the service user where appropriate.

Following assessment, a work plan will be drawn up which may be referred to in one of several ways: a care plan, individual care programme, individual programme plan or supervision plan. The way this is set out and documented will vary according to the carer's agency or work setting. The recording of events, happenings, actions taken and decisions made is of crucial importance and, again, will vary with each agency and type of worker. Some kind of periodic appraisal will take place in order to assess progress. Such progress reports may lead to the drawing up of a new work plan which may mean new or different approaches for the future.

Three case studies

We now turn to three case studies, each of which includes three possible strategies for helping. The case studies are composite portrayals, based on situations that could occur; they have been composed to illustrate different strategies. As we have already said, we would encourage carers to be eclectic in their approach. The case studies illustrate the fact that very rarely is there only one useful way to work with people. We also want to point out that each strategy could be used in a variety of situations and not just the one illustrated.

Case study 1

John, a 16 year old who has recently left school, has no job to go to. He has become frustrated and depressed – partly as a result of being unemployed, but also because of the tension that exists between his parents, who are on the verge of separating. Years of hostility (punctuated by violence) between his parents have taken their toll on him.

After a particularly bad row between his mother and father, John has taken (in the past three weeks) to staying out as much as possible and on some nights he does not return. When his mother questions him about where he has been, he becomes very aggressive and in desperation she contacts a social worker. She tells the social worker that she feels that John may get into trouble with the police – she describes some of his friends as 'undesirable', because, she says, they have 'been before the court on several occasions'. With the added pressure of marital problems, the mother feels 'near the end of her tether'. The social worker, after speaking with her for about an hour, says she would like to visit the whole family at home. This is arranged to take place in two days' time.

Unfortunately, when the social worker arrives at the house, John's father is not there, having stormed out earlier, saying to his wife that John is 'her problem' and she will have to 'sort it out'. The mother is tearful and distraught. In addition to John and his mother, John's two sisters, aged 12 and 14, are present.

Following this meeting, the social worker writes to John's father suggesting that she should meet him on a certain day, but he fails to turn up. After making an

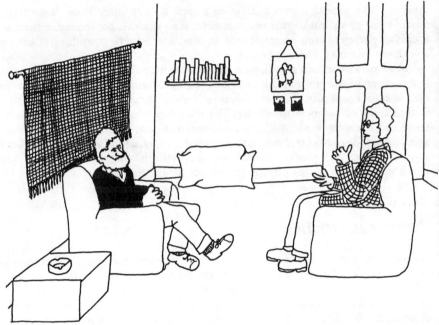

As well as listening, counselling involves the observation of non-verbal communication

assessment of the case, the social worker decides on the best plan of action in the given circumstances. She decides that there are three possible ways of intervening: counselling, Egan's 'skilled helper' model and family therapy.

Counselling

Counselling is basically a way of helping someone to explore a problem. The aim is to help a person to feel that they can either cope or live with the problem or find a solution to the problem. The basis of counselling is the growth of a relationship between the counsellor and client which is built on trust. Counselling involves *listening* effectively because, without a good understanding of the situation and the feelings of the person concerned, the counsellor will be unable to respond appropriately. A major requirement for listening effectively is a good understanding of *non-verbal communication*.

After making her assessment of John's case, the social worker begins to see him alone, twice a week, and to start to help him explore his feelings and problems. After an initial period of distrust and suspicion on John's part, they begin to make progress together and John begins to understand more clearly how he thinks and feels toward his own behaviour, his home and his family. Counselling gives him time and the 'friendly listening ear' of a sensitive adult. As a result, his behaviour changes – he becomes more aware of his mother's predicament and he begins to support her in what becomes an increasingly difficult situation where his father is concerned.

A note on styles of helping in counselling

A number of different ways of behaving or 'styles of helping' exist within the wider concept of counselling. It can be mildly or purposely directive, i.e. power is manifested to a lesser or greater degree. And at any one time there will be a power relationship between counsellor and client; each will be less or more in control of the interaction at different times.

Figure 8.1 shows a range of behaviours in counselling along an 'empowerment continuum'. On the far left hand side, the client is in control and as we move through the intervention styles, the counsellor takes more control; they take a more *directive* role.

Using behaviours to the right of the continuum may get things done, may get problems solved, but the risk is that the client will feel powerless, helpless or dependent. But using behaviours to the left should have positive, validating effects on the client, although they may be far more time-consuming.

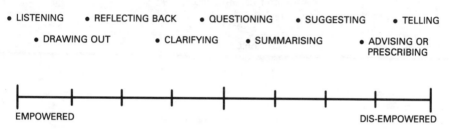

Fig 8.1   Styles of helping in relation to an empowerment continuum (based on an idea by CCDU, University of Leeds).

Gerard Egan's 'skilled helper' model

This is included here because it can be regarded as a model of counselling, but it differs in many respects from the conventional form of counselling dealt with above. The model was first published by Egan in 1975 in the USA but he has modified it since. It has three major stages. These could be termed: *exploration, understanding* and *action*. Some commentators on Egan's work add a fourth stage – *evaluation* – which, as the appellation suggests, is an appraisal of what has taken place.

Egan describes the function of the first stage, the present scenario (or current situation), thus: to 'help clients identify, explore and clarify their problem situations and unused opportunities' (p30). During this stage the counsellor aims to build up trust and establish a rapport, using skills such as active listening, reflecting and summarising preparatory to making an assessment. In Egan's words, the client should be helped to 'tell their stories. . . become aware of, and overcome, their blind spots and develop new perspectives on themselves and their problem situations' and to 'work on problems, issues, concerns or opportunities that will make a difference' (pp32–5).

In the second stage, which Egan entitles the preferred scenario, the counsellor aims to 'help clients develop goals, objectives or agendas based on an action-oriented understanding of the problem situation' (p31). This might involve helping the client to decide what they would like to do differently, using interpretative skills, noting themes and patterns in their behaviour and, to a certain extent, challenging or

---

You and I

I explain quietly. You
hear me shouting. You
try a new tack. I
feel old wounds reopen.

You see both sides. I
see your blinkers. I
am placatory. You
sense a new selfishness.

I am a dove. You
recognize the hawk. You
offer an olive branch. I
feel the thorns.

You bleed. I
see crocodile tears. I
withdraw. You
reel from the impact.

Roger McGough.

In Counselling, attentive, 'active listening' is essential.

---

confronting them about this.

The third stage, known as 'getting there', asks the counsellor to 'help clients develop action strategies for accomplishing goals, that is, for getting from the current to the preferred scenario' (p31). Egan calls this a 'transition stage'. It is one in which the carer uses their skills to set goals, provide support, ideas and resources and encourages the client to make decisions. Techniques such as brainstorming and role play may be applicable.

In Egan's 'skilled helper' model, the counsellor may play a more powerful role in influencing, advising and being an 'expert' authority than in mainstream counselling. In working with John in the case study, the carer would encourage him in the early stages, while building up trust and rapport, to 'tell his story', to explain how he sees his own situation and why he thinks, feels and behaves the way he does. The three stage process would then be followed through.

Family therapy

The social worker might have decided that neither individual counselling nor Egan's model was sufficient to deal with the problems presented by John's case. Assessment might have shown his problems to be fully rooted within his family relationships and the social worker might therefore have felt that *family therapy* would be more appropriate or effective.

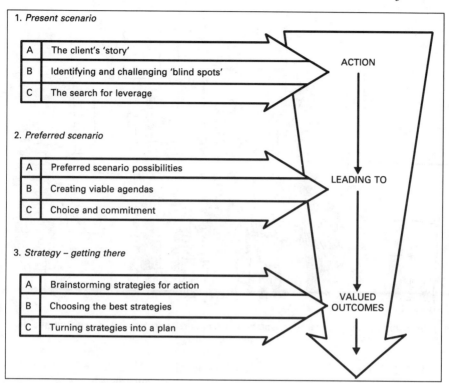

Fig 8.2 Egan's 'skilled helper' model.

This therapy treats the whole family, not just the member presenting a problem (in this case, John). Only very rarely is one particular individual solely responsible for problems – in fact, one person can take on the role of 'symptom-bearer', where his or her problem behaviour is a consequence of more fundamental family discord.

One of the advantages of family therapy is that it sees a whole family in operation or in interaction. It requires the use of skill, intuition and sensitivity on the part of the social worker to understand clearly the nature of a particular family's dynamics – the relationships between various members of the family and the blocks and hindrances to constructive interaction.

It will often take time to become effective. At first, meetings between the social worker and the family may be strained or artificial. However, the skilled practitioner will be able to help family members relax and encourage them to be more open and honest with each other. Much of the approach involves helping people to gain more insight into themselves and to better understand how their behaviour affects other members of the family.

A technique called *sculpting* is sometimes used as a device for clarifying relationships between family members. All members of the family in turn have the opportunity to visually represent their own perceptions of their relationships with the others. This will include non-verbal communication such as gestures, facial expressions and posture. This often enables people to see more clearly their own position and the position of others within the family.

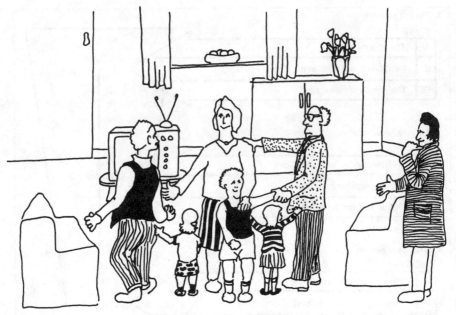

In sculpting, the physical representation of family relationships can provide insights for family members

In John's case, gaining the trust and co-operation of his father might have been very difficult, if not impossible, and the social worker would have borne this in mind when considering the usefulness of family therapy.

Case study 2

Joan is an elderly lady of 77 who lives with her daughter's family. The family consists of her daughter, her daughter's husband and their two children – a boy aged 18 and a girl aged 15. Joan is finding that mobility is becoming increasingly difficult and her condition of incontinence is becoming worse. This has put great pressure on the whole family. On one particular day, tired of assisting her mother upstairs, Mary, the daughter, leaves her mother to her own devices and Joan has a bad fall. The health visitor who visits Joan feels that the family needs the contact of a social worker, so she makes a referral to the local social services department.

Joan does not suffer from dementia – on the contrary, she is rather a lively and intelligent person. Recently, however, she has become depressed – a reaction to what she sees as the family's insensitivity to her problems. Her son-in-law works away from home most of the time, so Joan's daughter and the two children bear the brunt of responsibility for her.

When the social worker makes her first visit to Joan, she realises that the family is in a state of crisis – time has taken its toll on the goodwill which had once existed in the family and they now feel that they cannot go on much longer. When making her assessment, the social worker considers three different ways of approaching the problem: crisis intervention, residential care and task centred work.

Crisis intervention

Crisis intervention is not so much a distinct strategy for helping as a way of examining the situation of a person who is in a state of crisis and is undergoing much distress. It originated in psychiatry and it has often been applied in working with the bereaved. One of the factors central to it is that people in a state of crisis are usually more amenable to change. It therefore uses this openness to change as a basis towards reaching a desirable solution.

In Joan's case, the social worker attempts to help the family members to see that change can be positive and to encourage the growth of co-operation in reaching for a solution to their problem. This will involve not apportioning blame to anyone in particular (Joan cannot avoid the ageing process!). The social worker might well see Joan alone on some occasions, but will certainly want to see all the family members together in order to encourage them to see that the crisis involves them all, as does the finding of a solution.

Crisis intervention in this case will involve explaining the various alternatives to the family's present situation. It may involve practicalities such as introducing aids and adaptations to the home. Here are some possible examples: a chairlift for the stairs; rearranging rooms so that Joan can sleep downstairs and receive help with toileting; obtaining outside assistance with laundry services; and generally trying to spread responsibilities for assisting Joan more evenly among family members. This last will have the effect of involving the children more, thus reducing the pressure on the mother.

Fortunately, in this case, the family want Joan to remain with them at home – they do not wish to have her placed in residential care for the elderly. However, it is something which the social worker feels should at least be considered.

Residential care

Again, residential care should not be regarded as a distinct strategy for helping, but as a care setting in which a number of different approaches might be applied; for example, counselling or groupwork. Residential care is often automatically considered in a negative light because of its association with institutionalisation, but this is both unfair and not up to date. Not only can it be a positive resource that can offer asylum (in the true sense of the word) for individuals and a respite for their carers, but it is also increasingly realised that some people may well be 'institutionalised' in their own homes when they are trapped or isolated and have no contact with family, friends or neighbours.

One of the reasons why the social worker considers it in Joan's case is because the family is deemed to be in a state of crisis. The social worker may legitimately feel that a brief period in a residential setting – that is, respite care – may at some stage provide both Joan and the family with a desirable (if not essential) break from each other, to give them the opportunity to 'recharge batteries' and return to the situation with more energy. It would not, however, be wise to use the resource immediately, before the family has had a chance to formulate plans to deal with the current problem.

A period of separation may have the effect of actually strengthening the bond between Joan and the family, but the social worker would have to be aware that the opposite effect may unfortunately occur. The period of assessment is therefore extremely important. Equally important is that the social worker should have a good intuitive understanding of the likely consequences of intervention.

Task centred work

This is a modification of traditional *social casework*. It is an attempt to 'sharpen' it by tackling problems experienced by clients by means of specific achievable *tasks* which may be performed within a time limit, which will be specified and agreed by the carer in co-operation with the client. Assessment is very important and the approach usually involves the concept of a *contract* drawn up between the social worker and the client. One of the strengths of task centred work is that it concentrates on the client's own conception of their difficulties as the key to reaching a solution. It is similar to crisis intervention in that it holds that a breakdown in coping with problems can trigger off desires for change within the clients themselves. If used effectively, it will increase the clients' ability to cope in the near and distant future.

In Joan's case, the social worker would make an assessment which would break down the crisis that is facing the family into its component parts, first, by examining Joan's mobility and incontinence problems and then going on to examine how much and in what way these have caused wider difficulties in the family. Next, the social worker could encourage Joan and other family members to set simple and achievable tasks to help solve the problems. The achievement of one task – for example, rearranging rooms in the house to accommodate Joan downstairs – would generally have the effect of increasing the family's confidence and capacity to deal with others, for example Joan's toileting difficulties. As tasks are fulfilled, so family relationships would tend to improve and this would lead to an enhanced quality of life for all involved.

Ideally the tasks should be shared as equally as possible (within practical limitations) throughout the family. Joan's son-in-law would also be encouraged to take a greater part on his return home from working away.

Task centred work involves periodic assessment as tasks are achieved, or the setting of new tasks if problems occur along the way. Another strength of the approach is that, from the very start of a 'contract', the end is in view because all parties are fully aware of the tasks they have set in co-operation with the social worker. Contracts can be written or orally agreed as the approach is adapted to a particular case.

Case study 3

Jim is a 28 year old divorced man living alone in lodgings. He has a gambling problem which has caused his marriage to end in divorce. Money for the family had been scarce even when Jim was in work, but financial problems had got worse as his gambling habit increased. He and his wife parted two years ago. He has now been unemployed for a year and he is severely depressed. He has no social contacts apart from those in the local betting shop. He has recently sought the help of a social worker because he has begun to think that only suicide could bring an end to his problems. Obviously subconsciously he does not really want to end his life – only his problems – otherwise he would not have sought help.

The social worker, having made an assessment of Jim's case, considers three possible ways of tackling the problem: groupwork, behaviour modification and social or lifeskills training.

Groupwork

The social worker is aware of a group run by a colleague for people with problems concerning gambling. Jim is referred to this group and Jim, being desperate, is keen to take part in whatever is offered.

The initial focus of the social worker is to help the group to get to know Jim and to encourage Jim to share his problems with the group as a whole. Trust is an essential ingredient if this is to happen effectively and so too is a relaxed atmosphere.

Other group members are encouraged to share the various, often very personal, methods they have so far used to deal with the temptation to gamble. From the start, the social worker is pleased to observe that this gives Jim hope and an increased confidence that he can overcome his problem.

The group is an ongoing one – it does not set a time limit to its existence. However, after a period of some months, Jim may feel that he has accomplished something and will therefore try to manage without this form of support and assistance.

Note: Groupwork is so important and wide-ranging that there is an additional separate section on it below.

Behaviour modification

The social worker might have felt that behaviour modification would provide a more direct solution to Jim's gambling problem. Behaviour modification has its origins within psychology, from what is usually called *'learning theory'*. Central to this theory is the concept that behaviour is *learnt* in a social setting; therefore, when behaviour causes problems (in this case, Jim's gambling), it can be *unlearnt*. In other words, the client can learn new forms of more appropriate behaviour, in order to cope with life without gambling. The approach moves from the achieving of small, easy changes in behaviour to more difficult changes, perhaps involving more entrenched behaviour. Behavioural techniques can be used only if the client is willing to co-operate – in Jim's case, he would have to earnestly desire to give up gambling.

Gambling, like other forms of compulsive habit-forming behaviour – for example, smoking, overeating and drug addiction – is rewarding to the person who does it. The social worker using behavioural techniques must first of all have got Jim to look at those particular aspects of gambling which he finds especially enjoyable – for example, many gamblers are thrilled and stimulated by the tension and excitement they feel in a crowded betting shop when a race is about to be run.

The behavioural therapist would have helped Jim to work out in detail the stages that led up to his actively placing a bet – the time of day, the mood he was in, where he was in relation to the betting shop or telephone (if he was in the habit of telephoning bets) and so on – until he had a clear picture of all the behavioural steps that led up to the actual moment when Jim's money went across the counter. This information would then be used to design a programme in which alternative behaviours would be set up which were incompatible with Jim's placing a bet. For example, if it were discovered that Jim got the urge to gamble when he was alone and feeling miserable in the morning, it might have been suggested that at that time each morning he could arrange to attend an adult education class in a subject that he was interested in. Other alternatives would also have been important – such as avoiding walking past the betting shop, not listening to the racing on the radio or television and not buying racing papers.

Jim could also have been helped by deliberately calling to mind some of the more unpleasant experiences he had undergone as a result of his giving in to the temptation to gamble.

Jim would have been asked to keep a detailed record on a chart showing the number of times he felt like betting and the occasions when he managed to avoid giving in to this temptation. The social worker would have used this record to encourage Jim's effort by rewarding him with praise and offering suggestions of ways in which he could treat himself with the money he had saved. Most people in Jim's situation have lost their self-respect and consequently lack faith in themselves. This often causes them to give up if they have had a bad day – especially if there is no one near them to dissuade them – so measuring success in small steps and using record charts to point out the client's success is a very effective way of eventually overcoming the problem. Encouragement is an essential component of behaviour modification.

Social or lifeskills training

The behaviour modification approach in Jim's case would have focused on the particular behaviour patterns which led to compulsive gambling, but the social worker might have decided on a different way of tackling the issue. Jim was often bored and frustrated at having nothing to do during the day, owing to his being unemployed. He had been unemployed for a year and as time passed he was becoming more despondent about finding another job. His confidence was constantly being sapped and he was now at the stage where he did not even bother to look for jobs in local newspapers and Jobcentres.

Rather than focus on his gambling 'problem', the social worker might have thought that, if Jim could increase his chances of getting a job and in so doing inject more discipline into his lifestyle, then it might well have had the effect of diverting him from gambling.

The social worker might therefore have initiated a programme of *social skills training* (sometimes known as *lifeskills training*). It would have been very basic, but it might have had a powerful effect in increasing Jim's sense of self-worth and given him a sense of purpose. Jim would have been helped in looking for jobs, in scanning local papers and Jobcentre displays. He would have been helped to use the telephone more effectively and to address other people more pleasantly and positively. *Role play* might have been used to simulate a real interview to equip Jim with more confidence. Jim could have swapped roles in the scenario and thus have been helped to see other aspects of the interview situation. All this would have been aimed at helping Jim to feel better within himself, which in turn should encourage him to use his own initiative.

Groupwork and some other strategies for helping

As we said earlier, groupwork is such an important and wide-ranging approach it deserves to be treated in more detail. We do that here, in addition to introducing the reader to a number of other strategies that have not so far been mentioned.

Groupwork

Groupwork started to become properly established in the caring services in the UK in the 1960s. It was imported from the USA, where it had been developed by psychologists and psychotherapists. Today in the UK, an increasing number of carers are becoming involved in its use.

There are several different types of group. We can single out four important ones:

1. *Problem-solving groups* Social carers and social workers frequently run groups which help members who share a common problem to work through difficulties in co-operation with others. Discussion will take place, and the facilitator will be keen to see a build-up of confidence in the participants.
2. *Educational groups* The function of many groups is to teach members something which will be of use to them. We may include here *social skills training*, in which there has recently been a tremendous growth.

   Social skills (or *lifeskills*) *training* is well suited to group practice. Social carers and social workers may bring together, for example, groups of unemployed teenagers and work through the various problems and testing situations they are likely to meet in their efforts to find a job.

   Role play may be used, as we illustrated in our sample case study concerning Jim, to familiarise young people with job interviews. This can be an excellent group activity, involving all members of the group.
3. *Self-help groups* People who share a common problem will often form a group in order to provide mutual support. They can then work through their problems in co-operation with others. Examples of these are groups for the partners of men serving prison sentences; groups for the parents of drug abusers; groups for the parents of children with disabilities; and other groups too numerous to mention. Alcoholics Anonymous, of course, is a well-established, international, self-help group.

   Social carers and social workers can be instrumental in helping people to come together to start a group. Once it is established, the facilitator will withdraw from involvement completely so that it does literally become a self-help group.
4. *Activity-based groups* A wide diversity of activities takes place in activity-based groups (as the name implies) – for example, car repair or motorcycle building for groups of young offenders or those at risk of offending, and outdoor pursuits

(also known as 'Outward Bound') involving a group sharing the experience of living in the countryside for a weekend or a few days. Some of these can be very tough and tiring for all involved. Some activity groups may be designed to help young people use their leisure time more constructively, to stimulate or cultivate an interest – groups may go ice-skating or to the theatre, for example.

Note: The four types of groups mentioned here are not mutually exclusive – the same group may fulfil more than one function, even all four.

There are different styles of group leadership. An authoritarian leader will be very directive, but a democratic leader will endeavour to involve all group members as much as possible, at the same time. The style of leadership used will depend on the aims and objectives of the group and the task in hand.

Groupwork has become very popular because it is seen to be effective, although this is obviously very difficult to measure. In some ways groupwork simulates everyday life, thus the method is more natural than the one-to-one methods of intervention. (We spend much of our time with groups of other people – even if only with our family.) Groups often provide a more intense experience, because several people together generate more energy as they interact. Learning from others is a natural way of learning and carers believe it can be therapeutic.

Groupwork is not 'easier' than other strategies – it can involve more time and hard work, especially at the setting-up stage. However, if it is done well and it has the desired effect on the individuals concerned, the reward is considerable.

Psychodrama

Psychodrama is an active method of group psychotherapy that uses a dramatic format and theatrical terms to explore experiences, past and present, and sometimes even the future. It can have a number of uses: for example, to rid oneself of past hurt or trauma, to explore a current problem or to learn more about oneself. It is used in a wide range of settings: hospitals, day centres, schools and prisons. It can take place under the NHS or be funded by a general practitioner. A number of groups exist in the UK and they practise psychodrama regularly.

Classical psychodrama was developed from the 1920s on by Jacob Moreno, an Austrian psychiatrist. He watched children at play and considered psychodrama an extension of natural play and a useful practical alternative to the predominantly verbally based psychoanalysis (he was a contemporary of Freud). Moreno said of the technique:

> One of its objectives is to teach people to resolve their conflicts in a microcosm of the world (the group), free of the conventional restraints, by acting out their problems, ambitions, dreams and fears. It emphasises maximum involvement with others; in investigating conflicts in their immediate present form; in addition to dealing with the subject's early memories and perceptions.
> *'Psychodrama-Inspiration and Technique'* (Holmes and Karp, Routledge, 1991, p13)

Moreno said the approach had five elements:

1. the *protagonist* (from a Greek word meaning 'the leading or first actor') is the main focus, the person 'doing the work', in a particular session;
2. the *director* or therapist works closely with the protagonist and facilitates the drama and all that happens;
3. the *auxiliary egos* are members of the group who will play significant people in the protagonist's life or situation;
4. the *audience* comprises the remaining members of the group; they do not take part in the drama, but they remain actively involved;
5. the *stage* is whatever physical space the drama takes place in.

There were three stages to Moreno's original concept:

1. *warm-up*, in which the group comes together and interacts, hopefully building up trust, sharing experiences and becoming cohesive. From this process the protagonist will emerge by putting themselves forward to gain people's agreement for selection;
2. *enactment* is the drama itself. There is no script and no acting skills are needed. The enactment is spontaneous, with great stress on the director and others to be wisely intuitive;
3. *sharing* is the final stage in which all group members are encouraged to share views and feelings. People, particularly those playing leading roles, may need to literally 'de-role' at this time.

Group size will normally be from eight to 12. Only the most basic 'props' will be used, perhaps a table, TV set, chair. It is the 'action' that is of key importance. Various scenarios may be attempted, to try out a number of different ideas or behaviours. Particular techniques may be drawn upon: for example *role reversal*, in which the protagonist and one or more of the auxiliary egos swap roles. This may help the main actor to view themselves or their situation more objectively; *doubling* involves a member of the group standing alongside the protagonist, again with a view to helping the latter gain more insight and self-awareness; *mirroring* actually replaces the protagonist by another member of the group so that they can stand aside and observe the drama.

Psychodrama is a living strategy for helping and it is a field within which there has been much experiment and development. *Sociodrama* is another technique, also developed by Moreno, in which specific themes, for example, racism, masculinity, violence and so on, can be explored. Instead of acting as individuals in particular roles, group members represent certain attitudes or themes. In this way social issues can be focused upon and examined.

Key working

This may be best described as a good practice *style* of working rather than a strategy for helping. It brings together in a one-to-one association an individual client and a specific carer. The client knows that they can call on this person, 'special' to them, for a range of tasks, many of them of a very personal or private nature. These tasks could include co-ordinating the individual programme plan and regular reviews; meeting and arranging meetings with family and relatives; generally being a confidant(e); being an advocate for the client within the service or unit in which the carer works and generally helping the client in any way deemed necessary: To sum up – the key worker's role can be seen as providing an individualised service to a particular client.

Key working takes place in a variety of care settings; more recently it has grown in popularity within residential care. If a shift system of workers exists, then it may be that two or perhaps even three carers will be allocated as key workers to a particular client. The relationship should not be exclusive – it should be stressed that a client or resident should be able to call on any member of staff at any time.

If we are to achieve antioppressive practice, it is important when selecting a key worker, to bear in mind a range of compatibility characteristics. When considering both prospective client and carer the following (and this is not a comprehensive list) should be borne in mind: culture, social class, gender, race, religious belief, language, political allegiances, personality and shared interests. Whether or not the pair respect or like each other should also have some weight!

The main aim of the key worker arrangement is to support the client and if they are in residential care, to give the client a greater sense of belonging. The key worker will know 'their' client very well and may be able to act as a 'bridge' between the client and other carers in the agency or unit.

Life story work

This is a way of working directly with children, elders and other client groups that can be of considerable therapeutic value. It involves establishing a trusting relationship with a client, often through their key worker, in order to compile their life story. The carer and client usually agree to meet at a regular time, over an agreed period, in order to talk about the client's life.

Life story work was originally developed as a therapeutic device in work with certain children who had spent most of their lives in residential care and who therefore had little sense of personal history or of the value of their life experiences. It was recognised that many such children had 'lost' part of their childhood memories and this affected their sense of identity and consequently, perhaps, their sense of a quintessential self. A child who has had a series of carers in a number of different homes would not have had anybody personally responsible for recording, retaining and valuing the significant events in the child's life; experiences such as birthdays, favourite toys and animals, first day at school or learning to swim would often therefore be totally forgotten because they had not been specifically endowed with special meaning or interest by a particular person.

To counter this situation, life story work was introduced. Usually a large book was created, with the child's co-operation, and in it was recorded the child's life with such items as, say, the child's birth certificate and an assortment of photographs, letters, school reports, and so on. A written commentary of the child's life ran alongside this documentary material. With this aid it was hoped the child would gain a deeper sense of personal identity.

Subsequently, life story work was developed for use with elders and others; the process of going back over an adult client's life, whatever their age, proved to be a healing device in so far as it helped to resolve issues from the past in addition to building confidence in personal achievements and helping the person to achieve a sense of self-worth.

Sensitivity and care are of primary importance when using this strategy because very often, painful and traumatic memories surface. Skill is required to enable the client to feel safe enough to cope or deal with such memories and the emotions they invoke.

The life story can be retained by the client as an important record of their experience. The interaction between client and carer in compiling it usually builds a strong relationship in which real change and growth become possible because the client feels more valued and of more importance.

Welfare rights work and debt counselling

Over the past few years, much more attention has been given to the financial resources of clients and the way in which these will affect other aspects of the clients' lives. In fact some social workers have become specialists in this field and specific courses are run to equip carers with the necessary skills. The work of certain pressure groups such as the Child Poverty Action Group (CPAG) has encouraged this focus. This particular group publishes an annual national welfare benefits handbook which is invaluable for the amount of information it contains and its clarity of presentation. Another voluntary organisation, the CAB has been involved in a growing amount of welfare rights work in recent years.

The recipients of State benefits are not the only people that are assisted – the area of work has broadened to become known as 'debt counselling' and can involve dealing with any kind of financial problem.

Most carers do not specialise in this type of work – they incorporate it in their range of skills. They would only refer a case to a specialist if the problem was particularly difficult or complicated.

Networking

Along with approaches such as empowerment, advocacy and radical social work, networking has its origins in sociology and, specifically, in general systems theory or social systems theory. The network or social network is the social support system; the personal and social links that most of us have in the community in which we live. We should remember here that a growing number of people do not have any such support system – they are lonely and isolated.

As a strategy for helping, networking is an empowering device; it builds up interdependence between the client and others in the community and it has within it strong elements of self-help and mutual support.

Coulshed identifies three distinct strategies within networking:

1. *Network construction* This approach aims to create new networks in the community in addition to supporting and nurturing those that already exist. It originated as an aspect of community care when this type of support became

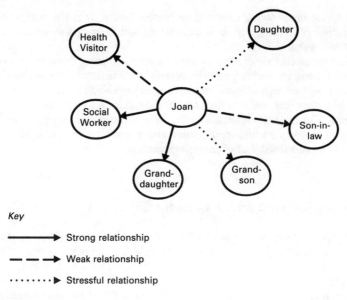

Fig 8.3   A network map, based on Joan (case study 2).

necessary for people with mental health problems who had been resettled in the community. Today the approach is used for a wider range of client groups, in particular older people who live in their own homes.

2. *Problem-solving network meetings* These bring together carers in the community, both paid and unpaid, to sort out problems; for example, an overlap in care service provision or an inadequate supply of care provision. It is important that care managers make themselves familiar with the existing network when assessing and formulating a programme of care.

3. *Network therapy* This is not unlike group therapy because to a large extent it draws on groupwork skills. This therapeutic approach aims to help families in crisis by bringing together their network to facilitate change. It may involve up to 50 people. A partial network assembly would be about 12 people. Coulshed refers to the 'network effect' as a positive outcome 'which is the result of simply bringing people together' op. cit (p57).

Community social work or community work

Networking is just one of a number of techniques drawn on by community workers, more commonly called community social workers today. It is essential that community resources, especially people, their skills, knowledge and experience, are valued and used.

Community social work is not strictly a strategy for helping but is a very important way of working which involves a whole range of specific skills. Some of these might be:

a) the ability to relate to a wide range of people who will vary in regard to age, ethnic origin, interests and political persuasion;
b) a good understanding of political issues – both locally and in a wider, someone national, context;
c) a thorough knowledge of local resources, groups, voluntary initiatives, local authority departments and a wide variety of other organisations;
d) some competence in group work skills because much of the job involves working with different groups of people – for example, council tenants, children, young people, pensioners;
e) an ability to help organise a range of different activities – for example, fundraising events or clubs catering for a wide diversity of interests;
f) good diplomacy – the community social worker will have to liaise with a wide range of different people, including various professionals, employees of local Government departments and those working for a large number of voluntary groups and organisations;
g) perhaps most important of all – an insight into how to empower people so that local residents can express their own views and do things for themselves.

A community social worker can be employed by a wide range of agencies, both statutory and voluntary. The focus of their work may be with young people; with certain special need groups (drug users, for example); or with whole communities, where the 'client' population will be a typical cross-section of society. The worker may have a specific task, for example, the setting up of play provision on a large council housing estate, or a general role – work in an area of a large city, assessing local facilities, resources and deficiencies and helping to meet social needs as they arise.

The range of skills utilised and the long working hours that are often required (frequently in the evening and at weekends) make the job a very demanding one. Nor is it glamorous. Bob Holman, who has worked as a community social worker for nearly 20 years, says of the worker's role: 'We should be concerned with ordinary activities that create trust and contact when more serious problems crop up' (Community Care 8.7.93).

Radical social work

Radical social work arose mainly as an ideological critique of traditional or psychodynamic social work in the mid-1970s. Its influence is not as strong today, but this is partly because much of its theory and practice have become part of mainstream caring. The emergence of antioppressive practice and the development of antiracist and feminist, or non-sexist, approaches, has to a certain extent developed from radical and Marxist approaches. Advocacy, empowerment and consciousness of oppression and discrimination are also now more prevalent, even commonplace.

A simplistic summary of the ideas behind radical social work would be: traditional social work individualises what are really socially created problems. People are blamed for their poverty or unemployed status, whereas these problems have their roots in the structure of society. Social workers collude with our capitalist State to 'blame the victim' and thereby support the present social order. Radical social workers aimed to reveal the unjust nature of society, with its unequal distribution of wealth and other resources. Social change to bring about a fairer society was the ultimate goal. This transition would be brought about by collective action with oppressed groups, including clients.

One of the weaknesses of this approach was that much of the literature was written by academics who had little or no experience of practice. Meanwhile hardpressed practitioners did not have the time to read, let alone write such material. As a result, there was much speaking (or writing) at cross-purposes, with academics often only having other academics as an audience.

Some people explain the decline in the influence of radical social work by the development of a growing concentration on single issues, such as racism, sexism and the pursuit of equality and the new emphasis on personal practice at the expense of the pursuit of more widespread social change.

Feminist social work and woman-centred practice

Feminist or non-sexist (or antisexist) approaches have their origins in the women's movement of the 1960s and 1970s. Their aim is to remove the effects of discrimination and oppression caused by sexism in society. In making women more 'visible' in the caring services, both as carers and clients, such approaches encourage collaborative action and consciousness raising efforts on the part of both groups. The dominance of men in most areas of life and work (including social work) means that they are usually defined by their status, while women are defined by their gender (e.g. as wives or mothers).

As well as stressing those aspects that women have in common, non-sexist approaches also draw attention to differences in and between women and their experiences. Some examples are differences between white and black women; differences in child care practices; differences in work patterns and status. It has also been noted that there is a link between sex discrimination and other forms of discrimination and oppression, particularly those relating to social class and race.

Jalna Hanmer and Daphne Statham have developed what they call a woman-centered practice or woman-centred social work. They did this because they felt women's lives and experiences were not well understood by either social work educators or practitioners and this had the knock-on effect of a poor service to women as clients. They want women to 'become valued in and for themselves' (*Women and Social Work*, 1988, p3). In order to move towards a woman-centered practice they say that 'new policies and practices are needed to alter the balance of power between women and men as colleagues and in professional relationships with clients' (P139).

More women are needed in senior positions in social work and all agencies should have 'whole-agency' antisexist policies. Hanmer and Statham's Code of Practice includes the following elements:

1. explore commonalities and diversities between yourself and women clients and between women clients when making assessments and during practice;
2. create situations in which social workers and clients can share and learn from each other;
3. believe the woman client, accept her and the problem she brings;

4. support and begin all-women groups for clients and social workers which recognise diversities as well as commonalities between women;
5. work in non-hierarchical ways with clients whenever possible.

The social systems model

The development of this model in the 1970s sprang from disillusionment with the then traditional tripartite division of social work methods into casework, groupwork and community work. Social work theorists and educators were keen to have more integration between these different approaches and also to go further and relocate 'problems' traditionally seen as being located in the mind of the individual. Social situations became the focus for change, rather than 'pathological' individuals.

This work was developed originally in the USA in the early 1970s. Allen Pincus and Anne Minahan (working together) and Howard Goldstein were instrumental in developing the model, but others have put forward similar theories. It was based on *social systems theory* which stresses the inter-relatedness of people, agencies and institutions in our society. The model of society that it proposes highlights how one institution is dependent on others for all to be able to function together and for society to be able to continue to exist.

When applied to relationships between people and organisations in our society, systems theory involves four levels of social system:

1. individual personality system (the individual);
2. interpersonal dyad system (two people in interaction);
3. interpersonal social systems (these can be families or groups of people relating together);
4. sociocultural social systems (this can refer to very large identifiable groups of people – for example, the homeless or single-parent families – or whole communities or even countries).

It can be seen that these systems include everyone from the individual to the nation State. All these groups of people or systems inter-relate (or interact) with each other and influence each other. Changes in one system will affect others, possibly causing changes in those too.

The model suggests that, if social workers see individuals as being part of a larger interacting social system, they will be aware of a wider range of variables, will see complex problems more clearly and will be aware of a greater range of possible solutions to people's difficulties. The model criticises casework for its concentration on individuals and their problems, because this focus may not be the best way of finding a viable solution. It may be more effective to look for a potential answer beyond the contact between social worker and client.

The model proposed by Pincus and Minahan recognises that, for individuals to live, they depend upon all kinds of people, agencies and organisations in society. They require material and emotional support. Those people or organisations that provide this are known as *resource systems*. The family is obviously crucially important in providing these resources, especially in an individual's early life.

Social workers should ensure that clients make the best possible use of the resource systems or network around them in society. In order to help social workers focus their intervention with clients, Pincus and Minahan identify four basic systems which interact:

1. *The change-agent system.* This refers to *who* is going to bring about change in a client's situation. It will be the social worker and also the agency employing them. If positive change is not occurring for a client, it may be the agency that requires changing. This illustrates the radical and wide nature of the model – it considers all possibilities.
2. *The client system.* This refers to the person, family, group, organisation or community that has 'engaged the services' of the social worker because assistance is required.
3. *The target system.* This describes those people whom the social worker (or change-agent) needs to influence in order to do their work and help to bring about change. Frequently the client system and the target system will be the same, but there will be exceptions – for example, when a social worker is attempting to get a family rehoused because of deplorable living conditions, the target system may well be influential employees of the local housing department.
4. *The action system.* Social workers do not work on their own: they involve all kinds of other people – for example, clients' families, friends and other professionals – in their efforts to find a solution. All these people, together with the social worker, are known as the action system.

Assessment is central to the systems model. Effective assessment will involve gaining a thorough knowledge of the client and their friends, relations and other social contacts. When examining the presenting problem, the social worker may well realise that the client should not be the target system for change. Many social workers have found the model beneficial for 'sharpening' their practice and useful in helping them to look more deeply into problems. It has also been discovered to be a good team-building activity when a complete social work team takes up and uses the model.

The approach is a useful assessment tool in that it involves a thorough investigation of the client's entire situation – i.e. all social contacts, etc. It involves indentifying four systems concerning the client's present situation. These four systems are inter-related. Part of the assessment process involves considering where the problem to be dealt with actually lies (the target system). It may be that the target system is not the client but someone or something else – for example, other people significant in the client's situation, the client's social setting, institutional care, etc. The following case involving two social workers illustrates this.

Susan is 14 years old. For the past two years she has been living in residential care in a small community home (Abbeycliffe House). You are a social worker in a social services department local office. You have recently taken over from Susan's social worker who has left the office. Before meeting Susan for the first time, you read through the case file. In it you come across the following passage which is part of the previous social worker's assessment of the case:

'Abbeycliffe House is ideally suited to Susan's needs, but she has so far proved difficult and unco-operative. Jim Kelly (officer-in-charge) has been very patient with her and has gone to great lengths to help her settle. She has not responded positively to this. Her behaviour has often been disruptive, upsetting other young people in the house. I believe Susan's new social worker should focus energies on modifying her behaviour and attitudes.'

Clearly, for this social worker, Susan's behaviour is 'the problem' – he has identified her as the target system.

Some time later. You have now met Susan three times at Abbeycliffe House and have gained a very different impression of her situation. As a result, you have made your own assessment. You find her quiet and you suspect that she is depressed. When seeing her along with the officer-in-charge, you have detected an intolerance in him for her. He has spoken curtly and impatiently to her. When speaking alone with her, you feel that she is unhappy at Abbeycliffe House and that it is not well-suited to her needs. You do not think you should focus on her as 'the problem' (target system): rather, you identify the target system as:

a) in the short term, the officer-in-charge and other staff at the home, who you feel are acting inappropriately towards Susan;
b) in the long term, the management within your own organisation, as (if things do not work out well) you may have to insist that Susan is moved to a home which would cater better for her needs.

Some of the positive factors about the social systems model are that it focuses on the social setting as well as the client and it can have integrated into it any strategy for helping which is suitable. Any of the approaches described in this chapter can be used.

Six-category intervention analysis

Finally, we look at an analytical tool by which we can examine our practice in caring – how we work, rather than the actual strategies we use. This is the work of John Heron which he developed at the University of Surrey in the 1970s. Heron analysed intervention in the helping professions and said that it could be examined in terms of six different categories. Whenever a carer is working with a client – especially in a one-to-one situation – they will be using interventions in one or more of the following categories, which are divided into two groups of three. The first group are *authoritative* interventions, meaning that the carer is being fairly dominant or assertive. The second group are *facilitative*, meaning that they are being less obtrusive and more enabling.

Authoritative

1. *Prescriptive* This involves giving advice, being critical or judgemental and generally aiming to direct the client's behaviour.
2. *Informative* Here the carer is acting as 'teacher' in giving new information or knowledge to the client.
3. *Confronting* The carer challenges the client, possibly by giving direct feedback about their behaviour.

AUTHORITATIVE	FACILITATIVE
1. Prescriptive	4. Cathartic
2. Informative	5. Catalytic
3. Confronting	6. Supportive

Fig 8.4   John Heron's six categories.

Facilitative

4. *Cathartic* This aims to help the client to release emotion – sometimes painful emotion – often signified by physical signs like crying, laughing and trembling.
5. *Catalytic* The carer here seeks to enable the client to learn and develop through self-discovery and self-direction. The onus for doing the 'work', in a one-to-one situation, is on the client.
6. *Supportive* This is extremely important in all helping situations as it affirms the worth and value of the client as an individual. The carer approves, confirms and validates the client.

Heron says of the above analysis that it aids 'the development of self-assessment and self-monitoring in the helping professions'. It helps carers to analyse what they do and to find out which particular parts of practice are helpful and which are not.

Heron makes the point that, in his experience, practitioners tend to be more skilled in the authoritative interventions than in the facilitative. He finds the least competence in cathartic intervention. All six categories are of equal importance – that is, none is better than the others. The skilled helper should possess expertise in all and be readily able to switch from one way of working to another.

It is important to remember that the six types of intervention are of value only if they are rooted in compassion, care and concern for the client.

Heron also speaks of 'degenerate' and 'perverted' interventions. Degenerate interventions are 'misguided, rooted in lack of awareness – lack of experience, of insight, of personal growth or simply of training' (Helping the Client, Sage, 1990, p144). They can affect any of the six categories and are of four kinds: unsolicited, manipulative, compulsive and unskilled. Perverted interventions are 'quite deliberately malicious; they intend harm to the client. Their purpose is to damage people' (p157).

Conclusion

The strategies for helping dealt with in this chapter are, in actuality, complex. In a sense, in trying to simplify them to make them speedily understood, they may well have been oversimplified. We would ask the reader to consult the 'further reading' section at the end of this chapter in order to obtain a fuller understanding of the various approaches.

As we have said, effective caring should be eclectic and should utilise a range of different approaches. Fashions in the use of strategies for helping are constantly changing and we should always question why this happens. Effectiveness in the helping process is notoriously difficult to assess: for example, how can we measure the extent to which an individual has been empowered? Whatever means are used to attempt to measure effectiveness, one thing is certain: carers should remain flexible in their use of different strategies and approaches, always adapting these to the client rather than vice versa.

Appendix 1 – an intervention checklist

Before intervention, possibly at the assessment stage, it may be helpful to consider the following questions:

WHO
- Is my agency/unit the correct one to be involved?
- Am I the right person?
- Do I possess the necessary skills?
- What are the implications of my own values/standards/ideology?

WHAT
- is the real nature of the problem?
- is being asked for?
- can feasibly be provided?
- are the implications of shortfall?
- are the implications for other clients?
- are the implications of non-intervention?

WHERE
- should I meet the client(s), e.g. office, home, neutral venue?
- can I locate necessary resources, e.g. colleagues, equipment, network?

WHEN
- should I intervene, i.e. how urgent? Is it a crisis?
- How long should intervention last, e.g. crisis, short term, long term?
- How much time do I have available?

HOW
- What strategy should I employ?
- Will it involve the individual client? Their family? Group? Network? Community?
- do I assess my own work practice using Heron's six categories?

. . . and a final question – *why* am I involved?

Exercise 1 – role play – a social work visit

Read case study 1 on p269. You are to role-play John's family situation from just before the social worker arrives at his home i.e. start with John's father leaving the house in an angry mood. Role-play through until the social worker leaves the house.

Roles

Father
Mother
John (aged 16)
Sister (aged 14)
Sister (aged 12)
Social worker

Think beforehand about the roles and what kind of personality you are going to take on. Think perhaps of some key things you intend to say as the role play progresses. Allow 30 minutes for the role play.

Following the role play, a discussion could take place examining what went on and any general issues raised with regard to family relationships, etc.

Exercise 2 – setting up a group

Groups are important tools in caring. By talking to people in your local community, by reading local and community newspapers and by speaking to key workers in your area – community workers, community centre wardens or youth workers, for example – isolate a particular 'live issue' in the area (anything you like, as long as it has a social component). Then plan the setting up of a pressure group or self-help group, or whatever type of group would be most appropriate for dealing with the matter. Ask yourself questions similar to the following:

a) How would I contact people I want to interest in my group?
b) Would I hold meetings?
c) What publicity would I need?
d) How should the group be organised?
e) Will it be a short term or an ongoing group?
f) What activity will the group need to involve itself in?
g) Where might I get funding?

Exercise 3 – case studies

Read the following two case studies. At the end of each, you have to decide which of the strategies explained in this chapter would be most appropriate to use. Firstly, do this on your own and then join up with others to compare and analyse the approaches you have chosen. Don't worry if you think that more than one strategy would be appropriate – just explain why you think this is the case. When you have decided, explain how you would actually set about using the technique(s) chosen in your work with the client. Plan your first meeting, using the method(s) you have decided on.

a) *The Afford Family* As a duty officer in a social services department local office you are meeting Mrs Afford for the very first time. She is distraught and you gain the overwhelming impression that she is overburdened at the present time. She tells you that three weeks ago her husband died, leaving her with her three children – two girls, aged 17 and 14 and a boy aged 12.

Sarah (the 14 year old) and Paul (the son) were both proving to be difficult a considerable time before their father's death, which was completely unexpected – the result of a serious accident at his workplace. Sarah spends a great deal of time out of the home, with a group of young people on the estate where the family lives. She seems to come home only to eat and sleep. She is insolent to her mother, who realises that Sarah was dreadfully upset by her father's death, being especially close to him. Paul spends most of his time indoors. What worries Mrs Afford is that he appears lethargic and depressed – not at all usual for him. She has great difficulty rousing him for school in the mornings and suspects he has played truant on occasions, going off on his own to amuse himself. Her older daughter, Jacqui, presents no problem and Mrs Afford describes her as having been supportive since her father's death.

Mrs Afford does not feel she can cope any longer on her own and her only relations live a long way away. She feels unable to share her problems with friends or neighbours, as she is worried that she will be thought of as 'inadequate' and a 'poor mother' (her own words).

After speaking with Mrs Afford for just over an hour, you feel that you have a fairly full understanding of her situation. You must now make an assessment as to how you will work with her and her family.

b) *Neil – a young offender* You are a probation officer in contact with Neil, aged 17. He has just appeared in court and was placed on probation for one year. He had committed a serious burglary at an electrical goods warehouse and you realised that there was a possibility of a custodial sentence. You are pleased that the court did not sentence him to custody but allowed him to remain in the community instead.

Neil lives with his mother (a single parent). He is an only child. His mother has struggled to manage financially over the last ten years since Neil's father left. The home is in a poor physical condition. His mother has found Neil difficult to discipline since he was about 13 and she feels that the lack of a father figure in the home has contributed to this. She certainly shows Neil affection, but his attitude to her is inconsiderate and he can be arrogant and aggressive.

He leads his life outside of the home, spending almost all his time hanging around with friends. He is unemployed, having dropped out of a training scheme some 18 months ago. He says he would like very much to work as a welder, but he does not have much idea about how to find a job. 'Scrambling' bikes are a great interest, but he cannot afford one of his own and so cadges rides on friends' bikes.

Neil seems to find his contact with you valuable and you feel it is important to build on this now. In three days' time you are to see Neil again. Plan your future contact with him.

Exercise 4 – life story work

Select a service user with whom you work closely in order to prepare an ongoing life story book. As mentioned earlier in the text, you will need to collect photographs, letters, certificates, school reports and other documents in order to build a foundation for the book. Together with your client you can now produce a written commentary to run alongside the documentary material. It is important to be imaginative with regard to presentation so that the product is meaningful to the service user and takes into account their cultural and personal needs and capabilities.

Exercise 5 – networking

Draw up a network map of yourself and your situation (see Figure 8.3 for guidance).

Exercise 6 – six-category intervention analysis

Analyse your own care practice using Heron's Six categories.

Questions for discussion

1. In working with people as a carer, do you think it is important that clients should *want* to change? Can anything be achieved if they resist the idea of personal change?
2. Measuring how effective we are as carers is extremely difficult in that there are so many criteria which we could choose to apply; for example, that clients are better able to manage their own lives; have more self-confidence; are able to form relationships more easily; have some control over an addiction; and so on. As a carer, how would you measure your effectiveness if you were working with one of the following:

   a) elders?
   b) people with learning disabilities?
   c) children?
   d) offenders?

   Do your answers encourage you to feel that effectiveness *can* be measured or is this an impossible task?
3. Some people think that social workers should concentrate on relationships and the interpersonal skills of clients rather than on practical and financial problems. Do you think that debt counselling and welfare rights work should be an integral part of a generic social worker's skills? Give reasons for your answer.
4. With reference to the concept of empowerment, power can only be taken, not

given. Discuss this in relation to the carer's role.
5. The two terms 'antidiscriminatory' and 'antioppressive' are used today inter-changeably. But are 'discrimination' and 'oppression' the same thing?
6. One of the original beliefs held by radical social workers was that social workers were agents of social control and that they should instead be agents of social change. To what extent is this true?

Further reading

There are two general texts on strategies for helping which stand out as being extremely useful. These are:

1. *Social Work Practice – An Introduction*, Veronica Coulshed (2nd edition, BASW/ Macmillan, 1991).
2. *Modern Social Work Theory – A Critical Introduction*, Malcolm Payne (Mac-millan, 1991).

In addition:

3. *The Casework Relationship*, Felix P. Biestek (Allen & Unwin, 1967). Despite its age and title, this is still an excellent and clear examination of the values which underpin good care practice.
4. *Brief Counselling: A Practical Guide for Beginning Practitioners*, Windy Dryden and Colin Feltham (Open University, 1992). A good introduction to counselling skills, which is not limited to any one particular 'school' of counselling.
5. *Groupwork*, Allan Brown (3rd edition, Ashgate Publishing, 1992). An excellent introduction, including material on antidiscriminatory groupwork.
6. *Working with Families*, Gill Gorell Barnes (BASW/Macmillan, 1984). A good overview of family work and some of the issues involved.
7. *Antidiscriminatory Practice*, Neil Thompson (BASW/Macmillan, 1993). Exam-ines each of the main areas of discrimination and what antioppressive practice means when implemented.
8. *Women and Social Work – Towards a Woman-centred Practice*, Jalna Hanmer and Daphne Statham (BASW/Macmillan, 1988). Examines the position of women in society and the practical steps needed for a woman-centred practice.
9. *The Skilled Helper – A Systematic Approach to Effective Helping*, Gerard Egan (4th edition, Brooks/Cole, 1990). Egan explains his 3-stage model of counselling in detail.
10. *Three Psychologies – Perspectives from Freud, Skinner and Rogers*, Robert D. Nye (4th edition, Brooks/Cole, 1992). An excellent introduction to the three main schools of psychology – psychoanalysis, behaviourism and humanistic psychol-ogy – through short biographies of their best known proponents.

9

Some Developments in the Caring Services

This book has explored the many fundamental changes to the caring services that have taken place during the last few years, the way they are organised and structured, the relative size and influence of the various sectors, whether statutory, private, voluntary or not-for-profit, and the way they are financed.

Those working in the caring services could be forgiven for feeling somewhat shell-shocked by the rate and pace of change. Developments following the introduction of the new community care arrangements – the new procedures for assessment and care management and the separation of the purchasing and provider functions of local authorities and health authorities – have accompanied the demands of substantial pieces of new legislation, such as the Children Act 1989 and the Criminal Justice Act 1991. Most of these changes have taken place against a backdrop of sustained economic recession, expenditure cutbacks, loss of jobs – both in and outside the caring services – and a growing feeling of insecurity about future work prospects.

Two factors should be borne in mind: firstly, resources are always finite where funding and personnel are concerned. Secondly additional money is also required in the caring services – welfare is, in effect, a 'bottomless pit' because unmet need is always to be found. This situation has led all three main political parties in Britain to re-examine, albeit for differing ideological reasons, their approach to the Welfare State and to consider new or different ways of organising services. In fact, whether or not we can actually afford a Welfare State has been called into question both in Britain and in a number of advanced industrial societies across the world. Given the escalating costs of welfare, most if not all countries have looked to find ways of cutting public spending.

It needs to be remembered, too, that the Welfare State was founded and consolidated on the principle of full employment. In fact, full employment only prevailed for some 30 years after the end of the Second World War. Since the mid-1970s widespread unemployment, with occasional fluctuations, has been a permanent feature of our economy. During the 1980s the Government actually encouraged the growth of unemployment as an economic means of controlling and lowering inflation. Furthermore, as a general trend, a large number of unskilled and semiskilled jobs have disappeared, many of them permanently, because of advances in production technology.

In addition, while the Welfare State is now seen to be in decline, it should be pointed out that there never was a 'Golden Age' in which the Welfare State catered for all social need. Beveridge's 'Five Giants' of 'want, squalor, ignorance, ill health and unemployment' have by no means been eradicated. In particular, the needs of poor people, women, black people and people with disabilities have not been catered for.

Demographic changes have resulted in there being a greater proportion of older people within the population. 'In 1952 the Queen sent telegrams to 200 people in the

United Kingdom to mark their 100th birthday. In 1990 she sent 2227' (*Big Issue*, 2 October, 1991, p4). It is estimated that by the year 2020 the number of people in Britain over the age of 85 will be 90 percent higher than in 1980 (ibid.). This age group naturally becomes increasingly dependent and costly in terms of service provision.

'New right' Conservative government ideology

Conservative party politics since the mid-1970s can be said to be 'radical' in the true sense of the word. They tackled the root of many policies and practices which had hitherto been taken for granted. This new approach has been so different and far-reaching that it has completely unsettled the status quo. Some have said that Government intervention has overturned the postwar consensus in British politics, particularly in relation to the position of the Welfare State, held by many to be permanent and sacrosanct.

During much of their time in power the Conservative party has enjoyed a large majority in the House of Commons and this has enabled them to push through a programme of reforms, some aspects of which have been highly controversial and have flown in the face of more traditional policies, especially in regard to welfare. Government policy has been informed by a consistent ideological commitment which may be summarised simply as a faith in the power of the marketplace to determine service provision.

Some of the key assumptions of this 'new' ideology are that the private sector is more efficient and therefore cheaper than the public sector; that efficiency and other economic factors should take precedence over equity; that the free market economy, unfettered by Government interference, will introduce competition between service providers and enhance choice; that as much human activity as possible should be privatised, thus making services more responsive to consumer preferences and economic conditions; that the public sector is unproductive and a burden on the economy and therefore its role and influence should be reduced; and that self-interest and self-reliance should be nurtured in order that individuals and families do not have to rely on public or collective services. It is also felt that these market principles are applicable to any area of Government activity including the provision of health and welfare.

The subsequent application of the ideology to practice has resulted in the shift from a largely State administered and provided service to a mixed economy of welfare in which agencies are either 'purchasers' or 'providers' of care. The roles of local authorities and health authorities, as public bodies, have been questioned, redrafted and curtailed with the result that the social services departments (and social work departments in Scotland), housing departments and education departments have been affected more than other agencies, for example, the Probation Service. The Probation Service is being required to work in partnership with the voluntary sector from whom it will purchase services. However it has been relatively protected in terms of funding because of government's concern with law and order.

As we have already mentioned throughout the book, social services authorities have been given a central role in relation to community care. They are required to assess and purchase rather than directly provide services. The Government's commitment to the free market and competition is reflected in their insistence that service providers should come increasingly from other sectors: private, voluntary and not-for-profit. In this way a mixed economy will be developed and incorporated into the Welfare State. The relationship between statutory authorities and the independent sector has been changed by the introduction of contracts and the 'contract culture' under which non-statutory agencies directly provide a service. As the overseer of the service provided, the local authority will be in a position to terminate or enhance contracts depending on the quality of provision.

The belief in individual rights and consumer choice is evident in the new community care arrangements that are intended to be needs-led or user-led, rather than, as in the past, resources-led. Resources are to be applied to service users' requirements rather than the other way round. Greater diversity of provision from a wider range of sources is expected to enhance clients' choice. It is hoped that quality assurance will be ensured by the existence of a rigorous complaints procedure. The care manager will monitor progress on the individual package of care.

Many of the principles behind this new system have widespread support. Perhaps the main strength of recent governments has been their commitment to questioning existing practices in order to see if there are not better, more cost-effective ways of providing and delivering services. However, there is deep concern that ideas may not work out in practice if sufficient resources are not provided to back them up and welfare is simply left to the vicissitudes of the market. There has been strong criticism of the Government's overall ideology not only from people of opposing political parties but from within the Conservative party itself. Ex-prime minister Edward Heath voices the fears of many: 'The truth is, as history has so often shown us, that unfettered market forces lead to the rich and the strong growing richer and stronger and the poor and the weak growing poorer and weaker' ('The *Growing Divide*'; Walker & Walker, p18).

The common good

The ideological restructuring of the Welfare State and the dependence upon a plethora of service providers generated by market forces is ostensibly aimed at improving efficiency, achieving value for money and encouraging individuals to make private arrangements for their own welfare and that of their immediate relatives. However, it can be shown that these identified goals have not yet been achieved; that the system is no less bureaucratic or evidently more efficient. For example, overall public spending has not been reduced: in 1979 it accounted for 2.4 percent of GDP but by 1993 it had risen to 2.6 percent. In relation to the NHS, Melanie Phillips has pointed out that 'doctors are drowning in bureaucracy' and that instead of 'slimming down the bureaucracy and channelling more money into patient care the reverse has happened. Some 18 000 *more* managers have been appointed, while more than 8000 nursing jobs have disappeared' (*Observer*, 27.6.93, p21, her emphasis). She adds that 'A system that was once the envy of the world for its relative efficiency and justice is being wrecked under the twin assaults of underfunding and ideology.'

It is argued that social policies over the last 15 years or so have called into question the idea of collective provision and in themselves have formed an assault upon the ideology of the 'common good'. Inherent in State-provided services is a sense of entitlement and belonging and of being valued as a member of society. Defenders of the Welfare State argue that people's health, social, educational and housing needs are too fundamental and important to leave to the free market. Furthermore some vulnerable members need protection by the State, otherwise they will not survive.

The central concept of an ideology that espouses the common good is that of equality; that all members of society are of equal worth and are entitled to respect and dignity. A practical expression of equality is the democratic right of all adults to elect their representatives and to have their own legal and personal rights upheld. It is in the interests of the common good to minimise wide social, political and economic differences between society's members and to ensure that provision is made for all those who are too vulnerable to manage by themselves. Power differentials are evened out so there is less likelihood of exploitation and stigmatisation.

An example of a policy that aims to reduce social difference and stigma is one that embodies the principle of universal provision. Universality means that each member receives basic benefits and services as of right, without the need for means testing, which can be stigmatising and sometimes degrading. The value of a society which promotes the common good is that its members feel that they belong and that they share a responsibility for others.

The effects of the diminished influence of public services' can be seen in relation to the provision of school meals. The Education Act 1980 removed existing nutritional standards on school meals and the obligation on schools to provide meals, except to children who qualified for free meals. The result is that today only 42 percent of children receive school meals. In schools where meals are provided they consist 'in 90 percent of cases, of crisps, sweets and hot snacks'. A recent report, *Nutritional Guidelines for School Meals*, points out that children's diets are 'high in fat and sugar and that children are suffering from weight problems, dental caries and nutritional anaemia' (*Independent*, 25.11.92). The introduction of compulsory competitive tendering has undoubtedly led to a reduction in the nutritional quality of meals which, when they were regulated, provided up to 40 percent of each child's daily nutritional needs. It is well known that one in nine children leave for school without having eaten breakfast and that one in six children have no hot meal when they return home.

The relationship between the provision of adequate nutrition and a child's ability to concentrate and benefit from education is obvious. Moreover, universally State-provided, regulated school meals carried with them, despite their notorious place in folklore, a sense of care of children being invested in and valued. Speaking on the television programme devoted to school meals ('Lumpy Custard', Open Space, BBC2, June 1993) one middle-aged contributor referred to society's need to provide minimum standards of care for all its members and outlined his own version of the common good. He himself valued highly the contribution of regular school meals in his own life and felt that they ought still to be available to all children. He said:

Most people given the choice of having a decent job at a decent wage with a reasonable amount of security and fending for themselves would choose to do that if they could. But in a world where there is a shortage of decent jobs and an abundance of not particularly well-paid jobs – often part-time – then it seems to me that we have got to care enough for those at the bottom of the ladder, not least the children, because whoever else may be at fault – it can hardly be them.

Other policies and practices devoted to the common good might be the universal provision of adequate child care resources, practical and emotional support for informal carers, genuinely preventive social work intervention, the re-establishment of a minimum wage and the provision of social security benefits, set at a decent level, in harmony with society's wealth (the basic unemployment benefit now represents about 12 percent of average male earnings – *Reconstructing the Welfare State – A Decade of Change 1980–1990*, N. Johnson, Harvester/Wheatsheat, p235). The costs of such provision would be higher than at present but the long term benefits in terms of savings in future expenditure and reduction of human suffering would be immeasurable. It has been estimated, for example, that:

> Unemployment is costing the NHS at least an extra £70 million pounds a year according to a report by the Office of Health Economics, *Impact of Unemployment on Health* (1993). The total includes £28.3 million for extra visits to the doctors by jobless people, £11.9 million for pharmaceutical services and £30.6 million for free prescriptions.

> (*Guardian*, 28.6.93)

Some recent developments

The Children Act 1989

Many of the changes introduced through legislation concerning the caring services during the 1980s and early 1990s have been broadly welcomed by those in the caring professions. Some, though, have been greeted with reservation and caution. In amalgamating previous child care legislation and aligning public and private law, the Children Act 1989 simplified a complex process. This simplification was long overdue. The Act aims to build upon the relationship between parents and children by emphasising the responsibilities of parents and the rights of children and young people. Partnership is stressed, not only between social workers and the families of children but between agencies concerned with the child so that a co-ordinated approach to the child's welfare can be undertaken. The 'paramountcy principle' emphasises the supremacy of the child's welfare over all matters. The child or young person's wishes are now to be listened to and acted upon where appropriate and for the first time in child care law, racial, cultural and religious rights have to be taken into account. This latter condition did not go far enough for many observers, who wanted it to be mandatory instead of being merely recommended practice. Social services provision has been extended to care-leavers and some homeless young people who are automatically included in the 'in need' category as are children and young people with disabilities, although a recent survey has shown that, 'three quarters of SSDs do not have enough accommodation to meet all young homeless peoples' needs' (*Community Care*, 18.3.93, p15).

Community Care

The principle behind the community care policy of enabling people to remain in their own homes, within their own communities, for as long as possible has universal support. This is something we would all want for ourselves and for all members of an advanced civilised society. However, the effectiveness of the policy depends on how well community care provision is resourced. There is a danger that people may be 'institutionalised' in their own homes where they are unable to do things for themselves and are not adequately supported by family, neighbours and health and social services provision. The same concern exists for people who have been discharged from long stay hospitals and are not properly supported.

> Many erstwhile mental patients have found themselves living in poverty and unable to cope with the new environment into which they have been plunged. For these people 'Community Care' has effectively reproduced, albeit in different form and intensity, the personal and social alienation of institutional life.
>
> *(Critical Social Policy.* P Levick, Issue 34, Summer 1992, p75)

Interagency collaboration was always an aspiration, which was practised in some areas, but now the community care legislation has imposed upon the local authority a 'statutory duty to co-ordinate services'. The policy guidance makes clear that the responsibility to provide a *seamless* service is shared by practitioners in all care agencies' (*Care Management and Assessment: Managers Guide*, HMSO, 1991, their emphasis). Once again, co-operation depends on resourcing. For example, 'A GP has described the impact of cuts in provision: "We used to see a social worker regularly at our weekly practice meeting. But now they have become an endangered species; rarely sighted and hard to track down".' (*BMJ*, Vol. 306, 15.3.93).

The purchaser/provider split introduced by the Act has not always been met with enthusiasm. On the one hand, care managers can look forward to creative ways of obtaining appropriate care for clients, through voluntary organisations within the community or through paid neighbourhood support, instead of having to rely solely on traditional local authority provision. Black voluntary care groups in particular, who have developed in response to unmet community need, have welcomed the prospect of the break-up of monopolistic local authority provision and the improved chance of operating culturally appropriate and sensitive services themselves.

On the other hand, the separation between the purchaser and provider functions has minimised some job roles and reduced job satisfaction for some care providers. For example, prior to the separation, home care organisers would attempt to 'match' appropriate home carers to service users when carrying out the initial assessment of clients' needs, so that the most appropriate worker in terms of culture, race, class, interest and personality could be allocated. Now, assessments are made by care managers and the service is provided in cold response to a request for provision. The deskilling of some home carers' roles coupled with the anxiety of being a part of a service unit, prone to privatisation and the fluctuating fortunes of the free market, has produced disquiet amongst local authority employees, many of whom have put in long service and are proud of the established and rounded care they provided. Similarly, local authority social workers are also having to undergo changes in role and have had to grapple with the demands of care management. Some have welcomed the opportunity to manage resources more directly and to endeavour to obtain appropriate and cost-effective care. Others are less comfortable in their new administrative role and question their current tasks in relation to their original motivation for entering the work.

The needs-led emphasis of the legislation has meant that services now have to be tailored to service users. Some day centres, for example, are providing services at the weekends and for longer hours during the week. In some areas, meals on wheels are provided at the weekends for housebound dependent people who need them. There are no longer grounds for refusing somebody a service merely because the local authority does not provide it or because there is a waiting list; purchasers may go elsewhere in order to obtain provision. However they will have to operate within the limits of the agreed budget.

The extended role given to private and voluntary agencies is an attempt to introduce more flexibility into the care system. The non-statutory organisations are seen to be more capable of adapting; they have undoubtedly been responsible for the introduction of areas of good practice in the past. In addition, voluntary organisations are often more accessible to service users who may be mistrustful of the local authority because of the bureaucratic officialdom it represents. Voluntary and community organisations have pioneered sensitive, responsive services to black families and to people with HIV in particular.

The production of jointly prepared local authority care plans involving all caring agencies have helped make services more comprehensive for and more accessible to the community. Their publication in all 'living' languages has ensured that all communities are aware of their entitlements. And the published complaints procedure is a way of drawing consumer feedback and giving service users a right to affect future delivery. Many authorities have produced newspapers and leaflets which outline services available, rights of clients and standards to be maintained; for example, they may pledge to publish and stick to the opening hours for all services or to respond to complaints within a maximum of 15 working days. Local authorities have been encouraged to become more accountable and responsible towards service users. They may obtain external validation of quality through independent organisations and be awarded with a quality assurance certificate for high standards of service.

The Health Service

The reorganisation and separation of the purchasing and providing functions within the health service has met with both support and criticism. Some GPs, given the opportunity to control their own budgets and generate income, have relished the opportunity of being able to buy their patients' care. Other GPs, who have so far resisted the financial incentives to become fund-holders, are concerned about their disadvantaged non-fund-holding status. For instance, 'A GP in Bath said he was attempting to get an operation for a patient with a crumbling hip brought forward. But a surgeon had said in a letter, "We are not allowed to expedite anybody unless they are the patient of a fund-holder" ' (*Pulse*, 16.1.93, p24). The introduction of fund-holding for some GPs has had the effect of damaging doctor–patient relations; some patients of non-fund-holding GPs feel that they are being given an inferior service and some patients of fund-holding practices believe they are being prescribed cheaper treatments and, as a result, develop feelings of being burdensome related to the perceived costs of their care. There is a fear, too, that potentially 'expensive patients', i.e. people who are chronically ill, may be discouraged from registering with fund-holding GPs or may be struck off existing lists, although in theory the existence of a complaints procedure should prevent this from happening.

There has been a greater reliance on technology in many surgeries as GPs have responded to legislative demands: computerised records have made it easier for GPs to carry out audits and discover more accurately the effectiveness of interventions and treatment programmes, as indicated by the assembled health information of patients. Against this, it needs to be said that some GPs feel that their jobs have become more bureaucratic and that their professional satisfaction has been reduced. One GP has commented, 'It is irritating that the new contract rewards GPs who do well at easily measurable tasks of doubtful validity rather than the intangible art and science of doctoring.' (*Retrospect – 10 years is a long time in general practice*. M. Safraner. British Medical Journal, No. 6888, Vol. 306, p. 1312)

Education

In the field of education the provider role of the local authority is diminishing as more schools are encouraged to opt out of local authority management and control. Some schools are happy with the freedom Local Management of Schools brings, but others criticise the lack of a consistent standard where all schools are adequately resourced. The publication of the performance-related league tables, designed to inform parental choice, does not tell the whole story and is regarded by many as a crude indicator based on raw assessment of exam results. The tests do not show the progress of each child and therefore cannot show parents how effective a school really is. League tables take no account of the wide variety of backgrounds and circumstances of pupils. Furthermore, schools at the bottom of the table may be doing a good job. League tables do not provide extra money but can damage the morale of teachers, parents and children. In the words of Katherine Whitehorn, speaking on Radio 4's Any Questions programme (broadcast 27.5.93), 'Any form of league table is a worship of measurement over quality'.

Fifteen years on from the Warnock Report, a document which revolutionised attitudes towards children with special needs, it is estimated that as many as 1 million children with special needs in ordinary schools are not getting the education they deserve. 'Statemented' children have attracted resources but less has been available for other children with special needs. 'Articulate parents can successfully argue the case for their child to gain a statement when his or her needs are less severe than those of a child in another part of the country whose parents lack such skills' (*Guardian*, 25.5.93). The absence of basic provision for all children with special needs, including mandatory nursery provision and parental education aimed at solving problems before children reach school, has led Robert Handcock, Director of the Spastics Society, to comment, 'The Government left special education needs provision to the ravages of the market economy. They have set it up to fail' (ibid.).

Housing

Perhaps the housing service has suffered most from the lack of adequate subsidy and dependence on the free market. Few council houses are now being built and the existing stock has been greatly diminished following the 'right to buy' legislation. Housing associations and private organisations are being encouraged to make up provision, but there remains a shortfall. Some people who purchased their own flats from the local authority in the late 1980s, having been drawn into the drive for owner occupation, are now being faced with the costs of communal maintenance; for lifts, roofs and window replacements. Their homes are worth less on the market than they paid for them at the height of the housing boom and now they find they are unable to pay the repair bills and keep up with mortgage payments. Other tenants of the public sector have seen their rent levels rise alarmingly in the last few years. Many are on fixed or low incomes and are finding this hard to bear. A record number of families have become homeless, having had their home repossessed because of their failure to meet regular payments, owing to changes in personal circumstances and fluctuations in the market. Some of these families have been forced to live in temporary accommodation.

At the end of March 1993, there was a total of 62 250 homeless households living in temporary accommodation in England, including an estimated 87 150 children. Temporary accommodation includes bed and breakfast hotels, hostels, private sector leased accommodation, short term housing and mobile homes. 'People who are most likely to experience living in temporary accommodation include members of minority ethnic groups, lone mothers, and those who speak little or no English, such as refugee or immigrant families (*Guardian*, 20.7.93).

There appears to be no consistency in the housing policy. The chief beneficiaries continue to be the owner occupiers whose position is subsidised by mortgage tax relief up to the amount of £30 000 on one property. 'The current mortgage relief means almost half the public money spent on housing goes towards subsidising high earners . . . an absurd situation which has fuelled past housing booms and helped to push up inflation' (*Guardian*, 1.6.92). Meanwhile the misery for people who are homeless continues whilst their basic right to shelter remains ignored. Nick Danziger, who spent a period sleeping rough preparing material for his television programme 'Down and Out in Paris and London' (Channel 4, 29.3.93), concluded:

> It is clear to me that only a few are homeless by choice. Most have lost jobs or never had a job. Others have had an accident or have suffered at the hand of a parent or a partner. The addiction to drink and drugs is an effect rather than a cause. I will never again judge homeless people by their appearance. Their wounds are internal.

Working in the caring services

Most of us are resistant to change: we prefer the comfort of familiarity and being able to practice in the way we have been used to. It is particularly reassuring when we act in ways that are consistent with our own ideological beliefs. The world of social and health care has been revolutionised, therefore it would not be realistic to expect that the pace and rate of change has not affected the morale of those who work inside the caring services.

The tensions and fears within social services authorities have centred mainly on the profound changes in community care arrangements. Bob Cervi recently wrote, 'Workers generally appear to be anxious about poor organisation, management and resourcing for community care' (*Community Care*, 25.3.93). One specific concern has been whether the new system is user-led or resouces-led. David Jones, BASW General Secretary, has said: 'What's needed for an effective and sensitive service is for staff to be treated better . . . (They) are told it has to be user-led and then that it has to be rationed and controlled' (ibid.).

Throughout all sectors and agencies, perhaps with the exception of the Probation Service, redundancies have been made and feelings of insecurity have grown regarding the safety of jobs. Increasingly carers are being appointed on short term contracts. The growth of the 'contract culture' has led to fears about the future. There is concern that there will be no guaranteed minimum standard level of service if the mixed economy does not generate satisfactory provision. With reference to the meals on wheels service, Catriona Marchant writes, 'What remains unanswered is what happens if the meals service run by the new contractors goes bust or is unsatisfactory and there is no in-house service to fall back on?' (*Community Care*, 1.7.93). Similar fears are expressed about the problems that would be created by a local hospital's failure to attract adequate income. Closure would certainly inconvenience the local community and would be wasteful of a capital asset.

Not everyone is depressed about the changes in their jobs. As mentioned earlier, many managers in various health and social care settings – hospitals, schools, social services authorities – welcome the opportunity to have more direct control over the management of resources. They appreciate, too, much of the increased profession-alism and raised standards established by recent legislation. The renewed emphasis on clients' rights and choices rests easily with many professionals. The aims of keeping clients in their own homes, keeping offenders out of prison and of involving service users and their families in their own care planning are readily endorsed by care workers. Their only concern is that of the availability of commensurate resourcing.

The gradual introduction of a systematic comprehensive assessment programme, based on National Vocational Qualifications (NVQs) and Scottish Vocational Qualifications (SVQs), has meant for the first time that carers may be formally recognised for their competence. For many workers, NVQs or SVQs represent a chance of progression as well as the opportunity to be valued for their current contribution. They may only be assessed as being competent if they demonstrate good practice. So this has implications for the establishment in which assessments take place: it is not possible for a worker to demonstrate 'good practice' unless good practice is the norm in the care setting.

It is too early to accurately assess the effect on the morale of health and social care workers although there is a temptation to say that concern and uncertainty outweigh optimism. A major worry is the move away from traditional social work to assessment and care management and the possible demotivation of the carer. The fear is that the new role of care manager will have too narrow a focus; a mere monitoring of the progress of the 'care package' at the expense of creative and innovative ways of working and preventive practice. Lesley Hayes and Robin Means write: 'One social worker feared her previous development role, albeit limited, would be squeezed out by care management work' (*Community Care*, 20.5.93).

Linked to this and representing the major ideological policy shift is the move from a 'holistic' model of care to a 'service' or 'consumer' model. Traditionally caring has been viewed as a dynamic two-way process in which both carer and client interact co-operatively to bring about positive change. In the consumer model a one-way service is provided by the agency *for* the client. This consumer model is reinforced in 'citizen's' or 'consumer' charters, within which there are complaints procedures which carry the threat of loss of contract by the providing agency. It is felt that there is a danger that this mode of working will contravene good practice. For example, residential care may become tantamount to a hotel service for residents with workers doing things for residents or waiting on them, instead of maximising people's autonomous functioning.

The wider social setting

The changes in the caring services are taking place within a society that has become more polarised. During the last 15 years or so, the gap between the rich and poor has widened mainly owing to high unemployment and low wages; poverty has deepened and deprivation has been extended. Furthermore inequality remains firmly structured along the lines of class, gender, race, age, disability and other factors. It is from these marginalised groups that the majority of clients of the caring services are drawn. For the purpose of briefly illustrating the continued existence of oppression and inequality we have selected three examples: race, gender and poverty.

Black people

It is well known that black people in Britain face discrimination in a number of different areas of their everyday lives. The education system has failed black people, both at school and with regard to access to training schemes. In the world of employment, black youths still find it disproportionately more difficult to obtain work and this pattern is sustained throughout adulthood. 'Considering . . . broad ethnic categories, black people suffer the highest unemployment rates, while Chinese and others display the lowest unemployment rates; though this is still well in excess of the rate for white people' (*Ethnic Minorities in Great Britain*, University of Warwick Centre for Research in Ethnic Relations, 1993, p6). When they do find work black people are not promoted at the same rate as their white counterparts and are therefore less likely to obtain managerial and supervisory positions.

There is evidence of both racism and sexism in the treatment of black women-headed households who have become homeless as a result of fleeing violence. Research has shown that black women and their children are waiting between 18 months and three years before they are rehoused (*The Hidden Struggle*, Amina Mama, 1989, p xiv).

It has already been noted, in Chapters 2 and 4, how social services and health care services have failed to meet the needs of black families. Specificallly with regard to mental health, 'Black people are far more likely to receive a diagnosis of schizophrenia than the indigenous population, and more likely to receive higher doses of psychotropic medication than counselling or psychotherapy' (*Health and Race*, Kings Fund Centre, 1992, p4). In relation to informal carers, the same report states, 'Black carers tend not to use respite care services for a break because most services do not cater properly for the person needing care' (ibid., p3).

In the field of criminal justice black offenders are more likely to receive harsher penalties at an earlier stage than white offenders; are more likely than white offenders to be remanded in custody rather than on bail; and are more likely to receive a custodial sentence rather than one which allows them to remain in the community. Black people are also under-represented as workers in the criminal justice system, particularly in senior and managerial positions.

Women

Single parents, the majority of whom are women, continue to experience poverty mainly because of the difficulty they have in obtaining well-paid work and adequate child care provision. The absence of available, accessible child care affects all families with young children and it is acknowledged that the UK remains second from bottom in the European child care league table (*Guardian*, 2.6.93, p4). Although the Government introduced workplace nursery tax allowance in 1990, in 1993 only one in 300 children under five attended a workplace nursery and less than 2 percent attended any form of nursery. Peter Moss, co-ordinator of the European Community Network, believes the issues involved in reconciling employment and child care are 'too important to leave to market forces and private endeavour alone' (ibid.). To do so would exacerbate labour market irregularities and 'make children's welfare dependent on the labour market value of their (parents)'. He adds that: 'Access to good quality, affordable services for children should be a public responsibility' (ibid.).

Despite the concern expressed about the needs of informal carers in the White Paper *Caring for People* (1989), no accompanying supportive measures have been produced to lessen their plight. Indeed, the development of community care policies may mean that more and more informal carers will be relied upon to provide caring tasks that range from cleaning and preparing meals to more intimate responsibilities such as bathing, dressing and toileting. It is mainly women who perform this role but men, too, act as informal carers, often tending their spouse. Furthermore, it is estimated that there are 1000 children and young people providing community care for parents or siblings, many of whom have as a result poor school performances, limited personal horizons and work aspirations.

Poverty

'In 1979 an estimated 5 million Britons were living in poverty' (*Observer*, 23.5.93). By 1993, Chris Pond, director of the Low Pay Unit, in a letter to the European Council stated that: 'A total of 20 million people in Britain, over a third of the population, have an income which leaves them in poverty or on its margins' including 'twenty five percent of British children living in poverty as defined by the EC' (a household income of less than half the EC average of £150 per week). Of other European countries only Portugal has more people living in poverty than the UK. Black people and their families are disproportionately represented in households with low incomes.

The financial limitations on the lives of people living in poverty are obvious and well documented. Latterly the concept of 'time poverty' has been introduced to describe the many practical ways in which poor people are excluded from full participation in society. Sue Ward has pointed out: 'Being poor takes up an enormous amount of time and energy' (*Power, Politics and Poverty*, in P. Golding, Excluding the Poor, CPAG; 1986, p37). She adds: 'Money also buys better housing and working conditions. These also affect the amount of time you have. Keeping clean, warm and fed – even just keeping going – in a damp council flat on the fourteenth floor, where the lifts don't work and the nearest supermarket is a mile away, is going to be a struggle anyway' (p38).

Kay Carmichael reiterates this, adding that: 'Travelling with small children, for example, is a much simpler exercise if one can bundle them into the back of the car, throwing mackintoshes into the boot in case it rains. The alternative of getting coats onto sometimes rebellious bodies, walking to the bus stop carrying bags, waiting, getting children and possibly a push chair onto the bus, keeping them happy on a crowded bus and after reaching one's destination knowing you have to do the whole thing in reverse is exhausting for anyone'. She adds: 'The financial ability to use taxis, telephones, restaurants, dry cleaners, offers a way of buying out of stress' (*Ceremony of Innocence – Tears, Power and Protest*, Kay Carmichael, Macmillan, 1991).

The relationship between poverty, deprivation and social work intervention is made clear by the findings of a piece of research on children entering care, carried out by Bebbington and Miles (*British Journal of Social Work*, Vol. 19, No. 5, October 1989, pp353–4). In a study of 2500 children admitted to care, this research found that before admission:

- only a quarter were living with both parents;
- almost three quarters of families received income support;
- one in five lived in owner occupied housing;
- over a half were living in a 'poor neighbourhood'.

The cumulative effect of these factors combined with others – overcrowding, large families, young mothers, parents of different racial origins – led the authors to compare two types of child and speculate on the likelihood of their admission to care:

Child A	Child B
Age 5–9	Age 5–9
No dependence on income support	Household head receives income support
Two parent family	Single adult household
Three children or fewer	Four or more children
White	Mixed ethnic origin
Owner occupier	Privately rented house
More rooms than people	One or more persons per room

The calculated odds of child A being admitted to care are 1:7000 whereas for child B they are 1:10.

Anti-discrimatory/anti-oppressive practice

The value of anti-discrimatory/anti-oppressive practice has been emphasised in recent years. It forms a central component of the value base of the Integrated Health and Social Care NVQ and SVQ Standards and has been fully incorporated into all Diploma in Social Work (Dip. SW) training programmes. Furthermore, antidiscriminatory/antioppressive practice has been rigorously promoted by CCETSW, who have published their own training materials for social care and social work students.

The increased awareness of the need for antioppressive practice has taken place against a constricting political backdrop. For example, section 28 of the Local Government Act 1988 forbade local authorities to intentionally 'promote' homosexuality and this has made people cautious, or at least self-conscious, about offering support to gay men and lesbians within the public sector. Similarly the rights and freedoms granted to people with disabilities in the Disabled Persons Act 1986 have not significantly altered their lives because so much of the Act is still, in 1994, not yet implemented.

There are signs that the progress towards equal opportunity, antiracism and antioppression made in the 1980s and early 1990s is now under threat. There seems to be a growing backlash against the equal opportunities strategies that have been established. Some critics claim that social work training has become too involved in 'trendy' doctrines and has been taken over by 'left wing extremists obsessed with politics of race, gender and class and that anyone who doesn't swear allegiance to their opinions is excluded from the profession' (*Guardian*, 2.6.93, p19). The Health Secretary, Virginia Bottomley, herself a former social worker, has written to the press stating that equal opportunities policies have gone 'too far' and 'to extremes'.

Tony Hall, the director of the CCETSW, has refuted these charges, arguing that: 'Part, but only part of our work involves training in antidiscriminatory issues. This is not at the expense of, but integral to, the skills that all social workers need if they are to work effectively in the social services of the nineties (ibid.). He was supported by David Jones, general secretary of the BASW: 'Social workers need a great deal more training in the "isms" that are being held up for ridicule, not less. But then the Government doesn't want to train people who can tell them about the armpit of society'. He adds: 'Forget about caring. It's all about control' (ibid.).

The backlash against equal opportunities is happening at a time when more is known about the harmful effects of past social and health care intervention on marginalised groups; black people and their families, particularly in the field of child care and mental health, and the assumption that they do not need services 'because they care for their own'; women who continue to bear the brunt of the responsibility of caring for children or dependent relatives; gay service users whose needs were often overlooked by the prevailing heterosexual orthodoxy of care regimes; people with disabilities and people with learning difficulties who have only relatively recently begun to be seen as individuals with the same rights as other people; and older people whose needs have often been ignored while health care resources have focused on younger people and social services provision has centred on child protection.

Professional social work training consists of two years of fulltime study in the UK (one year less than in the rest of Europe.) There are very few opportunities to qualify on a part-time basis so people with family or other commitments who cannot afford to undertake two years fulltime at college may not seek professional training. The bias towards predominantly middle-class white social work personnel will remain whilst barriers exist which make it difficult for working class people, black people and women and men with child care responsibilities to contribute to the planning and delivery of social care and social work. These are the very people who will share commonalities with service users. Social work and health care training cannot afford to relinquish its relatively recently developed commitment to equal opportunities and the promotion of antidiscriminatory practice since such issues are essentially about justice, equality, dignity and respect, core values of the caring professions. It is important that health and social carers continue to be mindful of these issues and actively promote antidiscrimination in their own practice.

Conclusion

Given that it is still too early to observe the effects of many of the changes introduced into the functioning of the caring services as they will require time to 'bed in', we must reserve judgement on their efficacy. As with all changes, their quality is always open to question; some we might feel are progressive, others not particularly helpful, if not damaging to welfare. In regard to community care in particular, many challenges lie ahead to see how well new assessment and care management procedures can be made to work. There is also the larger question of our country's further integration into the European community. The eventual adoption of the Social Chapter may have some effect in improving the conditions of workers in Britain, including those employed in the caring services. It is to be hoped that it would further reinforce equal opportunities.

Much debate has taken place about whether the changes of the last few years have fundamentally altered the nature of the Welfare State. The range of opinion stretches from those who believe that only a certain amount of transformation has taken place, through those who believe a more profound and radical restructuring has occurred, to those who express fears that what we are actually witnessing is the demise, by dismantling, of a co-ordinated welfare system. This debate is a thought-provoking one but, as can be seen, again it is too early to make a definitive judgement of it.

Many of us involved in the caring services have been concerned and saddened by what Michael Bayley describes as a 'form of individualism which appears to question any form of corporate responsibility above the level of the family' (*Welfare*, A *Moral Issue*, 1989, p33). Many people in other walks of life have likewise expressed anxiety on this feature of our society. Dr George Carey, Archbishop of Canterbury, has said, 'The pendulum . . . swung too far towards unbridled individualism in the 1980s. Our commitment to each other and to community, our faith in what we can build together as a society, was dangerously weakened' (*Independent*, 6.10.92).

However, there is a growing feeling of optimism, both within the caring services and in wider society, that the hold of such ideology is weakening. John Dossett-Davies has written, 'Empires and institutions come in cycles and we are near the bottom of one now. Social work's time will come again – the 'look after number one' era will pass and in another decade or two our profession will be moving towards a renaissance' (*Community Care*, 30.3.89, p21).

In the meantime, and as a way of hastening a new era, those of us involved in the caring services should acknowledge our strengths and the valuable contributions we make. Pessimism is disabling; remembering the worth of our skills and achievements, however small, can and should be enabling. David Divine provides thoughtful encouragement for us:

> We have a moral and professional obligation to expose the growing tide of human need but not to take on work which we cannot do. We have to set out our stall and make it clear what we can and cannot do. But we also have to nurture ourselves. We have so little time to think about the positive things we do because we are so busy responding to fire alarms. Without us many people would go to the wall and we should remember that.
>
> *(Social Work Today, 4.2.93)*

We must bear in mind that change is a continuous process in which we as individuals are all involved. It is therefore important that our practice standards reflect compassion, integrity and professionalism so that we can make a positive contribution, however small, to the future direction of the caring services.

Questions for discussion

1. Some areas of human need are too important to be left to the mechanisms of the free market. Discuss this statement.
2. The separation of the purchaser/provider functions will lead to a greater efficiency in meeting need. How true is this idea?
3. Only State-provided services will contribute to a sense of the 'common good': a mixed economy of care can never generate a sense of commitment and belonging. Discuss this statement.
4. People may be more institutionalised in their own homes than in residential settings. Comment on this.
5. Service users or their informal carers should be encouraged to take up the role of care manager. Present an argument either for or against this statement.
6. 'If social workers are to be perceived as agents of social change as much as agents of social control then issues of equality and rights must be firmly fixed on the agenda for policy and practice' (*All Equal Under the Act*, Ratna Dutt, p5). Discuss this statement.

Further reading

1. *Welfare, A Moral Issue*, Michael Bayley (Diocese of Sheffield Social Responsibility Commmittee, 1989). After an historical review of the Welfare State this short book reasserts the case for the common good.
2. *Changing Social Work and Welfare*, edited by Pam Carter, Tony Jeffs and Mark K Smith (Open University – 1992). This book looks at some current changes and dilemmas facing social work and social welfare through a series of essays by a range of authors.
3. *Social Work in an Unjust Society*, Bill Jordan (Harvester/Wheatsheaf, 1990).

Using case examples this book examines a variety of approaches to social work as well as anti discriminatory practice.

4. *The New Politics of Welfare – An Agenda for the 1990s?*, edited by Michael McCarthy (Macmillan, 1989). An examination of ideologies which have attempted to transform the Welfare State along with a robust defence of it.

5. *Community Care or Independent Living?*, Jenny Morris (Joseph Rowntree Foundation/Community Care, 1993). This report examines whether or not community care policies truly promote independent living.

6. *The Welfare State*, Dexter Whitfield (Pluto Press, 1992). This book analyses the effects of social deprivation and the privatisation of the Welfare State, as well as the true costs of promoting privatisation.

Annex 1

Training for work in the caring services

Introduction

Some people believe that effective carers are 'born and not made'. The implication of this is that no amount of education, experience and training will equip a person to function well if they do not have certain innate qualities. This may be considered an extreme view. Although individuals who earn their living working with people must have a liking for them and a wish to care for them, useful experience and relevant education on a training course are essential for effective caring. This chapter is concerned with the wide variety of training courses available to people who wish to pursue a career in caring. It does not cover social care and social work courses only – it also outlines the training that is available for those who wish to work in health, education, housing and youth and community work.

A definite requirement for a professional carer is a degree of maturity. For this reason, no one can practise as a professional social worker (or probation officer) before the age of 22. However, there are various ways of gaining experience before then. Voluntary work provides one method, as does work as a trainee social worker or work in a residential or day care setting.

Many people around the age of 16 have little if any idea of the kind of job or career they want to pursue. It is unreasonable to expect them all to be absolutely certain of what they want to do – individuals often need to have had some experience in a particular field of work before they can decide whether or not they will enjoy doing it. Those who go on from school into further or higher education have an advantage in that they can delay making a decision about a career.

There have been a number of important developments in training courses in recent years – they have become more flexible in running at times that are more convenient to some people such as evenings and weekends. The traditional college courses which started in September and ran through, in three terms, to June are largely a thing of the past. The development of National Vocational Qualifications (NVQs) has shifted the focus from what students or candidates *know* (passing exams or continual academic measurement) to what they can *do*, to whether or not they are competent practitioners. Some colleges are still involved in providing what is known, for NVQ purposes, as 'underpinning knowledge' but they do this in close partnership with practice agencies and they increasingly do it on a modular basis. Candidates can select which bits of knowledge they do not yet have and attend only to gain these.

In recent years there has also been a much heightened recognition in the caring services of the negative effects of prejudice, discrimination and oppressive practice. Being aware of these unhelpful processes and actively working in an antidiscriminatory or antioppressive way has been a requirement of all training at all levels; from preservice courses for 16 to 19 year olds to inservice courses and the professional level Diploma in Social Work (Dip. SW).

Apart form a small number of more specialised areas, the majority of young people and adults will proceed to qualification through the three routes of:

1. GCSE, A or AS levels, to degree and higher degree level;
2. National Curriculum Key Stage 4, through GNVQ (levels 1–4);
3. National Curriculum Key Stage 4, through NVQ (levels 1–5)

Leaving aside the first, more academic route, we now deal with GNVQs and NVQs.

GNVQ/Vocational A Levels

It is planned that in the next few years General National Vocational Qualifications (GNVQs) or Vocational Aa levels as they are to be known, along with the work-based NVQs, will replace most other vocational qualifications. GNVQs in Health and Social Care were introduced in September 1992. The purpose of GNVQs is to offer particularly the 16–19 age group (though they are open to other ages) a vocational alternative to A levels and a subsequent choice about whether to progress to employment or higher education. They therefore primarily suit young people in fulltime education who wish to keep their options open.

GNVQs will eventually exist at four levels (1–4). At present only levels 2 and 3 have been fully developed. Level 2 is considered to be of the same standing as four GCSE passes at Grade A–C, while level 3 is comparable, in its demands and coverage, to two A level passes. They are being offered in both schools and colleges. They provide a broad-based vocational education which includes a body of knowledge which underpins health and social care as well as a range of core skills such as communication and application of number and information technology. GNVQs are approved by the three awarding bodies, BTEC, City and Guilds and the RSA, and accredited by the National Council for Vocational Qualifications (NCVQ) (see figure 10.1 for more details of the content of the awards at levels 1, 2 and 3).

Assessment of GNVQ is based on the *outcomes* students must achieve. GNVQ's are made up of a number of *units*, credits in which may be awarded separately and accumulated for the award of a full GNVQ. They do not have to be completed in a certain time and the mode of learning can vary, e.g. fulltime or part-time attendance at school or college, open learning or private study, or a combination of these.

National Vocational Qualifications (NVQs)/Scottish Vocational Qualifications (SVQ's)

NVQs/SVQ's are a work-based qualification, recognised throughout the United Kingdom. A set of Integrated Competencies, made up of a number of units, prove competence for health and social care workers. These units of competence are known as National Standards. Each unit represents a co-ordinated piece of work performed in a normal working day. Units are further broken down into elements of competence and these in turn are broken down into performance criteria. Units can be claimed individually and accumulated until a complete qualification at whatever level (so far, levels 2 and 3 have been fully developed) can be gained. Joint awarding bodies for

Level 3 – Most commonly a 2-year programme for post-16 students

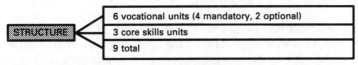

	12 vocational units (8 mandatory, 4 optional)
STRUCTURE	3 core skills units
	15 total

Educational Equivalents   Each 'vocational unit' is comparable (in its demands and coverage) to 1/6 of an A level or 1/3 of an AS level.

Note: Level 3 may be combined with *one* A level or *one or more* AS levels in a 2-year programme.

Level 2 – Most commonly a 1-year programme for post-16 students

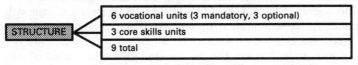

	6 vocational units (4 mandatory, 2 optional)
STRUCTURE	3 core skills units
	9 total

Educational Equivalents   Comparable to 4 GCSEs at grade C and above.

Note: Level 2 may be combined with GCSEs in a 1-year programme.

Level 1 – (At present not fully developed) Most commonly a 1-year programme for post-16 students. May be suitable for some pre-16 students and adults

	6 vocational units (3 mandatory, 3 optional)
STRUCTURE	3 core skills units
	9 total

Note: 2 of the 3 optional units can be chosen from different vocational areas.

Fig 10.1   GNVQ and educational equivalents.
Note 1: At all 3 levels, the 3 mandatory Core Skills Units are:-
1. Communication, 2. Application of Number, 3. Information Technology
Note 2: The development of problem-solving skills and personal skills is encouraged in all GNVQ's and although not formally assessed or certificated, they can be recorded along with all the above UNITS in the NATIONAL RECORD OF ACHIEVEMENT. (N.R.A)

NVQ are CCETSW and City and Guilds, and qualifications are accredited by the NCVQ.

There is no time limit to gaining NVQs. Assessment is usually carried out by the direct line manager to the candidate who is undergoing the award and in this capacity they are known as a 'work-based assessor'. Also integral to the system are 'internal verifiers' whose role it is to promote quality assurance across a number of units (perhaps a dozen or so) and to ensure that assessment is carried out in the same way in different settings. Thus it is intended that a national, consistent system of competency assessment will be set up. An 'external assessor' is an independent person, from another part of the country who has the task of overseeing the work of a complete assessment centre. Such centres are most commonly a partnership between a practice agency and a college base, but may involve several different organisations. Assessment takes place on the job, in the work unit, with a college base providing the so-called 'underpinning knowledge'.

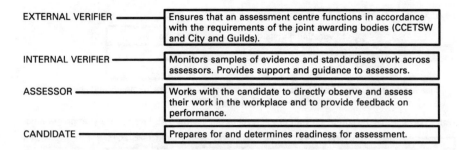

Fig 10.2   Functions within the NVQ/SVQ system.

There are a number of different awards: the general Integrated Competencies, also known as Care Awards, for a wide range of health and social care workers in a number of settings, such as day centres, health care support services and community care projects; Child Care and Education Awards for those working with children under seven years of age and their families; and the Criminal Justice System Awards for those working with offenders in community and residential settings, many of whom will be employed by the Probation Service.

At NVQ/SVQ level 3, the most popular award for health and social care workers who are not in management positions, there are eight mandatory units known as core units of competence. Seven of these, known as functional units, represent basic skills required by all carers, e.g. communication, dealing with distress and informing users about service delivery. The eight core unit, the most important of all, is the value base unit, coded the 'O' unit, which assesses the attitudes and values the individual carer holds towards the job. This aims to ensure that service users are respected as valued individuals with rights. As an important statement of anti oppressive practice, it requires carers to respect clients' personal beliefs and cultural identity, confidentiality, dignity and personal choices. In addition to the eight core units, candidates have to complete a number of further units which together make up an 'endorsement', which more closely relates to the specific nature of a candidate's role.

The Diploma in Social Work (Dip. SW)

The Diploma in Social Work is the professional qualification for all social workers (including probation officers) throughout the United Kingdom, in whatever sector or setting they work. It caters for non-graduates, undergraduates and graduates. The Dip. SW comprises at least two years of study and supervised practice, which includes direct observation of the student's social work practice skills. Dip. SW programmes are planned and run by colleges and social work agencies working co-operatively and is accredited by the CCETSW. The structure of courses may vary, depending on the specific needs of students and modular, 'open' and 'distance' learning arrangements are all permissible. Of central importance is the demonstration of anti oppressive practice. As the CCETSW state in their Handbook 9.3 – 'How to Qualify for Social Work', 'students are required to recognise, understand and confront racism and other forms of discrimination and to demonstrate their ability to work effectively in a multi racial society' (p5)

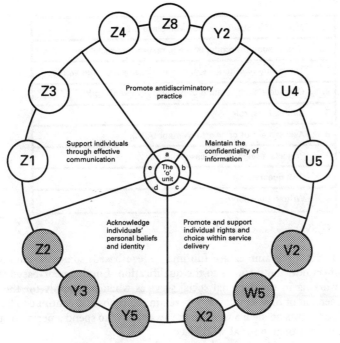

The 'O' unit (Value Base unit): Promote equality for all individuals.

The 7 Functional units (unshaded)	The 6 Endorsement units (shaded)
Z1 Contribute to the protection of individuals from abuse.	Z2 Contribute to the provision of advocacy for clients.
Z3 Contribute to the management of agressive and abusive behaviour.	Y3 Enable clients to administer their financial affairs.
Z4 Promote communication with clients where there are communication difficulties.	Y5 Assist clients to move from a supportive to an independant living environment.
Z8 Support clients when they are distressed.	X2 Prepare and provide agreed individual development activities for clients.
Y2 Enable clients to make use of available services and information.	W5 Support clients with difficult or potentially difficult relationships.
U4 Contribute to the health, safety and security of individuals and their environment.	V2 Determine the ways in which the service can support clients.
U5 Obtain, transmit and store information relating to the delivery of a care service.	

Note: The 8 'Core Units' are these 7 'Functional Units' plus the 'O' (Value Base) unit.

Fig 10.3 Composition of NVQ level 3 awards in Care – an example, 'Promoting Independence' (the eight core units plus six endorsement units).

Note 1: Other 'Awards in care' at level 3 include:-

Supported Living   Substance use
Rehabilitative Care   Support and protection
Continuing care   Self and environmental management skills
Supportive long-term care   Mental health care
Terminal care   Mobility and movement

Others have been, and are being, developed.

Note 2: A vert useful training package has been developed specifically on the 'o' **value base unit**. Details are:- **'Promoting Equality in Care Practice** – Preparation for the NVQ Unit O'. Written by **'Waterside Education and Training.'** Published by 'The Association for Social Care Training,' 1993.

1.	Naturalistic observation of workplace practice.
2.	Observation of 'products' – e.g. records, a 'made' bed.
3.	Testimony of others – e,g, clients, colleagues, other workers.
4.	Candidate's explanation of process/review of work.
5.	Simulations, role plays.
6.	Assessment of prior achievement (APA).
7.	Projects, assignments, case studies.
8.	Oral questioning.
9.	Written questioning.

Fig 10.4   NVQ/SVQ assessment methods.

Some Dip. SW programmes are fulltime college-based, some are employment-based and others offer both routes to the qualification. Employment-based students are already working in the personal social services when they apply for the course. With the agreement of their employer they retain their jobs and continue to have their salaries paid. Students on such a route to the award have to spend a period of assessed practice away from their normal workplace.

All candidates under 21 years on the date their course commences must have one of the following qualifications:

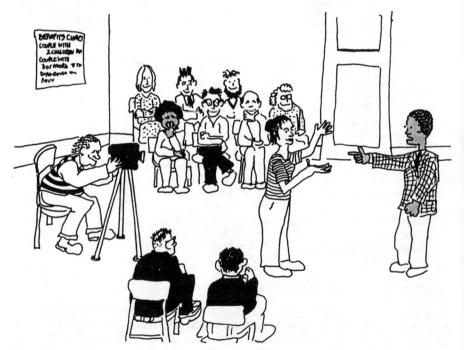

The training of social workers increasingly involves technology and experimental learning techniques

1. Two A level passes grade A–E and 3 GCSE passes in three other subjects, grade A–C;
2. Five passes in the Scottish Certificate in Education including three at the Higher Level;
3. Any other educational, vocational or professional qualification which the CCETSW considers to be equivalent.

Note: The CCETSW regards, amongst others, the following qualifications as equivalent to A Levels: NVQ Level 3, BTEC National Certificate/Diploma, SCOTVEC Advanced Certificate.

The Dip. SW cannot be awarded to anyone under 22 years. Where a student successfully completes the course under this age, the Diploma will show the 22nd birthday as the qualifying date.

For more information about the Dip. SW contact the CCETSW, Derbyshire House, St Chad's Street, London WC1H 8AD.

Employment in the health service

Nursing

Established nursing qualifications – Registered General Nurse (RGN), Registered Mental Nurse (RMN) and Registered Nurse for the Mentally Handicapped (RNMH) – are being replaced and a new education programme for nursing – Project 2000 – has been introduced. The Project 2000 course combines theoretical study with practical nursing experience. It is a three year course, the first half of which is taken up by the Common Foundation Programme (CFP). This is a general introduction to knowledge and core skills which is relevant to every field of nursing.

After passing this stage of the course, the student studies one of four specialities or 'Branch Programmes':

1. adult nursing;
2. mental health nursing;
3. 'mental handicap' nursing;
4. children's nursing.

Courses are based in colleges of nursing that have close links with colleges of higher education. Assessment is continuous throughout the three years and includes essays, projects and invigilated examinations. Successful completion leads to qualification as a registered 'first-level' nurse, as well as a qualification at higher education level. Future prospects might involve advanced clinical specialisms, research, management or education.

The normal requirement for nursing training is at least five GCSE passes or equivalent at grade C or above. Some vocational qualifications, e.g. BTEC or RSA II and III, may count towards entry. Your local college of nursing will advise you on this. The minimum age of entry to training is 17½, although you may apply from

16½. There is no upper age limit. Some colleges offer part-time courses for mature entrants.

To apply for nurse training contact Nurses' and Midwives' Central Clearing House (NMCCH), PO Box 346, Bristol BS99 7FB. For more information about nursing write to the relevant address:

England
Careers Advisory Service
English National Board
for Nursing, Midwifery and Health Vis-
iting
PO Box 356
Sheffield S8 OSJ

Wales
Welsh National Board for Nursing, Mid-
wifery and Health Visiting
13th Floor
Pearl Assurance House
Greyfriars Road
Cardiff CF1 3AG

Scotland
The Nursing Adviser
Scottish Health Service Centre
Crewe Road South
Edinburgh EH4 2LF

Northern Ireland
The Recruitment Officer
National Board for Nursing, Midwifery
and Health Visiting for Northern Ireland
RAC House
79 Chichester Street
Belfast BT1 4JR

Registered midwife (RM)

The majority of midwives are already qualified as general nurses or have completed the 'adult branch' of the Project 2000 course. Applicants for midwifery then go on to a postregistration programme, which lasts 18 months. This is based in a college or faculty of midwifery, to which your chosen application should be made directly.

However, there are also preregistration midwifery programmes which are of a minimum three years duration. For these programmes you must be 17½ years old and have at least five GCSE passes at grade A–C (or equivalents), including English Language and a science subject. Application for this programme should be made to the Nurses' and Midwives' Central Clearing House (address above).

There is also an advanced diploma in midwifery for those who want to take more clinical responsibility or to move on into management, research or education. Courses are provided on a taught or 'distance learning' basis.

District nurse

To become a district nurse, you must first be qualified in general nursing. Some experience is needed before applying for training as a district nurse. Applicants have to obtain secondment from a district health authority. Courses for the District Nursing Certificate last a minimum of 38 weeks and take place in a variety of colleges both at further and higher education level. The period of training includes three months of supervised district nursing practice. Application should be made directly to a training centre and a list of relevant centres can be obtained from national boards (addresses above).

Health visitor (HV)

To become a health visitor, you must first have qualified as a general nurse and have had some general nursing experience. Again, applicants need to obtain secondment from a district health authority. The course lasts one academic year and is followed by a period of supervised practice. A list of training centres can be obtained from national boards (addresses above).

Family planning nurse

Family planning nurses deal with issues such as contraception, smear testing, infertility and sexual health. They provide practical advice as well as counselling and health education. To become such a nurse requires qualification and experience in general nursing, midwifery or as a health visitor. Secondment to the course must be obtained from a district health authority. Courses are organised through a school of nursing or midwifery. They last a minimum of 20 weeks, of which the teaching programme represents a minimum of ten days, normally spread over the total period. Successful candidates are awarded a National Board Statement of Competence in Family Planning.

School nurse

School nurses deal with the health of children and adolescents in schools and aim to help them to achieve their full educational potential. School nurses monitor children's development and teach them about health issues. To become a school nurse requires qualification and some experience in general nursing. The course lasts 12 weeks and takes place in a range of college settings. For more information apply to your relevant national board (addresses above).

Physiotherapist

Physiotherapists use physical activity and exercise to help prevent and treat disease and injury. Most start work in a general hospital, but they can be employed in a wide variety of settings: schools, sports clinics, industry and the private sector. All physiotherapy students undertake a degree course in physiotherapy, validated by the Chartered Society of Physiotherapy. Courses last three or four years of full time study. Applications from mature students (over 21) are particularly welcomed. For more information, contact the Chartered Society of Physiotherapy, 14 Bedford Row, London WC1R 4ED.

Speech and language therapist

A speech and language therapist identifies, assesses and treats communication disorders in children and adults. They usually work as a member of a multi-disciplinary team which may include other caring professionals such as doctors, teachers and psychologists. Most work in hospitals and community clinics. Other settings include schools, special units, paediatric assessment centres, social education centres and language units. Courses are offered in a number of colleges and universities and are accredited by the College of Speech and Language Therapists. Undergraduate courses last for three or four years, postgraduate courses for two years. Most undergraduate courses require three A level passes or four Scottish Highers. Again, mature applicants (over 25) are welcomed. For more information contact the College of Speech & Language Therapists, 7 Bath Place, Rivington Street, London EC2A 3DR.

Occupational therapist (OT)

The minimum age to start training as an occupational therapist is 18 (17½ in Scotland). There is no maximum age limit. In order to become registered to work as an OT, you must successfully complete a degree in occupational therapy, which lasts three or four years fulltime. The degree is run in schools of occupational therapy, based either in hospitals or higher education establishments. One third of the course is practical placements in a variety of clinical settings.

Minimum academic qualifications for the degree are two A levels plus three GCSEs (at grades A–C) or, in Scotland, three H grades plus two S grades (1–3). Passes should include English and a science subject. BTEC and SCOTVEC national awards in relevant subjects, such as science or health studies, may be accepted as equivalents.

Occupational therapy helpers' who have qualified through further education or NVQ/SVQ courses or who have one year's supervised experience, may undertake a four year in service course leading to the Diploma of the College of Occupational Therapists and progress to eventual registration.

For further information on training as an occupational therapist, contact the College of Occupational Therapists, Education Department, 6–8 Marshalsea Road, Southwark, London SE1 1HL.

A range of other occupations

Nursery nurse

Training as a nursery nurse involves the broadest range of jobs with children up to seven years of age (eight in Scotland). In general they care for healthy children, but some do look after hospital patients, children with disabilities or children with special needs. A nursery nurse can work in a variety of settings – for example, day or nursery centres, nursery (or infant) schools, hospitals, colleges, town hall or private sector creches or as nannies in private houses.

The minimum age of entry to qualifying courses is 16 in colleges of further education, 18 in private colleges. In England, Wales and Northern Ireland, the recognised qualification is the Certificate awarded by the National Nursery Examination Board (NNEB). In Scotland the Scottish Nursery Nurses' Board (SNNB) is the awarding body.

For entry to training, most colleges require two or three GCSEs (grades A–C) or SCEs (grades 1–3). Private colleges may ask for at least three GCSEs/SCEs, including English. Competition for training courses is great and some applicants may have A levels/H grades. The fulltime course takes two years and assessment is continuous.

For more information about the course and about postqualifying studies offered, contact the National Nursery Examination Board, 8 Chequer Street, St Albans, Herts AL1 3XZ.

A BTEC National Certificate in Caring (Nursery Nursing) has also been developed. It is a two year part-time course for people who are already in work (whether paid or unpaid). For details of this contact your local college.

Further information

If you are interested in training in other areas of the caring services, you may find the following addresses useful:

Play training/playwork

The National Children's Play and Recreation Unit, 359–61 Euston Road, London NW1 3AL.

Youth and community work

National Youth Agency, 17–23 Albion Street, Leicester LE1 6GD.

Housing

There are a number of BTEC awards in housing. For details of what is on offer in your area, contact your local further education college. For details of professional qualifications in housing, contact the Institute of Housing, Octavia House, Westwood Way, Coventry CV4 8JP.

A general resource . . .

The most comprehensive annual guide to opportunities and trends in employment is *Occupations*, published by the Careers and Occupational Information Centre (COIC). It is available in public libraries, careers information and other advisory services offices.

Appendix 1 – GNVQ

GNVQ Level 2 – health and social care

Summary of the four mandatory units and elements

UNIT 1   PROVIDE EMOTIONAL SUPPORT
  1.1   Use conversational techniques to maintain social interaction
  1.2   Adapt conversational techniques to meet self-esteem needs of others
  1.3   Demonstrate supportive behaviour in individual and group situations
UNIT 2   INFLUENCES ON HEALTH AND WELL-BEING
  2.1   Identify ways in which individuals are affected by social factors
  2.2   Identify the effects of discrimination
  2.3   Identify lifestyle factors which influence health in social settings
UNIT 3   HEALTH EMERGENICES
  3.1   Identify health emergencies
  3.2   Respond to emergencies
  3.3   Explain health and safety principles relevant to emergencies
UNIT 4   HEALTH AND SOCIAL CARE SERVICES
  4.1   Identify the structure of health and care services
  4.2   Examine access to health and care services
  4.3   Identify client rights in health and care services

Summary of the four optional units and elements (of which the candidate must choose two units)

UNIT 5   THE CARE NEEDS OF INDIVIDUALS
  5.1   Investigate the needs of individuals in care settings
  5.2   Investigate methods used in meeting the needs of individuals in care settings
  5.3   Investigate client groups and resources in the care environment
UNIT 6   PROMOTING THE HEALTH OF THE INDIVIDUAL
  6.1   Investigate health-related leisure activities of interest to individuals and groups
  6.2   Identify the benefits of a balanced diet for promoting health
  6.3   Examine the promotion of individual well-being
UNIT 7   GROWTH AND DEVELOPMENT OF THE INDIVIDUAL
  7.1   Investigate growth and development throughout the human life span

7.2 Identify basic factors affecting the development of the individual at different life stages

7.3 Describe how the life changes of individuals are influenced by life stages

UNIT 8 SCIENCE IN HEALTH AND SOCIAL CARE

8.1 Identify the basic organisation and functions of human body systems

8.2 Investigate observation and measurement of individuals in care settings

8.3 Investigate the way science is applied in a care setting

GNVQ Level 3 – health and social care

Summary of the eight mandatory units and elements

UNIT 1 ACCESS, EQUAL OPPORTUNITIES AND CLIENT RIGHTS

1.1 Investigate attitudes and other social influences on behaviour

1.2 Investigate discrimination and its effects on individuals

1.3 Describe how equal opportunities are maintained

UNIT 2 INTERPERSONAL INTERACTION

2.1 Communicate with individuals

2.2 Promote communication within groups

2.3 Analyse clients' rights in interpersonal situations

UNIT 3 PHYSICAL ASPECTS OF HEALTH

3.1 Examine how body systems inter-relate

3.2 Investigate human disease

3.3 Investigate the components of healthy diet

UNIT 4 PSYCHOLOGICAL AND SOCIAL ASPECTS OF HEALTH AND SOCIAL CARE

4.1 Investigate the development of individual identity

4.2 Investigate threats to maintaining individual identity

4.3 Investigate the relationship of social and economic factors to health

UNIT 5 HEALTH PROMOTION

5.1 Prepare a plan of health promotion advice

5.2 Present health promotion advice to others

5.3 Identify different types of risks to health

UNIT 6 STRUCTURE AND PRACTICES IN HEALTH AND SOCIAL CARE

6.1 Investigate the structure of health and social care provision

6.2 Investigate the impact of legislation and funding on provision and priorities

6.3 Investigate ways in which services within health and social care operate

UNIT 7 CARE PLANS

7.1 Describe the development of care plans

7.2 Describe methods of assessing client need

7.3 Identify the purpose of monitoring and evaluation approaches within care plans

UNIT 8 RESEARCH IN HEALTH AND SOCIAL CARE

8.1 Investigate types of research used in health and social care

8.2 Construct a structured research instrument to survey opinion

8.3 Investigate methods of interpreting information

Summary of the eight optional units and elements
(of which the candidate must choose four units)

UNIT 9   WELFARE SERVICES AND SOCIAL CHANGE
9.1   Investigate the consequences of social change
9.2   Investigate the implications for welfare provision of changes in the population structure
9.3   Identify the impact of changing social attitudes on the provision of welfare services
9.4   Investigate social inequalities and assess their effect on access to welfare services

UNIT 10   HUMAN BEHAVIOUR IN THE CONTEXT OF HEALTH AND SOCIAL CARE
10.1   Investigate ways of explaining human behaviour
10.2   Investigate factors influencing human behaviour
10.3   Investigate the influences of personality and perception on human behaviour
10.4   Investigate emotional aspects of behaviour in relation to major psychological perspectives

UNIT 11   EQUILIBRIUM AND CONTROL IN HUMAN BODY SYSTEMS
11.1   Investigate and document equilibrium systems in the human body
11.2   Investigate control mechanisms in the human body
11.3   Investigate coping mechanisms in the human body

UNIT 12   SPECIAL NEEDS
12.1   Investigate special needs definitions
12.2   Investigate different models of special needs
12.3   Investigate the implementation of special needs provisions
12.4   Investigate the impact of service delivery on life experiences of people with special needs

UNIT 13   WORKING IN CARE ORGANISATIONS
13.1   Investigate the effective functioning of individuals as members of a care work group
13.2   Investigate work groups in care organisations
13.3   Investigate the ways in which care organisations function
13.4   Analyse the factors which influence the creation of a caring environment

UNIT 14   ENVIRONMENTAL HEALTH AND SAFETY
14.1   Investigate environmental health provision
14.2   Investigate processes and procedures for the maintenance of food hygiene
14.3   Identify the principles of first aid
14.4   Demonstrate the practices of first aid

UNIT 15   THE DEVELOPMENT OF SOCIAL POLICY
15.1   Investigate the development of social policy
15.2   Analyse the delivery of social services
15.3   Investigate social provision in the European Community

UNIT 16   INVESTIGATING AND MONITORING HUMAN BODY PROCESSES
16.1   Investigate the role of diagnostic testing in the monitoring of human body processes
16.2   Investigate tests used to measure chemical and microbiological function in the body
16.3   Investigate the use of physical tests to monitor body function

Appendix 2 – composition of NVQ/SVQ level 2 awards in Care

There are six awards in Care at level 2. These are:

1. developmental care;
2. direct care;
3. domiciliary support;
4. residential/hospital support;
5. postnatal care;
6. special care needs.

Each is made up of six core units, which consist of five functional units plus the 'O' (Value Base) unit, plus a number of endorsement units.

Summary of core units and elements

O	PROMOTE EQUALITY FOR ALL INDIVIDUALS
O.a	Promote antidiscriminatory practice
O.b	Maintain the confidentiality of information
O.c	Promote and support individual rights and choice within service delivery
O.d	Acknowledge individuals' personal beliefs and identity
O.e	Support individuals through effective communication
Z1	CONTRIBUTE TO THE PROTECTION OF INDIVIDUALS FROM ABUSE
Z1.a	Contribute to minimising the level of abuse in a care environment
Z1.b	Minimise the negative effects of disruptive or abusive behaviour
Z1.c	Contribute to monitoring individuals who are at risk from abuse
W2	CONTRIBUTE TO THE ONGOING SUPPORT OF CLIENTS AND OTHERS SIGNIFICANT TO THEM
W2.a	Enable clients to maintain their interests, identity and emotional well-being whilst receiving a care service
W2.b	Enable clients to maintain contact with those who are significant to them
W2.c	Support those who are significant to clients during visits to the client
W2.d	Enable those who are significant to the client to support the client
W3	SUPPORT CLIENTS IN TRANSITION DUE TO THEIR CARE REQUIREMENTS
W3.a	Support clients as they change from one care requirement to another
W3.b	Enable clients to become familiar with different care requirements
W3.c	Enable clients to transfer between different care requirements
U4	CONTRIBUTE TO THE HEALTH, SAFETY AND SECURITY OF INDIVIDUALS AND THEIR ENVIRONMENT
U4.a	Contribute to the promotion of client's health
U4.b	Contribute to maintaining the safety and security of clients and their belongings
U4.c	Contribute to maintaining the safety and security of the environment

U4.d   Maintain personal standards of health, safety and security
U4.e   Respond in the event of a health emergency
  U5   OBTAIN, TRANSMIT AND STORE INFORMATION RELATING TO THE DELIVERY OF A CARE SERVICE
U5a.   Obtain information relating to care service delivery
U5.b   Maintain, store and retrieve records
U5.c   Receive and transmit information to others on request

Summary of endorsement units

DEVELOPMENTAL CARE
  Z5   Enable clients to move within their environment
  Z13   Enable clients to participate in recreation and leisure activities
  X1   Contribute to the support of clients during development programmes and activities
  W8   Enable clients to maintain contacts in potentially isolating situations
  U2   Maintain and control stock, equipment and materials
DIRECT CARE
  Z6   Enable clients to maintain and improve their mobility
  Z7   Contribute to the movement and treatment of clients to maximise their physical comfort
  Z9   Enable clients to maintain their personal hygiene and appearance
  Z10   Enable clients to eat and drink
  Z11   Enable clients to access and use toilet facilities
  Z19   Enable clients to achieve physical comfort
DOMICILIARY SUPPORT
  Z7   Contribute to the movement and treatment of clients to maximise their physical comfort
  Y1   Enable clients to manage their domestic and personal resources
  W8   Enable clients to maintain contacts in potentially isolating situations
  U1   Contribute to the maintenance and management of domestic resources
RESIDENTIAL/HOSPITAL SUPPORT
  Z7   Contribute to the movement and treatment of clients to maximise their physical comfort
  Z10   Enable clients to eat and drink
  Z11   Enable clients to access and use toilet facilities
  U1   Contribute to the maintenance and management of domestic resources
  U2   Maintain and control stock, equipment and materials
POSTNATAL CARE
  Z10   Enable clients to eat and drink
  Z11   Enable clients to access and use toilet facilities
  Z16   Care for a baby in the first ten days of life when the mother is unable
  Z19   Enable clients to achieve physical comfort
  W6   Reinforce professional advice through supporting and encouraging the mother in active parenting in the first ten days of the baby's life
SPECIAL CARE NEEDS
  Z9   Enable clients to maintain their personal hygiene and appearance

Z10   Enable clients to eat and drink
Z13   Enable clients to participate in recreation and leisure activities
Y1   Enable clients to manage their domestic and personal resources
X1   Contribute to the support of clients during development programmes
      and activities
W8   Enable clients to maintain contacts in potentially isolating situations

Exercise 1 – what a job involves

Having decided on a caring agency (whether statutory, voluntary, private or not-for-profit) for which you would like to work, write a letter to the person with overall responsibility, asking if you can go and interview a member of staff who is doing a job which you yourself would like to do at some time in the future.

At the interview, find out:

a) what qualifications (if any) you require to get the job;
b) the experience required before taking up the job;
c) what the job actually entails – such as particular duties and responsibilities;
d) the authority structure of the agency and to whom you would be directly responsible;
e) any aspects of the job which give particular joy or satisfaction;
f) any aspects of the job which are particularly difficult or testing;
g) future promotion or career prospects.

Afterwards, ask yourself:

1. how well do your personal qualities equip you to do the job?
2. what experience do you need to gain in respect of the job?
3. how might you go about getting this experience?

Exercise 2 – role play – a college interview

In a group of three, you are to role-play an interview taking place in a college of further education.

Roles

1. A prospective student
2. A member of the college staff conducting the interview
3. An observer

Student

You are very keen to do a particular course (it can be one of your own choosing – pretraining, training, etc.) and feel that you have the ability, application and commitment to do it. You are keen to convey to the interviewer your personal qualities, strengths and capabilities. You also want to make it clear that you require certain things from the course in order to help you make progress in advancing your knowledge and skills. You want to find out a good deal about what the course can offer.

Interviewer

You want to find out if the student has the qualities that the college looks for in course members – persistence, concentration, a certain amount of maturity and a serious commitment. You will also want to try to assess academic ability and some familiarity with study skills, or at least the student's wish to improve what capability she or he already has.

Observer

You should merely observe and take no part in the proceedings. You should observe very carefully, noting the content of what is said, the mood of the participants and how it changes, and how well they set about the task. Anything else of interest should be noted. At the close of the role play, you should 'feed back' to the 'actors'.

Task

Allowing at least 20 minutes, role-play the interview. You will then need at least ten minutes for feedback. Total time – 30 minutes.
   Note: The roles can, of course, be reversed until all three have had a chance to play each.

Following the role play

A useful discussion could follow the role play around general issues in interviews, power and power relationships, the setting of 'agendas', who asks the questions, what questions were asked, etc. It will be useful to bring the whole group together to compare differing experiences.

Exercise 3 – course evaluation

Opinions vary a great deal as to whether training or experience is the more important in preparing for work in the caring services. Most agree that some form of training is essential but that it should of course be relevant to whatever the student intends to do in the future.

Examine a course you have completed in the past or one you are currently undertaking, in respect to the following criteria:

a) How relevant have you found the different parts of the course to the work in the caring services which interests you?

b) How well were vocational and academic studies represented? Were they balanced or not?

c) How well do you think it has equipped you for any physical skills you will require?

d) Comment on different teaching styles on the course. What have you found helpful and why?

e) How do you feel the course has contributed to your personal growth?

f) What improvements or innovations would you introduce to the course?

Annex 2

Practical work placements

An essential ingredient of all health and social care, social work and community care training courses, whether at a preparatory or professionally qualifying level, is the *practical placement*. The way in which placements are organised will depend on the nature of the course and the degree of involvement expected of the student. Most courses offer the student the chance to experience more than one placement.

Placements give students the chance to see the type of work they feel they would like to do and an opportunity to practise some of the skills learned in college.

Broad aims of a practical placement

a) To provide students with learning experiences within a practical setting which will help enhance personal characteristics such as reliability, sensitivity, practical ability, confidence and initiative.
b) To enable students to link theory and practice through practical work experience in a variety of placements.
c) To develop skills in communication and collaboration with staff and clients.
d) To give students an awareness of the work and range of the caring services.
e) To encourage the development of a critical capacity within the student, so that they may evaluate the standard of care.

Observational placements

Many students beginning social work preparatory courses may have had no experience of any working environment, let alone a social work setting. Other students may have done some voluntary work or have friends or relations who are social workers or they may have visited friends or relations who live in residential care establishments. Students on professionally qualifying courses are likely to have worked in only one particular setting.

Taking into account these mixed degrees of experience, the initial placement may be a short introductory one involving the student in an *observational* capacity, aimed at helping them to adjust to the working situation and begin to learn what can be expected of them in the future. Students will be able to watch carers at their work, observe the daily routine of the agency and learn to detect the needs of the people being cared for.

Types of placement

Placements may be undertaken within a whole range of health, social care and social work agencies. Initially it is more appropriate for students to be placed in practical work situations which are more familiar, where there is more structure and the student is not likely to be given too much responsibility and where the roles of the workers and the organisation are more easily comprehended.

Where possible, beginners are usually placed in day nurseries, playgroups or even special schools. Subsequent placements may take place in hospitals, probation hostels, public health authorities, children's homes, care homes, homes for people with learning difficulties, and other voluntary organisations. Some students may be placed with the Probation Service, the education social work department, social services or the health service and may accompany professionals as they go about their daily tasks.

Students who are undergoing professionals qualifying training will be given actual cases to work on by themselves, but students on preliminary courses will not have this opportunity.

Organisation of placements

Depending on the duration and level of the training course, practical placements may be undertaken on one or more days during the week, which may form part of a *block* experience of one or a number of consecutive weeks. A block placement enables the student to become more fully involved and it consolidates the experience gained over previous work visits. They will feel a more integrated member of the establishment and may appreciate more fully the day-to-day events and more easily observe the continuity of care. Furthermore, the student will have the opportunity to commit more deeply and also respond spontaneously themselves circumstances.

There now follows an outline of some important aspects of health, social care and social work placements. Many of these may perhaps seem obvious to some students – particularly to those who have worked in other settings and have an idea of what is expected from them – but these aspects are mentioned in order to help those who have had little adult life experience outside home and school.

A guide to practical placements

Introductory visits

The idea of an introductory visit is to allow you – the student – to make contact with the agency and to be introduced to the member of staff who will be supervising you during the placement. On your preplacement visit, you will be able to establish the expected hours of attendance, familiarise yourself with the setting and be informed of any special requirements of the agency. (For example, you may be required to wear a uniform – your course tutor should be able to provide the appropriate garment.)

First day of placement

You will probably be given an opportunity to meet other members of staff and be shown round the establishment. You may be allocated specific tasks or be expected to work alongside a particular member of staff. You will be made aware of fire drill and other safety procedures.

Keeping a diary

Not all courses insist on this practice, but keeping a diary of your day-to-day involvement can be a useful way of focusing and reflecting on your experience. You will also find the diary helpful as a source of reference when you are preparing the assignment which may be expected from you on completion of your placement. You may find it interesting to compare your initial impression with how you feel at the end of your placement.

Practical assistance on observational placements

There is a limit to the amount of time that can be spent simply observing others, so even when you are on an observational visit you may have the opportunity to assist in a practical way. The offer of help is always welcome in any work situation and observation can of course continue.

Practical placements

There is often a great deal of practical work to be carried out in a residential, day care or hospital setting and routine physical tasks form a high proportion of the carer's role.

Students should be prepared for *lifting*. In order to lift or raise a person in bed, you need to have been properly instructed – some people have seriously damaged their backs straining to move an adult on their own. Lifting takes two people – you will not be expected to lift anyone by yourself, and nobody will mind helping you.

Time keeping

Residential establishments involve shift work and staff change-overs – all activities are based on rotas. While on placement, although you will not actually be a member of staff, activities will be planned with you in mind. If you are late, organised events may have to be delayed or even postponed – taking a group of residents on a local outing will be more difficult if only one adult is able to supervise. Time keeping is important for any placement, because care workers and social workers will have appointments to keep.

Shift work

Normally your hours of attendance at a placement will be from 9 a.m. to 4 p.m. This is equivalent to the time you usually spend in college. However, in order to fit into the requirements of a residential placement, you may be expected to do shift work. Being available for the hours of a normal college day will be of no use in, say, a children's home or a probation hostel, as most of the residents will be out during this time. Obviously it is important to be around when the clients are there, so you could be asked to start work early in the morning (6 or 7 a.m.) or attend the later shift (from 1 or 2 p.m. until 9 or 10 p.m.).

The late shift may pose problems for some people – for example, older students with young families of their own and students who are unhappy at the prospect of making their own way home late at night. If you have such an objection, do not be afraid to express it – arrangements may be made to accommodate you. At the same time, it is as well to remember that shift work is an essential aspect of residential work – it is something you need to prepare for if you want to do this kind of work.

Attendance

Once you have been accepted by an establishment for whatever duration, you will be included in work plans and provision will be made for you. If you are ill or cannot attend for some reason, it is important to inform your placement supervisor and college tutor as early as possible. Even though your involvement is limited by the length of the placement, service users will be used to seeing you on a particular day of the week and may be disappointed if you fail to turn up – particularly if you have promised to do something for them or with them.

Being respectful

If you are placed in a residential establishment, it is important to remember that you are in someone's home. Naturally you need to observe basic politeness and to spend time learning how things are generally done in the home. At any place of work there will be accepted ways of behaving and it is important for you to try to be aware of them.

Being co-operative

Being somewhere on placement involves your being a member of a team, albeit in a restricted capacity. Teamwork involves sharing, supporting and co-operating with others, so naturally you should take your part in this process. There may be a number of tedious and routine jobs to perform, but you should be willing to undertake them. Similarly, doing your share of teamaking and washing up for other staff members is part of being a team member.

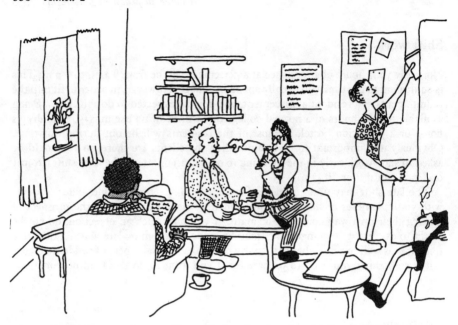

Staffrooms can often provide an ideal setting for relaxed informal discussion

Asking questions

People are generally willing to share their knowledge and expertise, especially if you express an interest, but they need to know what it is you do not understand or what you would like to know more about. Obviously you have to select an appropriate time to ask. At the same time, you need to be thoughtful about your enquiries and make sure that they are relevant. If you do not ask questions, it may give rise to doubts from the agency as to your degree of involvement.

Confidentiality

In most social work settings, you are likely to have access to clients' records – particularly those of the clients whom you deal with. You may come across information of a very sensitive nature and it is important to remember that such information is *strictly confidential*. You may know personally some of the families whose records you are reading, but it is vital that you use this information only to increase your understanding of a person's background.

Under no circumstances must you ever divulge confidential material to anyone other than those with whom you work. It is sometimes appropriate to describe circumstances of case histories to colleagues for academic reasons, but you should avoid mentioning any names, as this could cause embarrassment or suffering. Throughout a career in social work, as in any other life situation, you will be exposed to information which will require your judgement alone to help you decide whether or not you should be silent about it.

Representing your course and the college

Placements form a valuable aspect of any student training. They are made available through the co-operation of the agencies concerned. They take time and effort to set up and they can be used regularly thereafter by a series of students. Agencies will be keen to take interested and committed students, but a succession of poor students will discourage any organisation from making placements available for other students in the future. It is important to remember that during your time on placement you are contributing to the reputation of your course and the college you are attending.

The importance of reading

In order to increase your understanding of the work of the agency with whom you are placed, it will be beneficial to back up your experience with relevant reading. You may obtain some written information from the agency itself, which may have its own library or a stock of professional magazines and journals. Otherwise, you should be able to find sources of information about the particular agency or the service in general within your college library. You should do some reading on the special needs of clients with whom you are working or about different play or recreational activities which you might be able to put into practice. Information gained from reading will help you get more from your placement experience.

Placement supervision

Most agencies encourage students to be actively involved as much as possible, but there may be occasions when you will be preferred to be 'seen and not heard'. During your placement, you should receive regular supervision from a member of staff in order to obtain some direction and some feedback about the progress you are making. You will have an opportunity to express any anxieties you may have and to ask questions about the policy and practice of the organisation. For example, you may wish to establish the level of participation expected of students during agency staff meetings. Your supervisor may at some time ask you how you would run a residential home and what changes you would introduce. Your answer will be an indication of your commitment and interest in the work.

The standard and availability of supervision and the length of time devoted to it will vary according to the type and duration of the placement. A good supervisor will provide a student with time for considered reflection on social work policies and practices, will help them to see the relationship between theory and practice and will generally provide support and encouragement. If any difficulties have arisen during the placement, the supervisor may contact the tutor from college.

Some students, women and black people for instance, may wish to stipulate a preference for a woman or black person to act as their supervisor. These requests will be met whenever possible. It needs to be borne in mind that work placements are increasingly difficult to obtain owing to the pressure of work most people within the caring services are under. Not everyone is willing to carry the additional responsibility of supervising a student. Specific student requirements concerning distance, setting, service user group and supervision all make the placement finder's task even more difficult. There are times when an individual student's needs cannot be met. This eventuality can be used to advantage by students placed in settings not of their choice because all social care placements offer potential learning experiences. Even 'poor' placements, where practice is questionable, can generate learning and insight; the value of antidiscriminatory practice, for instance, can be identified by its very absence.

So for initial placements students may not always be placed in settings with the type of supervision they require. However, for major placements it is vital that student and supervisor are matched accordingly. Black supervisors can assist and challenge black students in a special way and women students may more readily accept supervision from another woman. These choices should be respected as far as possible.

Visits from college tutors

College tutors normally visit students at least once during their placement, but some will visit more often. Ideally they would like to have the opportunity of observing you working with clients, but this is not always possible – for example, when you are accompanying an education social worker who is visiting a family, or when you are engaged in bathing a resident in a home for physically disabled people. Tutors will have other college responsibilities and will be free to visit you only on certain days, but they will give you and your supervisor advance notice of their intention to come and see you.

The tutor will be concerned to observe how you put into practice the skills and knowledge you have gained during time spent at college. They will be interested in your understanding of the agency and its involvement with the rest of the community. A placement visit gives the tutor an opportunity to learn more about you as a person, your needs and your ambitions and a chance to consider appropriate future placements with you.

You may have the opportunity of showing your tutor around the establishment. This will be instructive and interesting for the tutor and will give you the chance to reverse your usual roles – you will be providing the information instead of being the recipient.

At some stage during the tutor's visit, they will spend some time talking to the head of the establishment, or your supervisor, about your attitude and involvement, in order to consider the progress you have made.

Assessment

At the end of the placement, students will usually be assessed by the supervisor and the college tutor. This assessment will have been going on throughout the placement and the views and opinions of other members of staff will have been sought and taken into account. Additionally, the student will be expected to contribute to the formal assessment.

Assessments made after initial placements will be regarded as tentative, but the final placement reports will more accurately reflect a student's suitability for the work and readiness to be considered for fulltime employment.

Assessment forms vary according to the level of the course. The example on page 340 has been devised to illustrate some of the basic aspects that assessors will be looking for. Some colleges will require a fuller assessment and reports, particularly for students completing final placements.

Comments

Placement supervisor's comments

Susan has been on placement for one day each week for ten weeks and has spent the last two weeks on block practice. She has been an outstanding student. She was very reticent at first and a little uncertain, but has since become very involved and has worked enthusiastically. She has shown a great deal of interest in and understanding of residents. I think they will miss her.

Signed: *W. Cross*

College tutor's report

Susan has matured during this, her second placement. She has overcome her tendency to stand back and await instruction and has involved herself fully and enthusiastically. I think she has enjoyed the setting and responded to the support given to her by various members of the home's staff.

Signed: *J. Brock*

Student's comments

I have enjoyed the placement and liked the atmosphere of the care home. I enjoyed working with the residents. I feel I am suited to this kind of work. This has been my best placement so far.

Signed: *S. McIntosh*

When they make their final assessment, the tutor and supervisor will be looking at how well you have managed to fit into the work placement. They will have considered your relationships both with clients and with members of staff and how you have you have used your time when not engaged in a specific task or activity. They will have observed whether or not you have gone about your job in a cheerful and co-operative manner and your reliability will have been judged by your punctuality and degree of efficiency in carrying out instructions. Above all, they will have gauged the interest you have shown and the commitment you have demonstrated.

The assessment reports can be a valuable source of information about how others see you – of points of weakness and areas of strength. You can compare these with your own thoughts and feelings about your experience.

Name of College

Name of student: Susan McIntosh
Duration of placement: Dates from Jan. 19- to April 19-
Name of organisation: Thomas Lottie Care home
Key to assessment: 1. Excellent. 2. Very good. 3. Good. 4. Below expectations. 5. Poor. 6. Very poor.
Please tick appropriate box.

	Tutor assessment						Supervisor assessment						Self assessment					
	1	2	3	4	5	6	1	2	3	4	5	6	1	2	3	4	5	6
1. Attendance	✓						✓						✓					
2. Punctuality		✓						✓						✓				
3. Initiative	✓						✓								✓			
4. Reliability		✓					✓								✓			
5. Manner and appearance			✓					✓							✓			
6. General attitude	✓						✓								✓			
7. Willingness and ability to help	✓						✓								✓			
8. Understanding of situation	✓						✓							✓				
9. Identification of clients' needs	✓								✓					✓				
10. Ability to relate to clients	✓						✓							✓				
11. Relationship with staff		✓							✓						✓			
12. Practical development	✓						✓								✓			
13. Communication skills	✓						✓							✓				
14. Practical caring skills		✓							✓						✓			
15. Response to guidance		✓							✓					✓				

A placement assessment form

It may now be possible for students to be assessed for competence against the existing integrated Care awards for NVQ and SVQ levels 2 and 3. This will depend on whether the establishment belongs to a consortium which is validated to carry out assessments.

Conclusion

Each placement experience is unique and contributes to the student's development and understanding of the work. However, the organisations themselves also can benefit from a student being placed with them, even though it makes added work – particularly for the supervisor.

Having somebody new around can be refreshing for both staff and residents alike. A new person has the opportunity to see the situation from an outside point of view, before they get used to the routine, and this may produce some new ideas. At the highest level, a student may be able to highlight redundant practices or make constructive suggestions for change. Essentially, though, the value of a student to an establishment is that they provide an extra 'pair of hands' and assistance which eases the load of existing staff.

Tutors too can benefit from a student's practical placement. Visits to and discussions with students can inform the tutor of current practices and date in their knowledge about the practical social work situation.

Finally, you may not always be able to be placed with the agency of your choice but you will often be given an opportunity to express a preference. It is not always practicable to arrange placements to suit each individual's choice. Sometimes a tutor will place a student in an agency distinctly not of the student's choosing, where the tutor feels that maturity and understanding could be gained. Sometimes students welcome the chance of an early placement in a field where they would not normally wish to work but where they can get experience and extend their knowledge of the caring agencies. It is normal, however, for students to undergo their final or major placement within an agency of their chosen field, so students undergoing professional training who have chosen community work or, alternatively, who have selected the probation option, will be placed in those fields. Wherever a student is placed, they always have an opportunity to develop skills and understanding of a kind which may be generalised to any health, social care or social work setting.

Appendix 1 – an account of a typical day's work for a student in an infant school

School begins at 8.55 with morning assembly – usually prayers and a hymn. The nursery nurse's first duty of the day is to usher the children into the hall and try to form some kind of orderly line with them. However, if the nursery nurse has strong convictions against attending the assembly, then do not have to be present.

After assembly, the children promptly walk to their appropriate classrooms and take off their coats and bags. The time is about 9.10 and the teacher does the register and various administrative tasks while the nursery nurse prepares for whatever activity the children are doing that day, such as painting/printing or modelling.

They usually have a small group of children to work with when they have finished their reading or mathematics, as the class works the integrated day.

If the children have any difficulties with their mathematics or English/reading, the will often break off from the creative activity to help alleviate the teacher's workload of hearing readers, etc. The nursery nurse also works with the teacher to organise the displays around the room and is often given the opportunity to do displays on their own while the teacher is occupied with the children's lessons.

The days are always varied, according to the class curriculum, and the nursery nurse generally helps with all activities such as dance, physical exercise, and reading stories. They are able to take on as much responsibility as the teacher feels they can cope with and is necessary at any particular time.

Typical school day

8.55 Assembly	12.00 Dinner
9.10 Mathematics/painting	1.30 Musical movement
10.30 Break	2.45 Break
10.45 Painting/constructive play	3-3.30 Storytime/prayer

Appendix 2 – account of a typical day's work for a student in a day nursery

9.00-10.00 The room has previously been set out as follows:
Basic play – sand, water, paint;
Constructive play – e.g. octagons;
Imaginative play – home corner;
Manipulative play – dough;
Creative play – collage;
Fine movements – puzzle, crayons;
Book corner.
'Free' play is the predominant theme of the first hour and during this time the student is expected to generally integrate with the children and encourage them to participate, but giving them freedom of choice.
There are intermittent chores such as changing children, cleaning up any mess in the room, taking soiled clothes to the laundry, as well as looking out for the general safety of the children.

9.30 Breakfast is served in the room.

10.00-10.15 Coffee break.

10.15-10.50 The children play outside with bicycles, scooters, baby trucks, etc. The student is expected to mix with the children and talk to them, pick up any who fall over and take any child inside who needs changing. They should be alert and able to cope with any accident or conflict.

10.50 Prepare the room for lunch – put away toys etc., clean the floor and set tables.

11.00 Continue outside supervision.

11.20 Take children to the bathroom
Bathroom routine: toilet (undress any children who cannot manage); encourage each child to get their own facecloth, to wash and to hang up their towel on the appropriate hook.

11.30 Sit down to lunch. Serve food. Ensure that children eat as much as possible. Eat own lunch with them.

12.00 Clean up room. Put children to bed. Set out toys (alternative choice to morning). For children who don't sleep – storytime.

12.30-1.15 Lunch break. (This is in fact 'time away from the children'. The student is expected not to leave the establishment without permission.) During lunch break, any preparation for afternoon must be done. One day a week the student undergoes a supervision session with their nursery nurse, when they are told of their negative and positive attributes and areas they must concentrate on.

1.15–2.00 Continue outside supervision.
2.00–2.30 Family time. The groups of children (known as 'families') are separate and the student supervises this time maybe two or three times a week, having chosen and prepared the topic beforehand – creative work, for instance. There are usually six to eight children and, while taking them alone, the student is also being observed by the training nursery nurse.
2.30–3.00 Clean up the room, set tables for tea, take children to the bathroom.
3.00–3.15 Tea.
3.15–4.00 Outside supervision.
In bad weather, outside play is replaced by continued free play with inside toys.
During the day the student is often asked to sing or read stories to the children. They are also expected to show interest in the children's background and to talk to their parents.

Exercise – role play – introductory placement visit

Situation
An initial visit to a placement in order for a student to introduce themselves and find out more about the agency and what is to be expected of them during the placement.

Roles
1. A member of staff of the agency
2. A student
3. An observer

Member of staff
You are the member of staff responsible for the student who is about to be placed with you. Your task is to explain the function of the agency and what will be expected from the student.

Student
You are about to undertake a placement with the agency or organisation. You need to ask pertinent questions and be able to explain about the course you are on and what you expect from the placement.

Observer
Observe the meeting between the member of staff and the student and make any relevant comments.

Task
Role-play the meeting. All the roles can then be interchanged.

Questions for discussion

1. You are placed with an organisation and you observe a member of the care staff being short and abusive to one of the residents. This is the second time you have seen this and you wonder whether you should mention the matter to your superior. What do you do?

2. If you had placements during a two-year course, what type of placements would you choose for yourself and why would you choose them? In what order would you prefer to experience them?

3. What do you expect from visits from your college tutor? Does the tutor visit the placement often enough and stay long enough, or does the tutor call too frequently?

4. Write up a week's placement. Categorise time you spent doing various activities. How much time did you spend talking to clients? Was this enough?

5. Write up a detailed case study of one of the people you have met on your placement.

6. How important is it to keep a diary during your placement? In what ways have you found the practice useful?

7. What is the value of supervision and why is it important that supervision should be made available at regular times?

8. Should students be able to stipulate the kind of work based study supervisors they would like – for example, a black person, a woman or a supervisor who is gay?

Index

Access courses, 181
Access teams, 22–3
Access to Personal Files Act (1987), 25
'Accommodated' children, 44–6, 49
Adoption, 42–4, 139
  agencies, 43
  panels, 40, 43–4
Adoption Act (1976), 44
Adult Training Centres (ATC's), (see Social
  Education Centres (SEC's)
Advocacy, 66–7, 213, 248, 268, 285
  citizen, 66, 248
  legal, 66
  self, 66, 69, 248, 267
After-care (of children and young people),
  53–4
Age Concern, 211, 218
Agenda for Action (see Griffiths Report)
Aids and adaptations, 60
Alcoholics Anonymous (AA), 213, 279
Alcohol misuse, 21, 160
  services for, 69, 127
Alzheimer's Disease Society, 218
Anti-discriminatory/anti-oppressive practice,
  2, 13, 101–02, 237–40, 253, 258, 267, 268,
  309–310
Apex Trust, 213
Approved Social Workers (ASW's), 28, 71
  role of, 71–2
Armitage, Simon, 111
Art Therapy, 69
Assertiveness, 69, 256
Assessment, 3, 19, 21–3, 57, 65, 73, 77, 158,
  268–9, 272, 276, 288
Association of Black Probation Officers
  (ABPO), 103
Asylum, 70
Attendance centres 115

Bail hostels, 126
Bail information schemes, 112–3, 145
Barclay Report (1982), 11–12, 18, 199, 200
Barnardo's 36, 212, 220
Behavioural psychology (behaviour

modification), 266, 277–8
Beveridge Report (1942), 10, 79, 214
Beveridge, William, 9, 296
Black Community Care Charter, 239, 248
Black people, 41, 306–7
  definition of, 1
Body Positive, 75
Booth, Charles, 9
British Association of Social Workers
  (BASW), 235, 241, 305, 309
British sign language, 74, 102, 248, 255
'Buddies' (See Terrence Higgins Trust)

Care (children in), 47, 253–264
  leaving, 53–4
  order, 47
Careers Service, 175–6
Care managers/management, 3, 19, 57
Care Officers/Assistants, 6, 20
Care Planning, 27
Carers National Association (Carers), 217–20
Caring for People (1989 White Paper), 13, 19,
  199, 216, 235, 307
Case Conferences, 85–8, 200–02
Casework (or Social Casework), 276
Catholic Children's Society, 36
Catholic Child Service (CCS), 43
Central Council for Education and Training
  in social work (CCETSW), 14, 92, 191,
  309, 315, 316, 319
  Paper 30, 14
Charity Commission, 211
Charity Organisation Society (COS), 8, 9, 212
Child Abuse, 23, 28, 31, 197–8, 202
Child Care Act (1980), 23, 29
Child guidance, 9, 174–5
Childminders, 32–3
Child Poverty Action Group (CPAG), 10,
  213, 283, 308
Child Protection, 12–13
Child Protection Register (CPR), 198–9, 201
Children Act (1975), 44
Children Act (Scotland) (1980), 23
Children Act (1989), 1, 13, 14, 17, 18, 20, 23,

29, 30, 32, 33, 34, 35, 37, 38, 40, 41, 44, 46,
47, 48, 53, 54, 55, 75, 79, 132, 136, 137,
138, 177, 185, 199, 200, 221, 222, 242, 243,
296, 300
  welfare checklist, 46–7, 136–7
children and families team, 28–9
Children and Young Persons Act (1933), 115–
16, 132
Children and Young Persons Act (1963), 29
Children and Young Persons Act (1969), 47,
48, 95, 120
Children's hearings, 122
Children's homes, 49–52
Church Army, 187
Church of England Children's Society, 212,
220
Citizens' Advice Bureau (CAB), 213, 224,
231, 232, 283
Cleveland (Child Abuse Inquiry), 13
Colleges of Further Education (Community
Colleges), 180, 182
Combination orders, 115, 119
Communication, 248, 255–6
Community care, 3, 25, 55–8, 68, 190, 236,
239, 247, 298, 301–02
  assessment, 3, 19, 21–3, 57
  housing and, 190
  mental ill-health, 68
Community drug teams, 195
Community education, 179–182
  adults with learning difficulties and, 181
  ethnic minority groups and, 181
  manual workers and, 180–1
  unemployed people and, 182
  women and, 180
Community Life, 234
Community mental health team, 68–9
Community psychiatric nurse (CPN), 68,
162–3
Community service, 95, 97, 98, 114–15, 117,
118–19
Community work (community social work),
190–6, 284–5
  relationship with social work, 191
  role of, 192–4
Complaints procedure (community care), 58
Compulsory admission to hospital
(psychiatric), 70–2
  to Residential Care, 63
Conciliation, 138
Confidentiality, 240–1
Contact order (Children Act 1989), 47, 137
Contracting/contract culture, 4, 223, 229, 298

Coulshed, Veronica, 267, 283, 284, 295
Councils for Voluntary Service, 212
Counselling, 194, 228, 267, 270–2, 275
Court Welfare Service (CWS), 134–9
Criminal courts, 110–27
Criminal Justice Act (1967), 95
Criminal Justice Act (1982), 96, 103, 120
Criminal Justice Act (1991), 1, 2, 54, 98, 101,
103, 111, 112, 115, 117, 119, 122, 125, 128,
130, 132, 139, 140, 144, 296
Crisis intervention, 275
Crown Prosecution Service (CPS), 109, 113

Davies, W H, 260
Day care, 6, 30, 31–3, 59, 60–1, 69, 73–4, 84–5
Day nursery, 342–3
Debt counselling, 283
Department of Health, 5, 16, 98, 202, 219
Department of Health and Social Security
(DHSS), 199, 215, 234
Department of Social Security (DSS), 5, 22,
177, 187, 195, 214, 215, 230, 259
Dignity, 247–8
Diploma in Social Work (DipSW), 6, 14, 92,
220, 309, 313, 316, 318–19
Directions hearings, 138
Disability, physical, 244
  children with, 34
Disability Alliance, 218
Disabled Persons (Services, Consultation and
Representation) Act (1986), 55, 73, 199, 309
Discrimination
  black people and, 306–7
  women and, 30
District nurse, 162
  training for, 320–1
Divorce, 135
Domiciliary Services, 6, 59–60, 73, 216
Downie, Bill, 125
Down's Syndrome, 64
Drug Misuse, 21, 160, 228
  services for, 69, 127

Education, 167, 303
Education Act (1944), 170, 173, 177
Education Act (1980), 34, 55, 299
Education Act (1981), 170, 171, 172
Education Act (1993), 173
Education department, 4, 6, 167–82 passim,
  education social workers, 176–8
  peripatetic teachers, 172
  school psychological child guidance
  service, 174–5

Education otherwise, 173–4
Education Reform Act (1988), 168
Education Welfare Service, 176–8
Egan, Gerard, 271–2, 273
Elders, 58–64
  confused, 60–1
  mentally infirm (EMI), 63
  service for, 58–9
  short stay care, 61–2
  telephones for, 61
  transport for, 61
Electroconvulsive therapy (ECT), 160
Emergency duty team, 78–9, 82–4
Emergency protection order, 46, 48, 197
Empathy, 253–4
Empowerment, 267, 268, 271, 285
Equal Opportunities, 102–3

Family assistance order, 48, 136, 137–8
Family centres, 30–32
Family courts, 134–9
Family court work, 134–9
Family planning nurse, training for, 321
Family Service Units (FSUs), 211
Family therapy, 272–4
Family Welfare Association (FWA), 212, 215
Feminist social work, 286–7
Field social work (fieldwork), 17–19 passim,
Foodchain, 76
Foster carers, 35–40
  emergency, 39
  training for, 37–8
Foster Placement (Children) Regulations, 36
Fostering, 35–42
Fostering and adoption panels, 40
Fostering services, 35–42
  adult, 42
  long-term (permanency), 39
  mixed race fostering, 40–2
  placement agreement meetings, 36
  respite care, 39
  same race placements, 40–2
  short-term/temporary, 38–9
  teenage, 39
Franks Report (1973), 178
Freud, Sigmund, 266, 280

Gambling, 277–8
Gay people, 75, 239–40, 309
General Practitioner (GP), 3, 5, 18, 68, 71,
  152, 153, 154–5, 156, 158, 161, 162, 163,
  164, 166, 167, 301, 302, 303

budget-/fund-holding, 3, 5, 152, 302, 303
Gingerbread, 213
General National Vocational Qualifications
  (GNVQs)/Vocational A Levels, 2, 6, 314,
  315, 324–6
Grendon Underwood (Psychiatric) Prison,
  Bucks, 129
Griffiths Report (Agenda for Action, 1988),
  19, 235
Groupwork, 275, 277, 279–80, 292
  in Probation Service, 123–5
  types of, 279
Guardian ad litem, 44, 48, 139

Health Service (*and see* NHS), 3, 302–3, 319–
  22
Health visitor (HV), 160–2
  specialist (HIV), 167
  training for, 321
Help the Aged, 194
Heron, John, 289–90, 291, 294
Hertfordshire, 93
Hill, Octavia, 9
HIV/AIDS, 21, 28, 36, 69, 72, 75–6, 124, 165,
  166, 167, 213, 226–8, 238, 240, 302
  services to people with, 75–6
Holman, Bob, 17, 31, 91, 285
Home care (homehelp(s)), 6, 59, 78
Homelessness, 185–8
  single homeless people, 187
Home Life, 62, 234, 241, 242
Homemaker schemes, 74
Home Office, 5, 92, 94, 96, 97, 98, 101, 102,
  103, 104, 108, 119, 120, 121, 123, 126, 132,
  133, 192
Hospital order (Mental Health Act, 1983,
  section 37), 116
Housing, 304, 323
Housing Act (1985), 186, 187
Housing aid, 189
Housing department, 183–90
  homeless families section, 186
  local estate offices, 188
  points system, 184–5
  tenant participation, 188
Housing (Homeless Persons) Act (1977), 186
Humanistic Psychology, 266–7

Identity, 245, 247
Ideology, 297–300
Independent sector, 4, 210–33 passim,
  future of, 229–30
Individual programme planning (IPP), 65

Institutionalisation, 70
Intake teams, 22
Inter-agency co-operation, 120, 198–202
    passim
Intermediate treatment (IT), 54–5, 95, 120–1
IT (*see* Intermediate Treatment)
Interpersonal skills, 255–8

Juvenile court (*see* Youth Court)

Keyworker/ing, 6, 27, 50, 281–2
King's Fund Centre, 219, 307

Law Centre Federation, 194
Law centres, 194–5
Learning difficulties/disabilities, 64, 159, 172,
    244
    day care for, 65
    residential care for, 67
    services to, 64–7, 181
    social work support to, 64–5
Learning theory (or social learning theory)
    (*see* Behavioural Psychology)
Legal Aid (Scheme), 195
Lifeskills training (*see* Social Skills Training)
Life Story work, 282–3, 294
Local Government Act (1988), Section 28 of,
    309
London Lighthouse, 75, 213
Love, 254

Makaton, 74, 248, 255
McGough, Roger, 272
McIvor, Gill, 99
Meals on wheels, 59
Medical social workers, 164–5
Mental Health Act (1959), 56
Mental Health Act (1983), 17, 70–1, 72, 79,
    116–17, 155, 158
Mental ill health (illness), 67–8, 158, 159–60
    causes, 6, 7–8
Midwife, registered, 320
MIND, 10, 68, 211, 213
Missing persons, 197
Mixed economy of welfare, 3, 210, 214–15,
    216, 229–30
Moreno, Jacob, 280, 281
Multi-disciplinary team (example of), 165–7

National Assistance Act (1948), 10, 62, 63
National Association for the Care and
    Resettlement of Offenders (NACRO), 102,
    103, 112, 113, 150

National Association of Probation Officers
    (NAPO), 94, 96, 103, 139
National Children's Bureau, 53, 215
National Council for Voluntary Organisations
    (NCVO), 212, 213, 214, 215, 218, 229
National Curriculum, 52, 173, 314
National Foster Care Association (NFCA), 37
National Health Service (NHS), 2, 5, 10, 68,
    69, 151–67 passim, 174, 235, 280, 298, 300
    history of, 151
    multi-disciplinary team, 165
    primary health care, 152, 153
    secondary health care, 152, 154
National Institute for Social Work (NISW),
    11, 194, 229
    Race Equality Unit (REU) of, 229, 235,
        238
National Society for the Prevention of
    Cruelty to Children (NSPCC), 6, 47, 199,
    211, 212, 217, 220–3, 230
    child protection teams, 222
National Vocational Qualifications (NVQs),
    3, 6, 20, 62, 181, 237, 250, 305, 309, 313,
    314–16, 317, 318, 319, 322, 327–9, 340
    assessment for, 315
Neighbourly help money, 59–60
Networking, 283–4, 294
Network therapy, 284
New Right ideology, 297–8
NHS and Community Care Act (1990) 1, 3,
    13, 17, 19, 20, 27, 55, 56, 57, 58, 62, 68, 69,
    75, 79, 199, 200, 235
Night shelters, 187
Non-verbal communication, 256, 270, 273
Normalisation, 63, 65–6, 268
Not-for-Profit organisation (sector), 4, 55,
    210, 216–17, 229, 237, 298
Nursery centres, 6, 169
Nursery nurses (nursery officers), 6, 7
Nursery nursing (training for), 322–3
Nursery schools/classes, 168–9
Nursing, training for, 319–20

Occupational therapy (OT), 77, 163
    assessment for, 77, 163
    rehabilitation and, 77–8
    training for, 322
Older people (*see* elders)
Open learning systems, 182
Orkney (child abuse inquiry), 13

Paediatrician, 166
Parker, Robin, 107

Parkinson's Disease Society, 218
Parole, 127, 130, 131
  Assessment Report, 127, 133, 146
Patch System, 11, 12
Pepper Pot Club, London (Kensington), 217, 224-5
Permanency principle, 34-5
Physical disability, people with a, 72-3
  services for, 72-4
  transport for, 74
Physiotherapy, 321
  training for, 321
'Piss on Pity', 268
Pitsmoor, Sheffield, 225
Playgroups, 33
Playtraining/Playwork, 323
Plowden Report (1967), 192
Police, 196-8
  Rape crisis/domestic violence units, 198
Police and Criminal Evidence Act (PACE) (1984), 55
Police court missionaries, 93, 94
Poor law, 8, 9, 10
Poor Law Act (1834), 8
'Positive Partners', 76
Poverty, 307-8
Power in the caring relationship, 267-8
Powers of Criminal Courts Act, The, (1973), 95, 103, 116, 117, 125
Practice nurse, 156
Pre-sentence reports (PSRs), 54, 96, 98, 110-12, 142-4
Preventive social work, 24-5
Primary health care (*see* National Health Service)
Prison, 116, 127, 128-34, 228
Privacy, right to, 241
Private agencies/sector, 4, 210, 215-16, 237, 298
Probation Service, 2, 6, 9, 11, 92-150 passim, 151, 155, 201, 202, 210, 211, 235, 297, 305, 316
  anti-oppressive practice in, 98, 101-2
  assistant chief probation officer (ACPO), 104, 106
  autocrime work, 108, 125
  bail hostels, 126
  bail information schemes, 112-13, 145
  black people and the, 103
  chief probation officer (CPO), 104
  crime prevention and the, 108
  deputy chief probation officer (DCPO), 104

equal opportunities in 102-3
family court work (court welfare service), 134-9
'gatekeeping', 112, 140
gender and the, 102
history of, 93-7
hostels, 126-7
intensive probation programmes, 125-6
national standards, 96, 97-8, 101, 112, 114, 119, 123, 126, 133, 139, 140, 144, 235
offence-based work, 99-100
pre-discharge report, 132-3
prisons, in, 127, 128
probation centres, 125-6
probation officer (PO), 106
probation order, 114, 119, 122-3
probation services' officers (PSOs), 95, 106
public interest case assessment (PICA), 109-10, 145
reparation and the, 95
senior probation officer (SPO), 106
specialisms in, 100-1
structure/organisation of, 103-7
'three year plan' (1992) for, 97
throughcare, 127-34
voluntary associates (VAs), 106-7
Prohibited steps order (Children Act, 1989), 48, 137
Project 2000, 319, 320
Psychiatrist, 157-60
  Child, 174
Psychoanalysis, 266
Psychodrama, 280-1
Psychologist, clinical, 156-7, 167
  educational, 171, 174
Psychology, 265-7
Purchaster/provider functions (of local authorities), 3, 55-6, 80, 214, 297-8, 301

Race Relations Act (1975), 237
Radical Social Work, 285-6
Reality Orientation Therapy (ROT), 60, 63
Recording, 25-6
Registered Homes Act (1984), 62, 217, 234
Rehabilitation of Offenders Act (1974), 142
Relationships, 243
'Release', 213
Reporting officer, 44, 139
Residence order, 38, 47, 137
Residential care, 61, 67, 70, 275-6
Residential social worker(ers) (RSWs), 6, 20, 27, 61, 62

Respite care, 39, 61
'Responsible adult', 79
Restriction order (Mental Health Act, 1983, section 41), 116–17
Rights, clients, 234–52
Risk, 242–3
Rogers, Carl, 266
Rowntree, Seebohm, 9
Rowntree Trust, 29
Royal National Institute for the Blind (RNIB), 75

Salvation Army, 187
Save the Children Fund, 194
Schizophrenia, 160
School nurse (training for), 321
Schools, 169–70, 171–2
    primary, 169, 341–2
    secondary, 169
Scotland, arrangements for young offenders in, 121–2
Scottish Vocational Qualifications (SVQs), 6, 20, 237, 305, 309, 314–16, 318, 322, 327–9, 340
Sculpting, 272, 274
Section 8 orders (Children Act, 1989), 47–8, 137
Seebohm Committee Report (1968), 10, 11, 17, 95, 100, 192
Sensory disabilities, people with, 72
    services for, 74–5
Sentencing in the criminal courts, 114, 117, 120
Sex Discrimination Act (1975), 237
Sexual offences, people who have committed, 132
Shelter, 10, 189
Sheltered workshops, 74
Six-Category Intervention Analysis, 289–90, 294
'Skilled Helper' Model (*see* Egan, Gerard)
Skinner, B F, 266
Social Care Association (SCA), 235
Social Care Methods (*see* Chap. 8 'Strategies for Helping), 265–95
Social Education Centres, 6, 65, 66
Social Inquiry Reports (*see* Pre-Sentence Reports (PSRs)
'Social Issues for Carers' (Webb & Tossell), 252, 265
Social Services Act (1970), 8, 10, 79
Social Services Department (SSD), 6, 8–91 passim, 210, 214

Social Skills Training, 278–9
Social Systems Model, 287–9
Social Work Assistants (SWAs), 19
Social Work Department (Scotland), 8, 10, 13, 15, 16, 21, 23, 25, 43, 95, 214
Social Work Methods (*see* Chap. 8 'Strategies for Helping') 265–95
Social Work (Scotland) Act (1968), 8, 10, 79, 121, 122
Sociodrama, 281
Special needs, 167, 170–5
Specific issue order (Children Act, 1989), 48, 137
Speech (or language) therapist, 322
    training for, 322
Statutory sector, 2, 4, 5, 151, 210
    administration of, 5
    definition of, 4
Strategies for helping, 265–5 passim
Supervision (of staff, professional), 26–7
Supervision order, 47, 119–21
System-induced old age, 245, 246

Task-centred work, 276
Teams/teamwork/meetings, 27
Terrence Higgins Trust (THT), 75, 76, 217, 226–8
    'Buddy' programme, 76, 227–8
Therapeutic communities, 52–3
'Time poverty', 308
Training, 314–31 passim
Transactional analysis (TA), 267

Under-fives, 84–5, 168–9
Under-eights, 6, 28, 30–3
Unemployed people, 182
Urban Aid Programme (Home Office, 1969), 192
User-involvement, 267

Value Base Unit (Unit 'O', NVQ, Levels 2 and 3), 250, 317
Voluntary agencies/sector, 4, 210–15, 217–28, 237, 298
    definition of, 4, 210–11
    history of, 211–13
    locally based, 223–6, 229
    range of, 213–14
Volunteer centre, 211
Volunteers, 211

Wagner Report (1988), 27, 62, 234, 235, 241
Ward sister, 166

Warnock Report (1978), 170, 181, 303
Welfare rights work, 283
Welfare State, 9, 192, 210, 213, 214, 229, 296, 297, 298, 299, 300, 310
history of, 10–11
Woman-centred practice, 286–7
Women's movement, 286
'Working for the Patients' (White Paper, 1989), 151–2, 199
World Health Organisation (WHO), 75, 226

Yemeni Community Association, Sheffield, 217, 225–6
Young offender institutions (YOI), 115, 127, 128, 130
Youth court, 119
Youth justice teams, 54, 55
Youth service, 178–9
detached youth workers, 179
outreach work, 179
training for, 323
youth centres, 178–9